Algorithmic Diagnosis of Symptoms and Signs: Cost-Effective Approach

Algorithmic Diagnosis of Symptoms and Signs: Cost-Effective Approach

R. Douglas Collins, M.D., F.A.C.P.
Diplomate, American Board of Internal Medicine
Diplomate, American Board of
Clinical Neurology
Consulting Neurologist
Lancaster Community Hospital
Lancaster, California

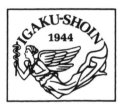

IGAKU-SHOIN   NEW YORK * TOKYO

Published and distributed by

IGAKU-SHOIN Medical Publishers, Inc.
One Madison Avenue, New York, New York 10010

IGAKU-SHOIN Ltd.,
5-24-3 Hongo, Bunkyo-ku, Tokyo 113-91.

Library of Congress Cataloging-in-Publication Data

Collins, R. Douglas.
    Algorithmic diagnosis of symptoms and signs : cost
effective approach / R. Douglas Collins.
        p.   cm.
    Includes bibliographical references and index.
    ISBN 0-89640-283-5 (New York). — ISBN
    4-260-14283-6 (Tokyo)
    1. Diagnosis—Handbooks, manuals, etc.   2. Medical
protocols—Handbooks, manuals, etc.   I. Title.
    [DNLM: 1. Diagnosis.   2. Algorithms.   3. Cost Sav-
ings. WB 141 C712a 1995]
RC71.3.C645   1995
616.07′5—dc20
DNLM/DLC
for Library of Congress   95-1040
                                                     CIP

ISBN: 0-89640-283-5   (New York)
ISBN: 4-260-14283-6   (Tokyo)

Printed and bound in the U.S.A.
10 9 8 7 6 5 4 3 2 1

Dedication

To my wife, Norie whose love and devotion for our Lord Jesus Christ has been an inspiration to me.

Acknowledgments

I'd like to express my appreciation to Clayton Reynolds M.D., FACP, Anil Kumar, M.D., FACC, and Tom Hamoui, M.D., FACP for their critical review of the manuscript. My thanks also to Cyndi Skelton who did the tedious job of typing most of the manuscript.

Finally to Lila Maron, vice president of Editorial of Igaku-Shoin goes the credit for the idea of a book like this.

Preface

The average textbook of medicine is not very useful to the busy practicing physician because all of the information in these texts is catalogued according to specific diseases. Until the physician has a diagnosis, he can not look up diagnostic tests or treatment that would address the patient's problem.

This book applies algorithms to the clinical diagnosis of symptoms and signs. It is aimed at organizing the approach to diagnosis and reducing the cost of a diagnostic work-up. To facilitate this procedure, the symptoms and signs are arranged alphabetically. Once the physician turns to a certain symptom or sign, he will find not just a list of diseases, but the diseases are arranged in an algorithm. At a glance he will be able to find what other historical and clinical data he needs to look for, to pin down the diagnosis. Then in the accompanying text he will find the tests to order for a diagnostic workup.

A highlight of this book is a discussion on when to refer to the appropriate specialist. Once a specific diagnosis has been established, the clinician can move on to treatment. I have written this book to provide primary care physicians and specialists with a useful tool in the rapid diagnosis of symptoms and signs that they can use in their offices, in the emergency room, or on the hospital wards.

Contents

INTRODUCTION

HOW TO USE THESE ALGORITHMS

The algorithms presented in these pages are at the very least a list of the most common disorders that may cause a given symptom or sign. As such, however, they are not all-inclusive. Rare or unusual conditions are excluded. The reader is referred to other treatises of differential diagnosis such as *French's Index of Differential Diagnosis* and *Handbook of Difficult Diagnosis*, edited by A.A. Louis, for a more complete list of diagnostic possibilities.

The list of diagnostic possibilities is broken down by the presence or absence of additional symptoms and signs. The reader should be aware that any specific patient may not present with an additional symptom necessary for this analysis and therefore the entire list of possibilities must still be entertained. Alternatively, the patient may present with the additional symptom, but still have one of the other disorders on the diagnostic tree; therefore, at all times the clinician should maintain an index of suspicion that the patient could have any one of the disorders listed on the page and not exclude any of the possibilities completely until he has a positive laboratory x-ray or tissue diagnosis. For example:

> A 47-year-old white female complained of progressive numbness and tingling and weakness of the lower extremities. Examination showed loss of vibratory and position sense in the lower extremities and positive Babinski's signs. A tentative diagnosis of pernicious anemia was made. However, tests for serum B_{12} and folic acid were normal. Magnetic resonance imaging (MRI) of the thoracic spine showed a neurofibroma at T6 to T7 level.

From this example, one can see that had the clinician not kept an open mind about the entire list of diagnostic possibilities, he would not have ordered

MRI of the thoracic spine and would have missed the diagnosis.

Finally, the text accompanying each algorithm contains valuable information on how to approach the patient with each presenting symptom and sign and how to proceed with the diagnostic workup. For example:

A 35-year-old white female presents to the emergency room with acute abdominal pain and diffuse tenderness and rebound.

The text on acute abdominal pain shows the routine diagnostic tests are a flat and upright plate of the abdomen, a complete blood count, urinalysis, amylase, and chemistry panel. Most clinicians would remember to order these tests without referring to this handbook. However, some clinicians might forget to order a chest x-ray or electrocardiogram and pregnancy test. Furthermore, there are additional tests to order in case the routine tests are unrevealing. The clinician is reminded to order x-ray contrast studies, ultrasound of the gall bladder and pelvis and he is reminded to do a peritoneal tap in order to diagnose a ruptured ectopic pregnancy.

Most of the time this little handbook is not presenting anything new to the experienced diagnostician. However, the materials presented here will jog his memory and help him proceed with a thorough workup.

ABDOMINAL PAIN, ACUTE

Ask the following questions:

1. Where is the pain located? If it is diffuse, one should consider pancreatitis, mesenteric artery occlusion, or ruptured peptic ulcer. In addition, another viscus may be perforated, such as a ruptured ectopic and there may be peritonitis. If it is focal, we need to know what quadrant it is in. For example, acute cholecystitis is in the right upper quadrant, while diverticulitis is usually in the left lower quadrant.

2. What is the nature of the pain? Colicky abdominal pain suggests intestinal obstruction, renal calculus and cholelithiasis or common duct stone, while constant pain is typical of pancreatitis, a ruptured peptic ulcer, appendicitis, diverticulitis, and a ruptured ectopic pregnancy.

3. Does the pain radiate? The pain of acute cholecystitis typically radiates to the right scapular or right shoulder. The pain of a ruptured peptic ulcer may also radiate to the shoulder. The pain of acute renal calculus may radiate to the testicle.

4. What are the associated signs and symptoms? Shock with generalized tenderness and rebound and diminished or absent bowel sounds should suggest a ruptured peptic ulcer or an acute pancreatitis. However, acute right upper quadrant pain with nausea and vomiting should suggest acute cholecystitis. On the other hand, appendicitis is more insidious in onset and is associated with anorexia and nausea, rarely vomiting, as well as constipation. Renal colic presents with hematuria.

5. Could this patient's abdominal pain be due to an extra-abdominal condition? Remember, lobar pneumonia, myocardial infarction, diabetic acidosis, and porphyria may be responsible for acute abdominal pain. There are numerous other conditions that need to be considered.

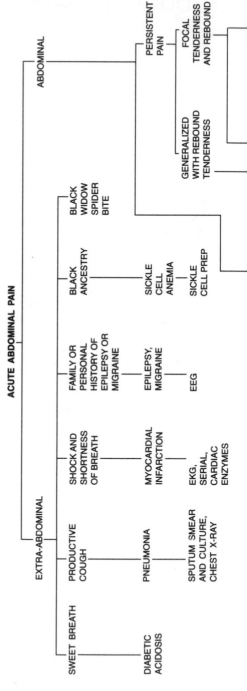

ACUTE ABDOMINAL PAIN

EXTRA-ABDOMINAL
- SWEET BREATH → DIABETIC ACIDOSIS
- PRODUCTIVE COUGH → PNEUMONIA → SPUTUM SMEAR AND CULTURE, CHEST X-RAY
- SHOCK AND SHORTNESS OF BREATH → MYOCARDIAL INFARCTION → EKG, SERIAL, CARDIAC ENZYMES
- FAMILY OR PERSONAL HISTORY OF EPILEPSY OR MIGRAINE → EPILEPSY, MIGRAINE → EEG
- BLACK ANCESTRY → SICKLE CELL ANEMIA → SICKLE CELL PREP
- BLACK WIDOW SPIDER BITE

ABDOMINAL
- PERSISTENT PAIN
  - FOCAL TENDERNESS AND REBOUND
  - GENERALIZED WITH REBOUND TENDERNESS

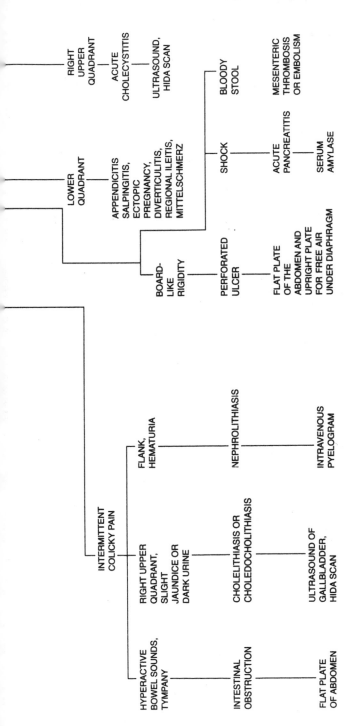

RIGHT UPPER QUADRANT — ACUTE CHOLECYSTITIS — ULTRASOUND, HIDA SCAN

LOWER QUADRANT — APPENDICITIS, SALPINGITIS, ECTOPIC PREGNANCY, DIVERTICULITIS, REGIONAL ILEITIS, MITTELSCHMERZ

BLOODY STOOL — MESENTERIC THROMBOSIS OR EMBOLISM

SHOCK — ACUTE PANCREATITIS — SERUM AMYLASE

BOARD-LIKE RIGIDITY — PERFORATED ULCER — FLAT PLATE OF THE ABDOMEN AND UPRIGHT PLATE FOR FREE AIR UNDER DIAPHRAGM

FLANK, HEMATURIA — NEPHROLITHIASIS — INTRAVENOUS PYELOGRAM

INTERMITTENT COLICKY PAIN

RIGHT UPPER QUADRANT, SLIGHT JAUNDICE OR DARK URINE — CHOLELITHIASIS OR CHOLEDOCHOLITHIASIS — ULTRASOUND OF GALLBLADDER, HIDA SCAN

HYPERACTIVE BOWEL SOUNDS, TYMPANY — INTESTINAL OBSTRUCTION — FLAT PLATE OF ABDOMEN

DIAGNOSTIC WORKUP

It is wise to consult a general surgeon at the outset. All patients with acute abdominal pain should have a stat, flat, and upright plate of the abdomen, a chest x-ray to rule out pneumonia, an electrocardiogram (EKG) to rule out myocardial infarction, and a complete blood count (CBC), urinalysis, amylase, and chemistry panel. Sometimes lateral decubitus films of the abdomen are necessary to show the step ladder pattern of intestinal obstruction. A pregnancy test is ordered when age and sex dictates it!

When these tests fail to confirm the clinical diagnosis, x-ray contrast studies or ultrasound may be necessary. For example, an intravenous pyelogram (IVP) can be done for a suspected renal calculus. Serial cardiac enzymes may confirm a myocardial infarction. Gallbladder ultrasound can be done to confirm cholecystitis and cholelithiasis. A nuclear scan of the gallbladder with iminodiacetic acid derivatives is very accurate in detecting acute cholecystitis. A peritoneal tap may diagnose a ruptured ectopic pregnancy. A double enema may help diagnose intestinal obstruction. A CT scan of the abdomen is the next logical step.

If the diagnosis remains in doubt, an exploratory laparotomy must be done before the patient's condition deteriorates. The only case where this might be risky is acute pancreatitis. If this is suspected and the serum amylase is repeatedly normal, a quantitative urine amylase or peritoneal tap may confirm the diagnosis. Endoscopy may need to be done to diagnose a peptic ulcer, gastritis, gastric tumor, or reflux esophagitis. In obscure cases of appendicitis and diverticulitis, a contrast barium enema may help confirm the diagnosis.

ABDOMINAL PAIN, CHRONIC RECURRENT

Ask the following questions:

1. Is there a family history of migraine or epilepsy? Migraine and epilepsy both present with abdominal pain.
2. Is the pain colicky or persistent? Chronic colicky abdominal pain may be due to chronic cholecystitis, cholelithiasis, renal calculus, or partial intestinal obstruction.
3. What is the location of the pain? If the pain is located in the upper abdomen, then one should consider peptic ulcer disease, pancreatitis, cholecystitis, and cholelithiasis. If the pain is located in the flanks, one should consider renal calculus and pyelonephritis. If the pain is located in the lower abdomen, one should consider diverticulitis, salpingitis, endometritis, and chronic appendicitis. Regional ileitis also may be located in the lower abdomen, particularly in the right lower quadrant.
4. What is the relationship to meals? Abdominal pain relieved by food may be due to a peptic ulcer. Abdominal pain brought on by food may be due to abdominal angina. If the pain comes on 2 to 3 hr after a meal, it may be due to a peptic ulcer. On the other hand, pain that comes on 1 to 2 hr after meals, especially if it's a fatty meal, may be related to cholecystitis and cholelithiasis.
5. Is there fever associated with the abdominal pain? Fever and abdominal pain may be due to pyelonephritis, diverticulitis, or appendicitis.
6. Is there a history of chronic alcoholism? The history of chronic alcoholism suggests acute and chronic pancreatitis.
7. Is there blood in the stool? The presence of blood in the stool would, of course, suggest peptic ulcer disease and diverticulitis.
8. Is there an abdominal mass? The presence of an abdominal mass, particularly in the midepigas-

trium, suggests a pancreatic cyst related to chronic pancreatitis. A mass in the right lower quadrant might be related to regional ileitis or salpingitis. In the left lower quadrant it may be related to diverticulitis and salpingitis.

DIAGNOSTIC WORKUP

Routine laboratory tests include a CBC, sedimentation rate, urinalysis, urine culture, sensitivity, colony count, chemistry panel, serum amylase and lipase, pregnancy test, stool for occult blood, and stools for ovum and parasites. A chest x-ray, EKG, and flat plate of the abdomen should also be done. A urine porphobilinogen will help exclude porphyria.

If these tests are negative, then an upper gastrointestinal (GI) series, esophagram, and gallbladder ultrasound would be done for upper abdominal pain; an IVP would be done for flank pain; and a barium enema and sigmoidoscopy would be performed for lower abdominal pain.

If these studies are inconclusive, a gastroenterologist should be consulted for endoscopic procedures. If there is upper abdominal pain, esophagoscopy, gastroscopy, and duodenoscopy would be performed. If there is lower abdominal pain, colonoscopy would be performed. A computed tomography (CT) scan of the abdomen and pelvis is a useful diagnostic tool also. Gallium scans may detect a diverticular abscess or other localized area of chronic inflammation. Pelvic ultrasound may be useful in lower abdominal pain, especially in females. Aortography and angiography will be useful in abdominal angina. Lymphangiography can be helpful in discovering retroperitoneal tumors. Ultimately, exploratory laparotomy may still be necessary in some cases.

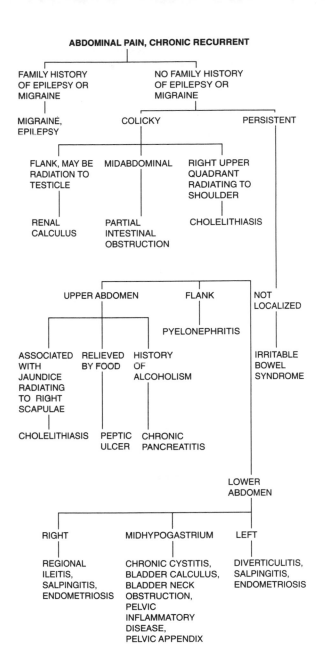

ABDOMINAL PAIN, CHRONIC RECURRENT

FAMILY HISTORY OF EPILEPSY OR MIGRAINE
→ MIGRAINE, EPILEPSY

NO FAMILY HISTORY OF EPILEPSY OR MIGRAINE

COLICKY

FLANK, MAY BE RADIATION TO TESTICLE
→ RENAL CALCULUS

MIDABDOMINAL
→ PARTIAL INTESTINAL OBSTRUCTION

RIGHT UPPER QUADRANT RADIATING TO SHOULDER
→ CHOLELITHIASIS

PERSISTENT

UPPER ABDOMEN

ASSOCIATED WITH JAUNDICE RADIATING TO RIGHT SCAPULAE
→ CHOLELITHIASIS

RELIEVED BY FOOD
→ PEPTIC ULCER

HISTORY OF ALCOHOLISM
→ CHRONIC PANCREATITIS

FLANK
→ PYELONEPHRITIS

NOT LOCALIZED
→ IRRITABLE BOWEL SYNDROME

LOWER ABDOMEN

RIGHT
→ REGIONAL ILEITIS, SALPINGITIS, ENDOMETRIOSIS

MIDHYPOGASTRIUM
→ CHRONIC CYSTITIS, BLADDER CALCULUS, BLADDER NECK OBSTRUCTION, PELVIC INFLAMMATORY DISEASE, PELVIC APPENDIX

LEFT
→ DIVERTICULITIS, SALPINGITIS, ENDOMETRIOSIS

ABDOMINAL SWELLING, FOCAL

Ask the following questions:

1. Is it in the right upper quadrant? A mass in the right upper quadrant is most often an enlarged liver. However, the liver may be pushed down by a subphrenic abscess and there may be an enlarged gallbladder due to cholecystitis or bile duct obstruction. There may be perinephric abscesses, tumors of the colon, renal tumors, adrenal tumors, hydrops of the gallbladder, fecal impaction, or an abdominal wall hematoma.
2. Is it in the epigastrium? A mass in the epigastrium also may be an enlarged liver, but other types of masses must be considered, including an omental hernia, pancreatic tumor, pancreatic cyst, gastric carcinoma, pyloric stenosis, aortic aneurysm, and retroperitoneal sarcoma.
3. Is it in the left upper quadrant? Left upper quadrant masses are often a splenomegaly, but abdominal wall hematomas occur in this area, as well as pancreatic tumors, pancreatic cysts, gastric tumors, colon tumors, kidney tumors, or enlargement and fecal impaction.
4. Is it in the right lower quadrant? A mass in the right lower quadrant is frequently a carcinoma of the colon, appendiceal abscess, psoas abscess, pyosalpinx, regional ileitis, intussusception, or an ovarian tumor.
5. Is it in the hypogastrium? A mass in the hypogastrium may be bladder, pregnant uterus, uterine fibroids, regional ileitis, urachal cyst, omental cyst, and rarely, endometrial carcinoma.
6. Is it in the left lower quadrant? A left lower quadrant mass is most often a palpable sigmoid colon, but pathological conditions such as diverticulitis with abscess, carcinoma of the colon, and ovarian tumors may be present.
7. Is the mass tender? The presence of a tender mass in the right upper quadrant often means

congestive heart failure, a tender liver from hepatitis, or a tender gallbladder from cholecystitis, subphrenic abscess, perinephric abscess, or an abdominal wall hematoma. A tender mass in the epigastrium may be a pancreatic cyst. A tender mass in the left upper quadrant may be an abdominal wall hematoma or a perinephric abscess. A tender mass in the right lower quadrant may be appendiceal abscess, psoas abscess, pyosalpinx, regional ileitis, or intussusception. A tender mass in the left lower quadrant may be a diverticulitis or pyosalpinx.

8. Is there blood in the urine or stool? The presence of blood in the urine, of course, would suggest a tumor of the kidney such as hypernephroma or Wilms' tumor. The presence of blood in the gastrointestinal tract would suggest either a gastric carcinoma or colon carcinoma, but may also be seen in intussusception, diverticulitis, and regional ileitis. Occasionally it is seen in carcinoma of the ampulla of Vater.

9. Is there fever? The presence of fever would suggest that the mass is an abscess such as subphrenic abscess, perinephric abscess, diverticular abscess, appendiceal abscess, or pyosalpinx. Fever also suggests hepatitis, cholecystitis, or cholangitis.

DIAGNOSTIC WORKUP

Routine diagnostic tests include a CBC, sedimentation rate, urinalysis, chemistry panel with electrolytes, amylase and lipase, stool for occult blood, EKG, chest x-rays, and a flat plate of the abdomen. If there are chills and fever, blood cultures ought to be done. Next in line are contrast radiographic studies such as upper GI series, barium enema, small bowel series, intravenous pyelogram, or cholecystogram.

An abdominal ultrasound will be helpful in differentiating cholecystitis and other cystic masses of the pancreas, kidneys, and reproductive organs.

Endoscopic procedures will help diagnose carcinoma of the stomach and colon and diverticulitis. Endoscopic retrograde cholangiopancreatography is useful in diagnosing carcinoma of the pancreas and bowel ducts.

Lymphangiography will help differentiate retroperitoneal tumors. CT scans of the abdomen and pelvis are useful in differentiating all types of masses. Gallium scans will help uncover subdiaphragmatic, perinephric, diverticular, and pelvic abscesses. Peritoneal taps will help differentiate ascites, pancreatitis, and peritoneal bleeding. A laparoscopy is useful in differentiating many types of masses also. Ultimately, exploratory laparotomy is still an excellent way of establishing a diagnosis.

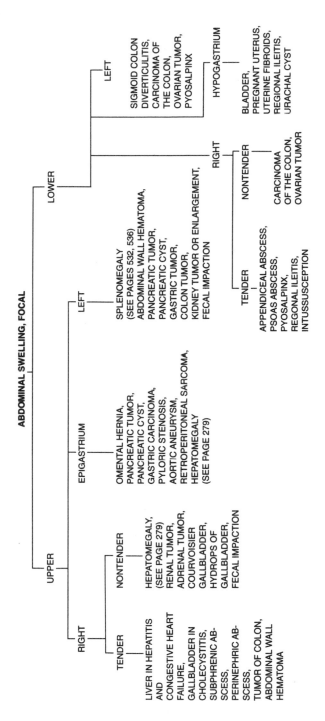

ABDOMINAL SWELLING, FOCAL

UPPER

RIGHT

TENDER

LIVER IN HEPATITIS AND CONGESTIVE HEART FAILURE, GALLBLADDER IN CHOLECYSTITIS, SUBPHRENIC ABSCESS, PERINEPHRIC ABSCESS, TUMOR OF COLON, ABDOMINAL WALL HEMATOMA

NONTENDER

HEPATOMEGALY, (SEE PAGE 279) RENAL TUMOR, ADRENAL TUMOR, COURVOISIER GALLBLADDER, HYDROPS OF GALLBLADDER, FECAL IMPACTION

EPIGASTRIUM

OMENTAL HERNIA, PANCREATIC TUMOR, PANCREATIC CYST, GASTRIC CARCINOMA, PYLORIC STENOSIS, AORTIC ANEURYSM, RETROPERITONEAL SARCOMA, HEPATOMEGALY (SEE PAGE 279)

LEFT

SPLENOMEGALY (SEE PAGES 532, 536) ABDOMINAL WALL HEMATOMA, PANCREATIC TUMOR, PANCREATIC CYST, GASTRIC TUMOR, COLON TUMOR, KIDNEY TUMOR OR ENLARGEMENT, FECAL IMPACTION

LOWER

RIGHT

TENDER

APPENDICEAL ABSCESS, PSOAS ABSCESS, PYOSALPINX, REGIONAL ILEITIS, INTUSSUSCEPTION

NONTENDER

CARCINOMA OF THE COLON, OVARIAN TUMOR

LEFT

SIGMOID COLON DIVERTICULITIS, CARCINOMA OF THE COLON, OVARIAN TUMOR, PYOSALPINX

HYPOGASTRIUM

BLADDER, PREGNANT UTERUS, UTERINE FIBROIDS, REGIONAL ILEITIS, URACHAL CYST

ABDOMINAL SWELLING, GENERALIZED

Ask the following questions:

1. Is there hepatomegaly? If there is hepatomegaly, one should suspect congestive heart failure, emphysema, constrictive pericarditis, hepatic vein thrombosis, and cirrhosis of the liver.
2. Is there dyspnea or cardiomegaly? If there is dyspnea or cardiomegaly, one should suspect congestive heart failure or emphysema.
3. Is there hypertension or proteinuria? The presence of hypertension or proteinuria should arouse suspicion of nephritis or nephrosis.
4. Is there diffuse abdominal tenderness and rebound? These findings are suggestive of tuberculous peritonitis, ruptured viscus, pancreatic cyst, advanced intestinal obstruction, mesenteric thrombosis or embolism, acute pancreatitis, and ruptured ectopic pregnancy.

DIAGNOSTIC WORKUP

Routine diagnostic tests include a CBC, sedimentation rate, urinalysis, microscopic examination of the urine sediment, chemistry panel, amylase and lipase, tuberculin test, stool for occult blood, chest x-ray, EKG, and flat plate of the abdomen with lateral decubiti. In women of childbearing age a pregnancy test should be done.

The presence of ascites or smaller amounts of fluid can be established by ultrasonography or CT scan. If peritoneal fluid is established, a peritoneal tap is done and the fluid analyzed and cultured. Cultures should be done for both routine and acid-fast bacilli. The fluid may be spun down and a Papanicolaou smear made or cell block study done. Contrast radiographic studies may identify a primary neoplasm or primary source for infection. Gallium scans may be utilized to identify a source for infection. Laparoscopy or exploratory laparotomy are useful in establishing the diagnosis. A general surgeon or gastroenterologist should be consulted early in the diagnostic evaluation.

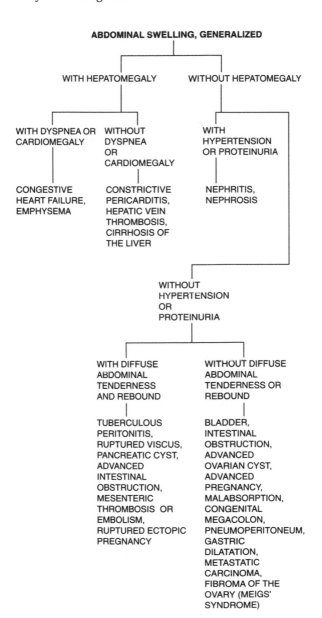

ABSENT OR DIMINISHED PULSE

Ask the following questions:

1. Is it in the upper or lower extremities? Diminished pulse in the upper extremities should suggest dissecting aneurysm, embolism, fracture, arteriovenous fistula, coarctation of the aorta, aortic aneurysm, thoracic outlet syndrome, and subclavian steal syndrome. Diminished pulse in the lower extremities should suggest embolism, fracture, arteriovenous fistula, peripheral arteriosclerosis, Leriche's syndrome, and coarctation of the aorta, as well as dissecting aneurysm. Diminished pulses in all four extremities would suggest shock or constrictive pericarditis.

2. Is it unilateral or bilateral? The presence of unilateral absent or diminished pulse should suggest dissecting aneurysm, embolism, fracture, arteriovenous fistula, some cases of coarctation of the aorta, aortic aneurysm, thoracic outlet syndrome, and subclavian steal if it is in the upper extremity. In the lower extremities, unilateral decrease in the pulse may be due to arteriosclerosis. Bilateral diminished pulses would suggest Leriche's syndrome, saddle embolism, dissecting aneurysm, and coarctation of the aorta if it is in the lower extremity, and if it is in the upper extremity it may also be related to a dissecting aneurysm and rarely arteriosclerosis.

3. Is it sudden in onset? The presence of a sudden onset in diminished pulse should suggest an embolism or dissecting aneurysm regardless of where the diminished or absent pulse may be. However, if it is just the lower extremities, it could be Leriche's syndrome as well. If all four extremities are involved, of course, it could be shock.

DIAGNOSTIC WORKUP

Routine tests include a CBC, sedimentation rate, urinalysis, chemistry panel, VDRL, EKG, and chest x-ray. If there is a history of trauma, x-rays of the involved extremity or extremities should be done. If it is acute onset with fever, a blood culture should be done to rule out bacterial endocarditis. Since an acute onset suggests an embolism, a search for the embolic source should be undertaken. This would include serial EKGs and cardiac enzymes to rule out myocardial infarction, echocardiography to rule out a thrombus in the atrium or ventricle, and 24-hr Holter monitoring to rule out auricular fibrillation of the paroxysmal variety. A cardiologist should be consulted for further guidance in determining if there is an embolic source.

If there are transient ischemic attacks, four-vessel angiography should be done to determine if there is a subclavian steal. If a dissecting aneurysm is suspected, aortography is the diagnostic procedure of choice and this must be done without delay. Doppler studies are of assistance in diagnosing the peripheral arteriosclerosis regardless of where it is, but angiography will ultimately need to be done to determine the exact location of the blockage and whether surgery could be effective in alleviating the condition.

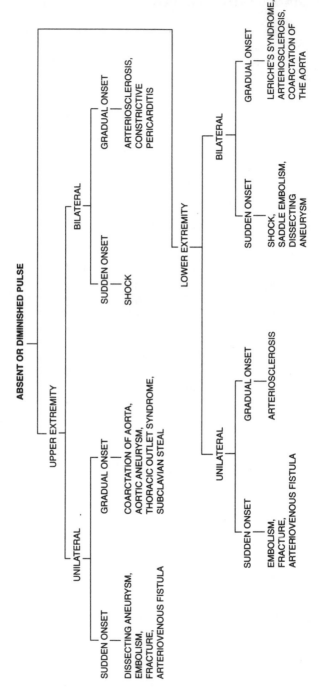

ALOPECIA

The clinician faced with a patient with hair loss must decide whether it is focal or diffuse. If it is focal, he should determine whether or not there is a rash in the area of hair loss. If there is a rash, one should consider conditions such as tinea capitis, lupus erythematosus, psoriasis, and seborrheic dermatitis. If there is no rash, then one should consider alopecia areata, syphilis, burns, and other injuries to the skin.

If the area of hair loss is diffuse, one must consider that it might be male pattern baldness, as well as female pattern baldness in later years. If it is not typically a male pattern baldness, then one must consider that it might be due to a systemic disease like myxedema, hyperpituitarism, hyperthyroidism, anticoagulant drug therapy, or cancer chemotherapy.

DIAGNOSTIC WORKUP

If you are looking for pyoderma or a fungal infection, then a smear and culture of the scrapings for bacteria and fungi should be done. If these are negative, a skin biopsy should be performed. The skin biopsy will help identify lupus erythematosus, psoriasis, and alopecia areata. Systemic disorders may need to be ruled out with thyroid function tests, ANA, VDRL, CBC and serum iron and ferritin. A dermatologist should be consulted in difficult cases.

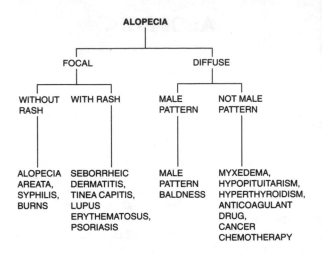

ALOPECIA

FOCAL — DIFFUSE

WITHOUT RASH — WITH RASH

MALE PATTERN — NOT MALE PATTERN

ALOPECIA AREATA, SYPHILIS, BURNS

SEBORRHEIC DERMATITIS, TINEA CAPITIS, LUPUS ERYTHEMATOSUS, PSORIASIS

MALE PATTERN BALDNESS

MYXEDEMA, HYPOPITUITARISM, HYPERTHYROIDISM, ANTICOAGULANT DRUG, CANCER CHEMOTHERAPY

AMENORRHEA

Ask the following questions:

1. Is there galactorrhea? Of course, the most common cause of galactorrhea would be the galactorrhea following pregnancy and delivery. However, if there is galactorrhea, one should consider the possibility that the patient is taking drugs, including contraceptive pills and marijuana. Also, one should consider pituitary tumors and hypothalamic tumors.
2. Are there abnormal or absent secondary sex characteristics? If there is masculinization, then an adrenal or ovarian tumor or polycystic ovaries should be considered. If there is simply absence of female secondary sex characteristics, one should consider Turner's syndrome or Simmonds' disease and other pituitary disorders.
3. Are there abnormal findings on the vaginal examination? The amenorrhea may be due to an imperforate hymen, an imperforate vagina, absence of the vagina, a cervical stenosis with hematometra and absence of a uterus, as in testicular dysgenesis. If there are normal female secondary sex characteristics and a normal vaginal examination and no galactorrhea, then some systemic disease such as anemia, leukemia, or Hodgkin's disease must be considered as well as psychogenic causes. Perhaps the amenorrhea is secondary to a neurologic disorder.

DIAGNOSTIC WORKUP

The first thing to do is a pregnancy test, as pregnancy is the most common cause of secondary amenorrhea. If the pregnancy test is negative, referral to a gynecologist may be done at this time. If a specialist is not handy, one may proceed with the workup. A trial of medroxyprogesterone acetate (Provera®) may be done by intermuscular injection or by mouth. If bleeding occurs upon withdrawal of the progesterone, then it is established that the uterus is functional. It also establishes that the cervix and vagina are patent.

If there is no galactorrhea and the patient is a teenager, one may simply discontinue studies at this point and observe for the normal onset of the menstrual cycle.

If the patient with primary amenorrhea has already reached her twenties or if there is definite secondary amenorrhea, then further diagnostic studies should be done. If there is galactorrhea, a serum for prolactin should be done. If that is elevated, then a CT scan of the brain should be done to look for a pituitary tumor or hypothalamic tumor. If there is no galactorrhea, then you should still order a prolactin, but also order tests for follicle-stimulating hormone (FSH), luteinizing hormone (LH), and serum estradiol. If the FSH and LH are elevated and the estradiol is decreased, primary ovarian failure must be considered. A buccal smear for sex chromogens should be done to rule out Turner's syndrome. Other causes of primary ovarian failure are ovarian agenesis and resistant ovary syndrome.

If the FSH, LH, and estradiol are all decreased, then hypopituitarism should be considered, as well as hypothalamic disorders. Referral to an endocrinologist is wise at this point. When an adrenocortical tumor is suspected, then a serum cortisol and cortisol suppression test should be done.

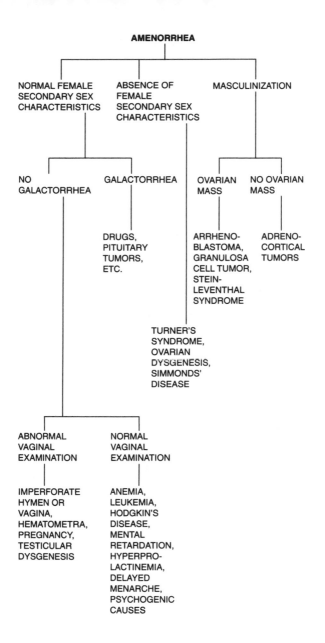

AMNESIA

Ask the following questions:

1. Is the amnesia transient or persistent? If it is transient, one should look for evidence of a head injury. If there is no evidence of a head injury, then one should consider epilepsy, transient ischemic attacks, and migraine. If there is evidence of a headache injury, one would consider concussion and some of the other more serious conditions of the brain that occur with a head injury.
2. Is there a fever? If the amnesia is persistent and there is a fever, one needs to consider encephalitis, meningoencephalitis, cerebral abscesses, and encephalomyelitis. If there is no fever, then one must ask if there is a reduction of memory for recent events. If there is reduction of memory for recent events, one should consider some of the more serious diseases of the brain such as cerebral tumors, chronic drug or alcohol use, Alzheimer's disease, cerebral arterial sclerosis, and neurosyphilis. If there is no reduction of memory for recent events, then a psychiatric disorder such as hysteria, dissociated reaction, or schizophrenia must be considered.

DIAGNOSTIC WORKUP

All patients with a history of amnesia deserve a computed tomography (CT) scan or magnetic resonance imaging (MRI). The CT scan would be more cost-effective and would be the diagnostic test of choice because it also helps detect acute brain hemorrhages. Patients with fever should have a spinal tap as well as CBC, urinalysis, and chemistry panel. These patients also probably deserve a blood culture. An electroencephalogram should be ordered to rule out epilepsy and toxic metabolic inflammatory diseases of the brain.

If all these studies are negative and an organic

cause is still considered, then referral to a neurosurgeon or neurologist is in order. If these studies are negative and a psychiatric disorder is suspected, a psychiatrist should be consulted.

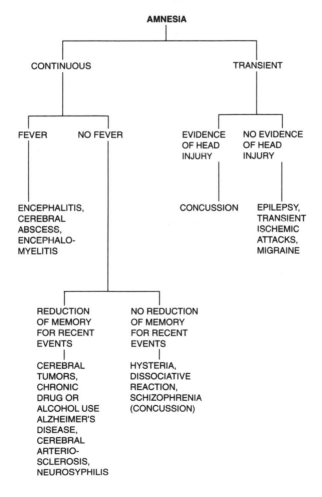

AMNESIA

CONTINUOUS

TRANSIENT

FEVER   NO FEVER

EVIDENCE OF HEAD INJURY

NO EVIDENCE OF HEAD INJURY

ENCEPHALITIS, CEREBRAL ABSCESS, ENCEPHALO-MYELITIS

CONCUSSION

EPILEPSY, TRANSIENT ISCHEMIC ATTACKS, MIGRAINE

REDUCTION OF MEMORY FOR RECENT EVENTS

NO REDUCTION OF MEMORY FOR RECENT EVENTS

CEREBRAL TUMORS, CHRONIC DRUG OR ALCOHOL USE ALZHEIMER'S DISEASE, CEREBRAL ARTERIO-SCLEROSIS, NEUROSYPHILIS

HYSTERIA, DISSOCIATIVE REACTION, SCHIZOPHRENIA (CONCUSSION)

ANOSMIA OR
UNUSUAL ODOR

Ask the following questions:

1. Is it acute or chronic? Acute loss of smells would certainly suggest an acute upper respiratory infection. It would also suggest recent exposure to toxic fumes or recent head injury. If the anosmia or unusual odor is intermittent, then one should consider psychomotor epilepsy.
2. Is there a history of trauma? A skull fracture, particularly if it involves the cribriform plate, may interrupt the olfactory nerves and cause anosmia.
3. Is there a history of drug use or overuse of nasal sprays? Captopril and penicillamine may cause anosmia. Overuse of alcohol or tobacco may also be the problem. Antirheumatic and antiproliferative drugs are also known to cause anosmia.
4. Is the anosmia unilateral or bilateral? If there is unilateral anosmia, one should consider an olfactory groove meningioma.
5. Are there other neurologic signs? Multifocal neurologic signs should suggest multiple sclerosis and additional neurologic signs such as memory loss should suggest an olfactory groove meningioma or parietal lobe tumor.
6. Are there signs of a systemic disease? Many systemic diseases may cause anosmia, including hypothyroidism, diabetes, renal failure, hepatic failure, and pernicious anemia.

DIAGNOSTIC WORKUP

If the disorder is acute and associated with an upper respiratory infection, nothing need be done. However, if the condition has been of gradual onset and the nasopharyngeal examination is negative and the history of drugs is negative, then a CT scan of the brain should be done. If this is negative, a workup for systemic disease should be done and that should include a CBC and chemistry panel, thyroid profile, serum B_{12} and folic acid, glucose tolerance test, and liver profile. If the anosmia or unusual odors are intermittent, a wake-and-sleep electroencephalogram (EEG) should be done.

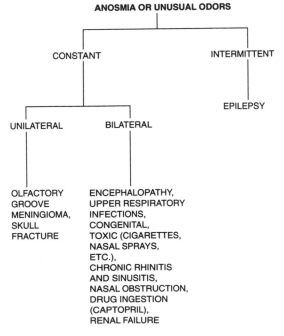

ANOSMIA OR UNUSUAL ODORS

CONSTANT

INTERMITTENT

EPILEPSY

UNILATERAL

BILATERAL

OLFACTORY GROOVE MENINGIOMA, SKULL FRACTURE

ENCEPHALOPATHY, UPPER RESPIRATORY INFECTIONS, CONGENITAL, TOXIC (CIGARETTES, NASAL SPRAYS, ETC.), CHRONIC RHINITIS AND SINUSITIS, NASAL OBSTRUCTION, DRUG INGESTION (CAPTOPRIL), RENAL FAILURE

ANKLE CLONUS

Ask the following questions:

1. What other symptoms and signs are present? Ankle clonus rarely occurs by itself. Usually, there are pathologic reflexes such as a Babinski's sign on the lower extremities. The patient usually also will complain of weakness and may be found to have weakness when the muscles are tested. If the ankle clonus is longstanding, there will be atrophy. There will also frequently be sensory findings, as well as sensory complaints. Finally, with bilateral ankle clonus there will often be hyperactive reflexes throughout the lower extremities and sometimes in the upper extremities.

2. Is the ankle clonus unilateral or bilateral? If it is unilateral, then it is a sign of either hemiparesis or monoplegia and if it is hemiplegia or hemiparesis, one should consider the possibility of a cerebral disorder. If there is headache and papilledema, that disorder is most likely a space-occupying lesion of the brain such as a brain tumor, abscess, or hematoma. If there is hemiparesis and it is acute onset, there is most likely an occlusion of one of the cerebral arteries, whereas if the hemiparesis is gradual in onset, one should consider multiple sclerosis and, once again, a brain tumor. Ankle clonus associated with monoplegia is more likely related to a spinal cord tumor, but a parasagittal tumor could also be present. Bilateral ankle clonus is more likely due to a disorder of the spinal cord such as a spinal cord tumor, amyotrophic lateral sclerosis, or multiple sclerosis. Syringomyelia and Friedreich's ataxia may also present with bilateral ankle clonus. However, if there are cranial nerve signs, one must consider a brain stem tumor as well as other degenerative diseases of the brain and brain stem.

DIAGNOSTIC WORKUP

Ankle clonus is a significant clinical sign, especially when it is unilateral. Therefore, if a brain disorder is suspected, a CT scan of the brain or MRI of the brain should be done. If a spinal cord lesion is suspected, then a CT scan at the appropriate level of the spinal cord should be done. If there are no findings on the examination to indicate a level, then of course the entire spine would have to be covered. MRI is a more cost-effective method for the cervical and thoracic levels of the cord. The spinal tap with analysis of the fluid for myelin basic protein and gamma globulin levels should be done if multiple sclerosis is suspected. In addition, somatosensory evoked potentials and visual evoked potentials should also be done if multiple sclerosis is suspected. Finally, the most cost-effective approach to a patient with ankle clonus is to refer the patient to a neurologic specialist.

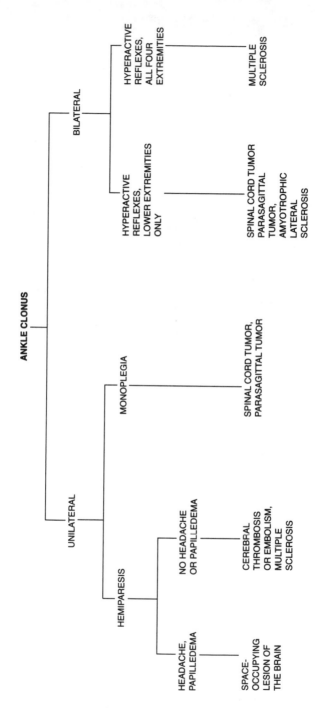

ANKLE CLONUS

UNILATERAL

HEMIPARESIS

HEADACHE, PAPILLEDEMA

SPACE-OCCUPYING LESION OF THE BRAIN

NO HEADACHE OR PAPILLEDEMA

CEREBRAL THROMBOSIS OR EMBOLISM, MULTIPLE SCLEROSIS

MONOPLEGIA

SPINAL CORD TUMOR, PARASAGITTAL TUMOR

BILATERAL

HYPERACTIVE REFLEXES, LOWER EXTREMITIES ONLY

SPINAL CORD TUMOR PARASAGITTAL TUMOR, AMYOTROPHIC LATERAL SCLEROSIS

HYPERACTIVE REFLEXES, ALL FOUR EXTREMITIES

MULTIPLE SCLEROSIS

ANOREXIA

Ask the following questions:

1. Is it acute or chronic? Acute anorexia would most likely be due to an acute febrile disease or acute psychiatric disturbance.
2. Is there a history of drug or alcohol ingestion? Alcoholics frequently have a loss of appetite. Patients on aspirin and digitalis and many other drugs may lose their appetite.
3. Is there an abdominal mass? The abdominal mass may be either an enlarged liver or other mass. The most likely abdominal mass to produce anorexia as the only symptom would be an early pancreatic neoplasm. When the neoplasm advances, then jaundice should be present. Other neoplasms may be felt and/or metastasize to the liver and cause hepatomegaly.
4. Is there a cough? If there is a chronic cough, one should consider tuberculosis or carcinoma of the lung.
5. Is there hepatomegaly? Hepatomegaly without any other masses present in the abdomen would certainly bring to mind a cirrhosis. This could be of cardiac origin so congestive heart failure should be ruled out. Also, the hepatomegaly may be related to a collagen disease or metastatic carcinoma.

DIAGNOSTIC WORKUP

All patients with anorexia as the major sign should have a CBC, sedimentation rate, chemistry panel, thyroid profile, (FT_4I and S-TSH) and a chest x-ray. A referral to a gastroenterologist may be wise if these are negative. However, if the clinician wishes to proceed on his own, then a search for a neoplasm should be conducted and should include an upper GI series, barium enema, abdominal CT scan, and bone scan. If these are negative, a gastroscopy or colonoscopy may be required.

A complete endocrinological workup may be indicated if all the above studies are negative. Patients with a normal physical examination and normal diagnostic studies should be referred to a psychiatrist.

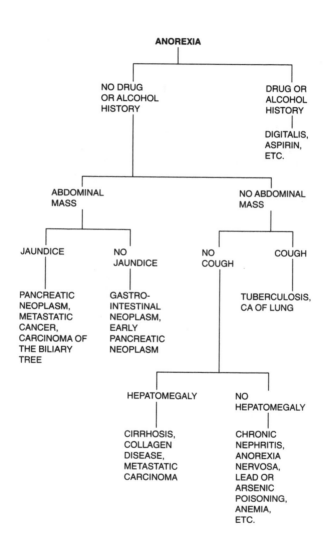

ANURIA OR OLIGURIA

Ask the following questions:

1. Has the patient been on any drugs? Sulfonamides are notorious for causing renal failure, but we must also consider amphotericin B, gold compounds that might be administered in arthritis, and lead and other drugs or heavy metals.
2. What is the blood pressure? If there is hypertension and anuria, one should consider acute or chronic glomerulonephritis, polycystic kidneys, and acute tubular necrosis. If there is a low blood pressure, one should consider prerenal causes of anuria such as dehydration, blood loss, the acute abdomen and other causes of shock.
3. Is there cardiomegaly or chest pain? If there is an enlarged heart, one should consider congestive heart failure. If there is chest pain, one should consider myocardial infarction or pulmonary infarction. If there is chest or abdominal pain with hypertension, then one should consider dissecting aneurysm.
4. Is there enlargement of the kidneys? Enlargement of both kidneys should suggest bilateral hydronephrosis or polycystic kidneys. Unilateral enlargement of the kidneys is not usually associated with anuria.
5. Is there bladder enlargement? Enlarged bladder would make one think of bladder neck obstructions due to prostatic hypertrophy or carcinoma or a urethral stricture. Occasionally what is thought to be an enlarged bladder is actually a pelvic mass that is obstructing the ureter.
6. Is there hematuria? Hematuria would suggest glomerulonephritis, acute tubular necrosis, intravascular hemolysis, and nephrolithiasis.
7. What has been the patient's recent intake of fluid? Dehydration is a frequent cause of oliguria and anuria.

DIAGNOSTIC WORKUP

The first thing to determine is whether the patient really has anuria or oliguria. A Foley catheter should be passed and attached to drainage to determine the urine output. If there is obstructive uropathy due to bladder neck obstruction, obviously this will determine the diagnosis, as there will be a large volume of urine and it should be taken off gradually. Then studies of obstructive uropathy can be done, including cystoscopy and retrograde pyelography. If the obstructive uropathy is due to obstruction of the ureter, then renal ultrasonography can be reliable in detecting the dilated calyces or dilated ureter.

If the patient presents with anuria and hypotension, the most important thing is to reestablish the blood pressure. If the anuria does not cease at this point, then high-dose furosemide or a mannitol infusion can be started. Meanwhile, a CBC, chemistry panel, urinalysis, spot urine sodium, serum protein electrophoresis, an antinuclear antibody (ANA) assay, an EKG, and chest x-ray should be done. A flat plate of the abdomen should give an idea of the kidney size. The clinician should examine the urinary sediment himself and this will identify cases of acute glomerulonephritis, lupus erythematosus, and acute tubular necrosis with considerable accuracy. The BUN and creatinine ratio is helpful in distinguishing pre-renal from renal azotemia.

If intravascular hemolysis is suspected, serum haptoglobins and serum hemoglobin should be done. Eosinophilia of the blood or urine will be found in drug induced nephritis. Renal angiography and aortography should be done in cases of suspected dissecting aneurysm or bilateral renal artery stenosis. Abdominal ultrasound will also be helpful in diagnosing polycystic kidneys and pelvic masses that may be obstructing the ureter. A CT scan may be necessary as well.

In difficult cases, a renal biopsy may be necessary to diagnose the various collagen diseases and the various forms of glomerulonephritis. Referral to a nephrologist would be best at this point.

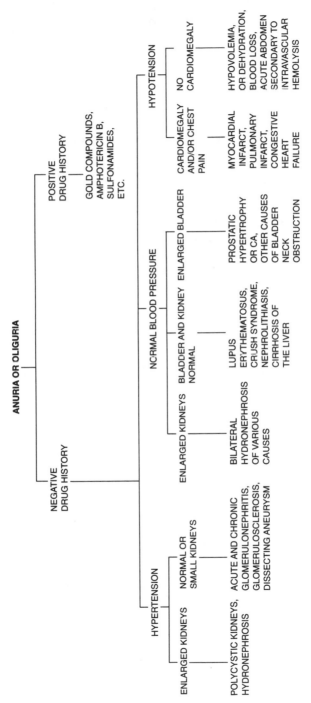

ANURIA OR OLIGURIA

NEGATIVE DRUG HISTORY

HYPERTENSION

ENLARGED KIDNEYS
POLYCYSTIC KIDNEYS, HYDRONEPHROSIS

NORMAL OR SMALL KIDNEYS
ACUTE AND CHRONIC GLOMERULONEPHRITIS, GLOMERULOSCLEROSIS, DISSECTING ANEURYSM

NORMAL BLOOD PRESSURE

ENLARGED KIDNEYS
BILATERAL HYDRONEPHROSIS OF VARIOUS CAUSES

BLADDER AND KIDNEY NORMAL
LUPUS ERYTHEMATOSUS, CRUSH SYNDROME, NEPHROLITHIASIS, CIRRHOSIS OF THE LIVER

ENLARGED BLADDER
PROSTATIC HYPERTROPHY OR CA, OTHER CAUSES OF BLADDER NECK OBSTRUCTION

POSITIVE DRUG HISTORY
GOLD COMPOUNDS, AMPHOTERICIN B, SULFONAMIDES, ETC.

HYPOTENSION

CARDIOMEGALY AND/OR CHEST PAIN
MYOCARDIAL INFARCT, PULMONARY INFARCT, CONGESTIVE HEART FAILURE

NO CARDIOMEGALY
HYPOVOLEMIA, OR DEHYDRATION, BLOOD LOSS, ACUTE ABDOMEN SECONDARY TO INTRAVASCULAR HEMOLYSIS

Anuria or Oliguria   35

ANXIETY

Ask the following questions:

1. Is the anxiety intermittent or constant? Intermittent anxiety suggests the possibility of psychomotor epilepsy, a pheochromocytoma, or insulinoma. It is also possible that the patient is suffering from an intermittent cardiac arrhythmia such as paroxysmal supraventricular tachycardia or atrial fibrillation.
2. What is the patient's age? The young or middle-aged patient is more likely to be suffering from a psychiatric disorder, while the older patient may be suffering from cerebral arteriosclerosis or some other type of dementia.
3. If there is tachycardia, is it sustained during sleep? Tachycardia that is sustained during sleep would suggest hyperthyroidism, caffeine effects, or other drug effects.
4. Is there associated weight loss? Sustained tachycardia with weight loss makes hyperthyroidism a very likely possibility.

DIAGNOSTIC WORKUP

Patients with intermittent anxiety with long periods of calmness in between should have a wake-and-sleep EEG and possibly a CT scan to rule out a cerebral tumor. A 24-hr urine collection for catecholamines should be done also to rule out a pheochromocytoma. Twenty-four hour Holter monitoring may be necessary to rule out a paroxysmal cardiac arrhythmia. In difficult cases, a 24-hr EEG or an EEG with nasopharyngeal electrodes inserted may be necessary.

Patients with constant anxiety should have a thyroid profile and an EKG. If these are not revealing, perhaps 24-hr Holter monitoring may be of some value. With a negative workup, a referral to a psychiatrist is in order. It may be even wiser to consult a psychiatrist before undertaking an expensive workup.

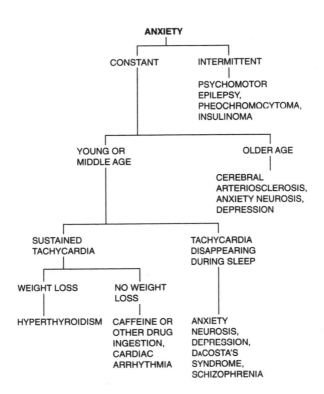

APHASIA, APRAXIA, AND AGNOSIA

Ask the following questions:

1. Is it intermittent? Episodic aphasia, apraxia, or agnosia would suggest epilepsy, transient ischemic attacks, migraine, or hypertensive encephalopathy.
2. Is it acute or gradual in onset? Acute onset of aphasia, apraxia, or agnosia would suggest a cerebral vascular accident, or if there is fever, the onset of a cerebral abscess. It may also mark the onset of acute encephalitis. The gradual onset of aphasia, apraxia, and agnosia would suggest a tumor or other type of space-occupying lesion.
3. Is there associated headache or papilledema? Headaches with aphasia, apraxia, and agnosia might suggest migraine, but we should not forget a brain tumor. Obviously, papilledema is a sign of a space-occupying lesion.
4. Is there significant dementia? The development of dementia along with the aphasia, apraxia, and agnosia suggest Alzheimer's disease, Pick's disease, herpes encephalitis, multiple sclerosis, or Korsakoff's psychosis.

DIAGNOSTIC WORKUP

All patients should have a CBC, sedimentation rate, chemistry panel, a VDRL test, and a CT scan of the brain. The CT scan may demonstrate an infarct, a space-occupying lesion, a degenerative disease, or multiple sclerosis. If this is negative, then a neurologist should be consulted before ordering MRI or a spinal tap.

If the patient presents with intermittent aphasia, apraxia, or agnosia, an electroencephalogram should be done to rule out epilepsy and a carotid scan should be done to rule out carotid stenosis or carotid plaques with ulceration. Four-vessel angiography may need to be considered, but a neurologist should be consulted before this is done.

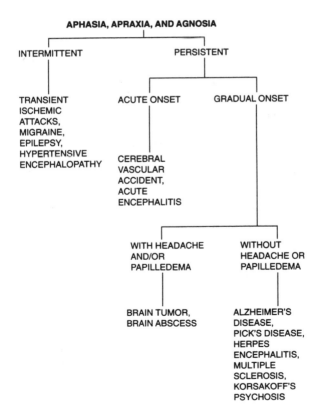

APHASIA, APRAXIA, AND AGNOSIA

INTERMITTENT

PERSISTENT

TRANSIENT ISCHEMIC ATTACKS, MIGRAINE, EPILEPSY, HYPERTENSIVE ENCEPHALOPATHY

ACUTE ONSET

GRADUAL ONSET

CEREBRAL VASCULAR ACCIDENT, ACUTE ENCEPHALITIS

WITH HEADACHE AND/OR PAPILLEDEMA

WITHOUT HEADACHE OR PAPILLEDEMA

BRAIN TUMOR, BRAIN ABSCESS

ALZHEIMER'S DISEASE, PICK'S DISEASE, HERPES ENCEPHALITIS, MULTIPLE SCLEROSIS, KORSAKOFF'S PSYCHOSIS

ASCITES

Ask the following questions:

1. Is there associated dyspnea? If there is associated dyspnea, one should look for congestive heart failure, pulmonary emphysema, and other cardiopulmonary conditions.
2. Is there hepatomegaly? If there is associated hepatomegaly, certainly cirrhosis of the liver has to top the list of possibilities, but additional causes of ascites with hepatomegaly are constrictive pericarditis, the cardiomyopathies, Budd-Chiari syndrome, metastatic carcinoma, and hydatid cyst.
3. Is there edema of the lower extremities or significant proteinuria? Edema in the lower extremities along with significant proteinuria certainly suggests a nephrotic syndrome, whether it be due to glomerulonephritis, diabetes, or a collagen disease. It also suggests end-stage nephritis. If there is no significant proteinuria, then a primary peritoneal condition such as tuberculous peritonitis or peritoneal carcinomatosis must be considered. Remember, a large ovarian cyst can simulate ascites.
4. Is there a history of a primary tumor elsewhere? Gastrointestinal tumors may spread to the peritoneal surface and cause ascites, but a malignant melanoma may do the same thing.

DIAGNOSTIC WORKUP

A peritoneal tap with analysis of the fluid to determine whether it is a transudate or exudate and cell block studies as well as amylase, culture and sensitivity should be done. A CBC, chemistry panel, urinalysis, and sedimentation rate need to be done on all cases and the urinary sediment should be examined under the microscope.

To rule out congestive heart failure, venous pressure and circulation time, EKG, pulmonary function studies, and chest x-ray should be done. To rule out pulmonary emphysema, pulmonary function studies and chest x-rays should be done. To rule out liver disease, a liver profile may be done along with a serum protein electrophoresis and a CT scan of the liver. A tuberculin test can be done to rule out tuberculous peritonitis, but the ascitic fluids should be studied with an acid-fast smear and culture. Guinea pig inoculation is sometimes necessary for a positive diagnosis. A CT scan of the abdomen should be done to determine if there is peritoneal carcinomatosis or a primary malignancy of the GI tract and other structures in the abdomen. An upper GI series and barium enema may need to be done. Also, colonoscopy and gastroscopy may need to be done.

As the diagnostic tests become more expensive, the clinician should consider a referral to a gastroenterologist, nephrologist, or hepatologist beforehand.

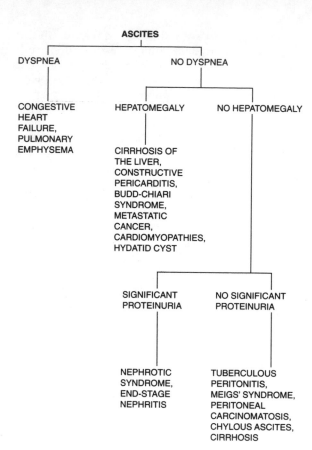

ASCITES

DYSPNEA

CONGESTIVE
HEART
FAILURE,
PULMONARY
EMPHYSEMA

NO DYSPNEA

HEPATOMEGALY

CIRRHOSIS OF
THE LIVER,
CONSTRUCTIVE
PERICARDITIS,
BUDD-CHIARI
SYNDROME,
METASTATIC
CANCER,
CARDIOMYOPATHIES,
HYDATID CYST

NO HEPATOMEGALY

SIGNIFICANT
PROTEINURIA

NEPHROTIC
SYNDROME,
END-STAGE
NEPHRITIS

NO SIGNIFICANT
PROTEINURIA

TUBERCULOUS
PERITONITIS,
MEIGS' SYNDROME,
PERITONEAL
CARCINOMATOSIS,
CHYLOUS ASCITES,
CIRRHOSIS

ATAXIA

Ask the following questions:

1. Is there vertigo, tinnitus, or deafness? Any one of these three signs and symptoms should suggest Ménière's disease or other labyrinthine disease as well as eighth nerve pathology.
2. Are there headaches, nystagmus, or papilledema? These signs should suggest a cerebellar tumor or acoustic neuroma.
3. Are there other neurologic signs? If there are long tract signs such as hyperactive reflexes and loss of vibratory or position sense, one should consider multiple sclerosis, pernicious anemia, or basilar artery insufficiency. If there are glove and stocking hypesthesia and hypoactive reflexes, one should consider peripheral neuropathy or tabes dorsalis.
4. Is the ataxia worse in the dark? This is a sign that the dorsal column or peripheral nerve is affected and one should look for peripheral neuropathy, pernicious anemia, multiple sclerosis, and Friedreich's ataxia. One should also look for tabes dorsalis.
5. Is there a secondary gain? Hysterical patients and patients who are malingering will often show a completely normal neurologic examination, but be unable to walk or stand without staggering. The author has been particularly impressed with patients applying for long-term disability who stagger a great deal without support, but as soon as support in the form of a cane is given, their ataxia completely clears up.

DIAGNOSTIC WORKUP

The wise clinician should consider a neurologic referral at the outset. If there is vertigo, tinnitus, or deafness, then an audiogram and caloric testing should be done. If these suggest eighth nerve damage, then a CT scan or MRI of the brain should be done. Headaches, sustained nystagmus, or papilledema are other indications for a CT scan or MRI. If multiple sclerosis is suspected, MRI of the brain is very useful, as well as spinal fluid for gamma globulin and myelin basic protein. Perhaps visual evoked potentials, brain stem evoked potentials, or somatosensory evoked potential studies should be done. Patients with hypoactive reflexes and glove and stocking hypesthesia and hypalgesia will need a neuropathy workup (see page 425). When there is ataxia in the presence of a normal neurologic examination, referral to a psychologist for psychometric testing should be done.

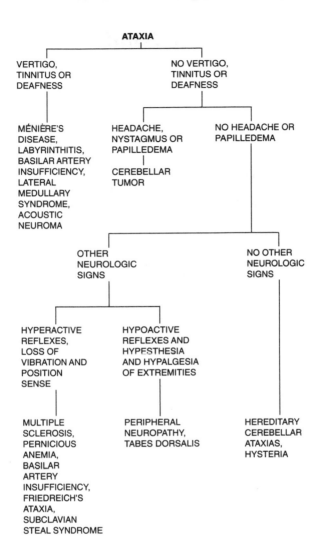

ATHETOSIS

Athetosis is an involuntary, smooth, sinuous, writhing movement of the upper limbs and, less commonly, the face and lower extremity. The pill-rolling of Parkinson's disease is an example. Athetosis is due to a lesion of the basal ganglia. It may be the result of cerebral palsy, encephalitis, Wilson's disease, Parkinson's disease, dystonia musculorum deformans, or a cerebral infarct.

DIAGNOSTIC WORKUP

Patients presenting with this complaint should have MRI, a serum copper and ceruloplasmin, a CBC, and liver function tests. A spinal tap should be performed if central nervous system lues is suspected.

AXILLARY MASS

Ask the following questions:

1. Is it unilateral or bilateral? Unilateral masses are usually enlarged lymph nodes due to some infectious process in the extremity served by the axillary nodes or the breast served by the axillary nodes. The unilateral mass may also be a tuberculous abscess, lipoma, a sebaceous cyst, metastatic carcinoma, or Hodgkin's disease. Rarely it is due to an aneurysm. When the masses are bilateral, one should consider a systemic infection, leukemia or advanced lymphoma. Rheumatoid arthritis and tuberculosis may be associated with bilateral axillary nodes.

2. Is it painful or painless? A painful axillary mass is usually an acute abscess or an acute inflammation of the lymph node due to infection on the extremity or breast supplied by the lymph node or hidradenitis suppurativa.

3. Is there a discharge from the mass? A discharge from an axillary mass usually means hidradenitis suppurativa.

4. Is there fever? Fever with a bilateral axillary mass would suggest an acute systemic infection or infectious mononucleosis. Fever with a unilateral axillary mass would suggest that there is mastitis, a breast abscess, or lymphangitis of the extremity supplied by the axillary lymph nodes.

5. If the mass is unilateral, are there signs of an infection on the extremity or breast supplied by the axillary nodes? In tularemia there will be a bubo on the extremity supplied by the axillary nodes and in lymphadenitis there should be an infectious lesion on the extremity involved. If the lymphadenitis is due to mastitis, there should be a breast discharge or extreme tenderness and enlargement of the breast.

6. Does the mass pulsate? A pulsatile mass in the axilla is usually an aneurysm.

DIAGNOSTIC WORKUP

If the mass is fluctuant or exudes a discharge, then needle aspiration should be done and the material retrieved in order to have culture and sensitivity performed on it. The discharge may also be cultured for an organism. All patients with bilateral axillary masses should have a CBC, sedimentation rate, chemistry panel, and urinalysis. Skin testing for tuberculosis, sarcoidosis, and various fungi should be done. A chest x-ray should be done to look for tuberculosis or malignancy. Mammography should be done in cases of unilateral axillary masses that suggest lymphadenopathy. In the final analysis, a biopsy of the mass may need to be done to make the diagnosis.

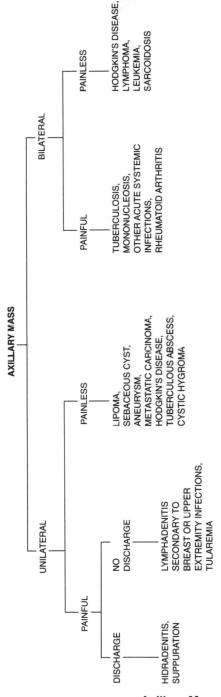

AXILLARY MASS

- **UNILATERAL**
  - **PAINFUL**
    - **DISCHARGE**
      - HIDRADENITIS, SUPPURATION
    - **NO DISCHARGE**
      - LYMPHADENITIS SECONDARY TO BREAST OR UPPER EXTREMITY INFECTIONS, TULAREMIA
  - **PAINLESS**
    - LIPOMA, SEBACEOUS CYST, ANEURYSM, METASTATIC CARCINOMA, HODGKIN'S DISEASE, TUBERCULOUS ABSCESS, CYSTIC HYGROMA
- **BILATERAL**
  - **PAINFUL**
    - TUBERCULOSIS, MONONUCLEOSIS, OTHER ACUTE SYSTEMIC INFECTIONS, RHEUMATOID ARTHRITIS
  - **PAINLESS**
    - HODGKIN'S DISEASE, LYMPHOMA, LEUKEMIA, SARCOIDOSIS

BABINSKI'S SIGN

Ask the following questions:

1. Is the onset acute? A Babinski's sign of acute onset is due to trauma or vascular diseases in most cases. If there is a fever, one should consider an infectious process, most likely a cerebral abscess. Multiple sclerosis may also cause a Babinski's sign of recent or acute onset.
2. Is the Babinski's sign unilateral or bilateral? Unilateral Babinski's signs suggest a space-occupying lesion of the brain such as hematoma, abscess, or tumor. It also suggests a cerebral vascular accident. If the Babinski's signs are bilateral, it may be due to a toxic or degenerative condition of the brain such as encephalitis. It may also be due to a spinal cord tumor or other space-occupying lesion of the spinal cord.
3. Are there associated cranial nerve signs? If there is associated central facial palsy on the ipsilateral side, one should consider an infarct or a space-occupying lesion of the opposite cerebral hemisphere. If there are cranial nerve signs besides a facial palsy, one should consider a brain stem lesion, especially if they are contralateral.
4. Are there hypoactive reflexes? Babinski's signs with hypoactive reflexes, if it is acute onset, would be considered a traumatic or vascular lesion of the brain if it is unilateral and an acute vascular or traumatic lesion of the spinal cord if it is bilateral. Hypoactive reflexes of relatively insidious onset should make one think of pernicious anemia or Friedreich's ataxia.
5. Are there hyperactive reflexes? Unilateral hyperactive reflexes of the upper and lower extremity with cranial nerve signs should bring to mind middle cerebral artery thrombosis or hemorrhage, carotid stenosis, and a space-occupying lesion of the brain. Hyperactive reflexes of the upper and lower extremities with no cranial nerve signs should suggest a high spinal cord tumor or a herniated disk, especially if it is unilateral.

Unilateral hyperactive reflexes of the lower extremity only would suggest an anterior cerebral artery thrombosis or parasagittal meningioma. Hyperactive reflexes of all extremities with cranial nerve signs should suggest a basilar artery thrombosis, brain stem tumor, or other lesion of the brain stem. Weakness and hyperactive reflexes of all four extremities without cranial nerve signs and without any sensory changes should suggest a primary lateral sclerosis, although multiple sclerosis may occasionally present in this manner.

6. Are there sensory changes? Hyperactive reflexes with sensory changes confined to the trunk and extremities would make one think of a spinal cord lesion such as multiple sclerosis, pernicious anemia, or Friedreich's ataxia and especially if it is unilateral one would consider a space-occupying lesion of the spinal cord. Other considerations are transverse myelitis and anterior spinal artery occlusion.

7. Is there involvement of the lower extremity only? This is an important question to ask, as this would suggest a spinal cord tumor of the thoracic level or a parasagittal meningioma.

8. Is there radicular pain? The association of radicular pain in the cervical or thoracic area would make one think of a spinal cord tumor or other space-occupying lesion of the spinal cord.

9. Is there associated fever? The finding of fever along with a unilateral Babinski's sign should make one think of a cerebral abscess or an epidural abscess somewhere in the spinal column. The finding of fever with bilateral Babinski's signs should make one think of an encephalitis, particularly if there are disturbances of consciousness. However, fever may be associated with a cerebral vascular accident, so don't be misled.

DIAGNOSTIC WORKUP

The diagnostic workup depends on other symptoms and signs that help the physician determine what level the neurologic lesion might be. If there are acute unilateral Babinski's signs with hemiplegia and cranial nerve signs, a space-occupying lesion or vascular lesion of the brain must be considered. In that case, a CT scan or MRI of the brain should be done and this may be followed with a spinal tap and carotid scans if a vascular lesion is suspected. A spinal tap would not be done if there is any possibility of increased intracranial pressure.

If a cerebral vascular disease is suspected, then a source for an embolism should be looked for. Useful studies include echocardiography and possibly blood cultures and an EKG. If the patient's condition had an insidious onset and there are no cranial nerve signs, then an MRI of the cervical or thoracic sign should be done to look for a tumor, multiple sclerosis, or degenerative diseases.

A Babinski's sign associated with trauma and without cranial nerve signs should prompt one to do x-rays of the cervical, thoracic, and lumbar spine for fracture and other traumatic lesions. If there are associated disturbances of consciousness, we must look for a cerebral lesion and MRI of the brain must be done in these traumatic conditions.

The fact that a Babinski's sign is a definite sign of neurologic disease is reason enough to call a neurologic specialist in before undertaking any diagnostic studies. A neurologic consultation is much less expensive than a CT scan or MRI.

BABINSKI'S SIGN

UNILATERAL

HYPERACTIVE REFLEXES OF UPPER AND LOWER EXTREMITY AND CRANIAL NERVE SIGNS
MIDDLE CEREBRAL ARTERY THROMBOSIS OR HEMORRHAGE, CAROTID STENOSIS, SPACE-OCCUPYING LESION OF THE BRAIN

HYPERACTIVE REFLEXES OF UPPER AND LOWER EXTREMITIES, NO CRANIAL NERVE SIGNS
HIGH SPINAL CORD TUMOR OR HERNIATED DISK

HYPERACTIVE REFLEXES OF LOWER EXTREMITY ONLY
ANTERIOR CEREBRAL ARTERY THROMBOSIS, PARASAGITTAL MENINGIOMA, EARLY SPINAL CORD TUMOR OR OTHER SPACE-OCCUPYING LESION

BILATERAL

WEAKNESS AND HYPERACTIVE REFLEXES OF LOWER EXTREMITIES ONLY
SPINAL CORD TUMOR, PARASAGITTAL MENINGIOMA, AMYOTROPHIC LATERAL SCLEROSIS, SYRINGOMYELIA, TRANSVERSE MYELITIS, ANTERIOR SPINAL ARTERY OCCLUSION, HYPOGLYCEMIA

WEAKNESS AND HYPERACTIVE REFLEXES OF ALL EXTREMITIES WITH CRANIAL NERVE SIGNS
PSEUDOBULBAR PALSY, BASILAR ARTERY THROMBOSIS, BRAIN STEM TUMOR

WEAKNESS AND HYPERACTIVE REFLEXES OF ALL EXTREMITIES WITHOUT CRANIAL NERVE SIGNS

PARESTHESIA AND SENSORY CHANGES
MULTIPLE SCLEROSIS, POSTERIOR FOSSA TUMOR, PERNICIOUS ANEMIA, FRIEDREICH'S ATAXIA, SYRINGOMYELIA, HIGH SPINAL CORD TUMOR, TRANSVERSE MYELITIS, ANTERIOR SPINAL ARTERY OCCLUSION

NO PARESTHESIAS OR SENSORY CHANGES
PRIMARY LATERAL SCLEROSIS

HYPOACTIVE REFLEXES
PERNICIOUS ANEMIA OR FRIEDREICH'S ATAXIA

BACK PAIN

Ask the following questions:

1. Is the pain of acute onset or gradual onset? If it is acute onset, one must consider the possibility of epidural abscess, pyelonephritis, or other abdominal conditions as the cause of the back pain. If it is gradual onset, one should consider that it may be a tumor, particularly of the spinal cord or cauda equina, a pelvic tumor, or an aortic aneurysm that is compressing one of the nerve roots. In addition, chronic conditions such as lumbar spondylosis, rheumatoid spondylitis, and prostatitis must be considered.
2. Is there a history of trauma? If there is a history of trauma, one should consider a compression fracture of the spine, a sprain or herniated disk, as well as spondylolisthesis. Without a history of trauma, one should consider a tumor, herpes zoster, or dissecting aneurysm. Lumbar spondylosis might be silent for a while only to cause pain after a significant traumatic event.
3. Is there radiation of the pain around the trunk or into the extremities? Radiation of the pain would certainly be more likely to signify a space-occupying lesion of the spinal column such as a tumor, an epidural abscess, or a herniated disk. If there is no radiation, one would consider osteoarthritis or lumbar spondylosis and rheumatoid spondylitis.
4. Finally, are there bladder symptoms associated with the pain? If there are, then one must consider the possibility of a spinal cord tumor, cauda equina tumor, or kidney disease.

DIAGNOSTIC WORKUP

All patients with back pain need to have a CBC, urinalysis and probably a urine culture, as well as a chemistry panel. A sedimentation rate should be done if rheumatoid arthritis is suspected. All patients should also have plain x-rays of the thoracic and/or lumbar spine. It is very important to get anterior posterior views, as well as oblique and lateral views. If there is doubt about the diagnosis at this point, a neurologic or orthopedic specialist may be consulted. If there is radiation of the pain into the extremities or around the trunk and definite neurologic findings, one should proceed to a CT scan or MRI immediately. The CT scan costs about half as much as the MRI and usually will show any significant herniated disks, primary or metastatic tumor. Even without radiation of pain into the extremities or definite neurologic findings, a patient with persistent back pain should have a CT scan or MRI. Electromyography will be useful in identifying radiculopathy.

When all these studies are negative, it might be wise to get a bone scan because this will show the increased uptake of the sacroiliac joints in rheumatoid spondylitis. Also, one should test for the HLA B27 antigen. In the event that all the above studies are negative, the possibility of a non-neurologic condition or nonorthopedic condition causing the back pain should be considered. Perhaps abdominal ultrasound should be done to rule out an aortic aneurysm. Perhaps a pelvic tumor or prostatic tumor should be reconsidered. Perhaps there is a pancreatic tumor that is causing the back pain. Occasionally, combined myelography and CT scan is the only way to identify a lesion. Exploratory surgery is rarely necessary. Older patients should have a serum protein electrophoresis (for multiple myeloma) and acid phosphatase or prostate specific antigen (PSA) to rule out prostatic carcinoma.

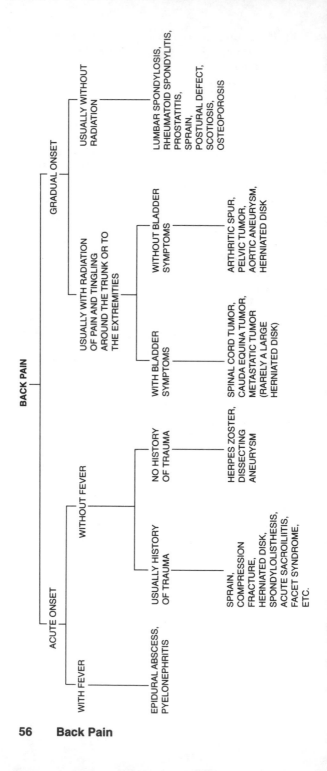

BACK PAIN

- **ACUTE ONSET**
  - **WITH FEVER**
    - EPIDURAL ABSCESS, PYELONEPHRITIS
  - **WITHOUT FEVER**
    - **USUALLY HISTORY OF TRAUMA**
      - SPRAIN, COMPRESSION FRACTURE, HERNIATED DISK, SPONDYLOLISTHESIS, ACUTE SACROILIITIS, FACET SYNDROME, ETC.
    - **NO HISTORY OF TRAUMA**
      - HERPES ZOSTER, DISSECTING ANEURYSM
- **GRADUAL ONSET**
  - **USUALLY WITH RADIATION OF PAIN AND TINGLING AROUND THE TRUNK OR TO THE EXTREMITIES**
    - **WITH BLADDER SYMPTOMS**
      - SPINAL CORD TUMOR, CAUDA EQUINA TUMOR, METASTATIC TUMOR (RARELY A LARGE HERNIATED DISK)
    - **WITHOUT BLADDER SYMPTOMS**
      - ARTHRITIC SPUR, PELVIC TUMOR, AORTIC ANEURYSM, HERNIATED DISK
  - **USUALLY WITHOUT RADIATION**
    - LUMBAR SPONDYLOSIS, RHEUMATOID SPONDYLITIS, PROSTATITIS, SPRAIN, POSTURAL DEFECT, SCOLIOSIS, OSTEOPOROSIS

BLEEDING GUMS

Ask the following questions:

1. Are there abnormalities on examination of the teeth or gums? The gums may be swollen, as in phenytoin use and early scurvy and bleed on slight pressure, as in pyorrhea or other conditions. There may be ulceration of the tongue, gums, and buccal mucosa. There may be an isolated dental caries which is causing bleeding. Excessive tartar may be noted on the teeth.
2. Is there an enlarged spleen or a systemic rash? The presence of an enlarged spleen should bring to mind Hodgkin's disease, leukemia, lupus erythematosus, thrombocytopenia purpura, and aplastic anemia. A systemic rash which is due to petechiae is common in any disorder that might cause thrombocytopenia.
3. Is there a positive Rumpel-Leede test? This would test for capillary fragility and it may be positive in scurvy, thrombocytopenia purpura, leukemia, and other disorders which depress the platelet count. It will also be positive in disorders of platelet function such as von Willebrand's disease.

DIAGNOSTIC WORKUP

A CBC, sedimentation rate, chemistry panel, antinuclear antibody titer, and coagulation profile are basic studies that need to be done. X-rays of the teeth need to be done to look for dental caries, abscesses, and pyorrhea. X-rays of the teeth will also help identify scurvy. A plasma or platelet ascorbic acid level needs to be done if scurvy is suspected. If syphilis is suspected, then a VDRL test needs to be done.

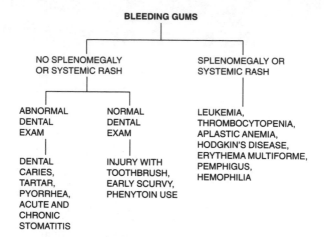

BLEEDING GUMS

NO SPLENOMEGALY OR SYSTEMIC RASH

ABNORMAL DENTAL EXAM

DENTAL CARIES, TARTAR, PYORRHEA, ACUTE AND CHRONIC STOMATITIS

NORMAL DENTAL EXAM

INJURY WITH TOOTHBRUSH, EARLY SCURVY, PHENYTOIN USE

SPLENOMEGALY OR SYSTEMIC RASH

LEUKEMIA, THROMBOCYTOPENIA, APLASTIC ANEMIA, HODGKIN'S DISEASE, ERYTHEMA MULTIFORME, PEMPHIGUS, HEMOPHILIA

BLINDNESS

Ask the following questions:

1. Is it transient? Transient blindness may occur in transient ischemic attacks, epilepsy, migraine, and hypertension.
2. Is it a sudden onset? The sudden onset of blindness may occur in optic neuritis, retinal vein thrombosis, central retinal artery occlusion, vitreous hemorrhage, detached retina, carotid artery thrombosis, temporal arteritis, injuries to the optic nerve, retrobulbar neuritis, fracture of the skull, glaucoma, posterior cerebral artery occlusion, multiple sclerosis, and hysteria.
3. Is it unilateral or bilateral? Unilateral blindness may occur in glaucoma, vitreous hemorrhage, optic neuritis, retinal vein thrombosis, central retinal artery thrombosis, carotid artery thrombosis, temporal arteritis, injury to the optic nerve, fractured skull, brain tumors, retinoblastomas, and sphenoid ridge meningiomas. Bilateral blindness may occur in posterior cerebral artery occlusion, pituitary tumors, retinitis pigmentosa, hereditary optic atrophy, uveitis, toxic amblyopia, cataracts, glaucoma, multiple sclerosis, and iritis.
4. Is there papilledema? The presence of papilledema should make one suspect optic neuritis, retinal vein thrombosis, and space-occupying lesions of the brain.
5. Are there abnormalities on ophthalmoscopic examination? Besides papilledema, there may be changes on the ophthalmoscopic examination in iritis, glaucoma, papillitis from optic neuritis, retinal vein thrombosis, central retinal artery occlusion, vitreous hemorrhage, detached retina, and retinoblastoma.

DIAGNOSTIC WORKUP

Referral to an ophthalmologist is usually the first step in a good workup. If one is not available, a careful eye examination including slit lamp examination, visual acuity evaluation, tonometry, and visual field studies should be done. If these are unrevealing, a referral to an ophthalmologist or neurologist should be done without further delay. Additional studies would include a CT scan or MRI of the brain and orbits, carotid scans, spinal tap, visual evoked potential studies, and four-vessel cerebral angiography.

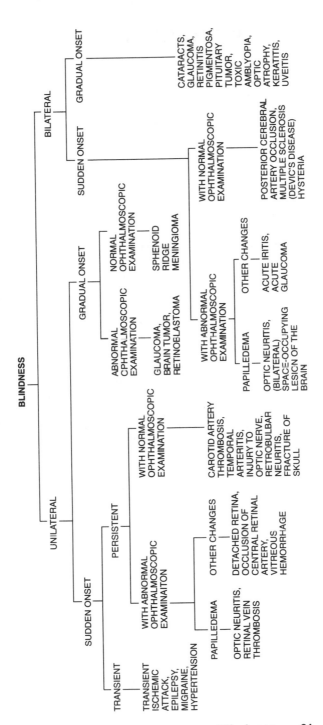

Blindness 61

BLURRED VISION

Ask the following questions:

1. Is it unilateral or bilateral? The presence of unilateral blurred vision should suggest such local ocular conditions as cataract, refractive error, iritis, glaucoma, keratitis, retinal detachment, foreign body, and optic neuritis. Transient blurred vision may occur in migraine and carotid artery insufficiency. Orbital fracture and vitreous hemorrhage may cause unilateral blurred vision also.

   Bilateral blurred vision may result from cocaine use, methyl alcohol poisoning, tobacco, barbiturates, quinine, and other drugs. However, cataracts, glaucoma, chorioretinitis, retinitis pigmentosa, optic atrophy, papilledema, papillitis, optic neuritis, refractive error, pituitary tumors, posterior cerebral artery occlusion, concussion, migraine, and hysteria must also be considered.

2. Is there a positive history for drug or alcohol ingestion? If this history is positive, then cocaine, tobacco, barbiturate methyl alcohol, quinine, and other drugs may be responsible.

3. Is it sudden in onset? Sudden onset of blurred vision should make one suspect migraine, optic neuritis, vitreous hemorrhage, iritis, keratitis, glaucoma, retinal detachment, foreign body, retrobulbar neuritis, orbital fracture, carotid artery insufficiency, and hysteria.

4. Is the eye examination abnormal? Local ocular diseases such as cataracts, refractive errors, iritis, keratitis, glaucoma, retinal detachment, foreign bodies, retinitis pigmentosa, chorioretinitis, and papilledema should be detected by the primary care physician.

DIAGNOSTIC WORKUP

A referral to an ophthalmologist is usually the first step in a workup. If an ophthalmologist is not available, a careful eye examination including slit lamp evaluation tonometry, visual acuity evaluation, and visual fields should be done. If these studies are unremarkable, referral to a neurologist may be made. Further studies would include a CT scan or MRI of the brain, carotid scans, spinal tap, visual evoked potentials, and four-vessel cerebral angiography.

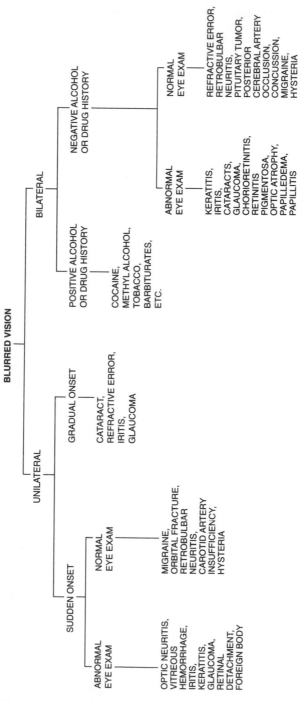

BLURRED VISION

UNILATERAL

- **SUDDEN ONSET**
  - **ABNORMAL EYE EXAM**
    - OPTIC NEURITIS, VITREOUS HEMORRHAGE, IRITIS, KERATITIS, GLAUCOMA, RETINAL DETACHMENT, FOREIGN BODY
  - **NORMAL EYE EXAM**
    - MIGRAINE, ORBITAL FRACTURE, RETROBULBAR NEURITIS, CAROTID ARTERY INSUFFICIENCY, HYSTERIA
- **GRADUAL ONSET**
  - CATARACT, REFRACTIVE ERROR, IRITIS, GLAUCOMA

BILATERAL

- **POSITIVE ALCOHOL OR DRUG HISTORY**
  - COCAINE, METHYL ALCOHOL, TOBACCO, BARBITURATES, ETC.
- **NEGATIVE ALCOHOL OR DRUG HISTORY**
  - **ABNORMAL EYE EXAM**
    - KERATITIS, IRITIS, CATARACTS, GLAUCOMA, CHORIORETINITIS, RETINITIS PIGMENTOSA, OPTIC ATROPHY, PAPILLEDEMA, PAPILLITIS
  - **NORMAL EYE EXAM**
    - REFRACTIVE ERROR, RETROBULBAR NEURITIS, PITUITARY TUMOR, POSTERIOR CEREBRAL ARTERY OCCLUSION, CONCUSSION, MIGRAINE, HYSTERIA

BONE MASS
OR SWELLING

Ask the following questions:

1. Is there a history of trauma? Trauma, of course, may cause fractures and subperiosteal hematomas.
2. Is the patient a child or an adult? Children are more likely to have Ewing's tumors, scurvy, rickets, syphilis, battered baby syndrome, osteosarcoma, osteomas, and osteochondromas. Adults are more likely to have a giant cell tumor, metastasis, osteomyelitis, osteogenic sarcoma, fibrosarcoma, multiple myeloma, generalized fibrocystic disease, Paget's disease, acromegaly, and chondromas.
3. Are the lesions single or focal or are they multiple or diffuse? Multiple and diffuse lesions in children are often due to scurvy, rickets, syphilis, and the battered baby syndrome. Multiple lesions or diffuse lesions in adults are often due to metastasis, multiple myeloma, generalized fibrocystic disease, Paget's disease, acromegaly, and chondroma. Single lesions in children are more likely to be fracture, osteomyelitis, hematoma, Ewing's tumor, osteosarcoma, osteomas, and osteochondromas. Single lesions in adults are often due to a giant cell tumor, osteomyelitis, fracture, hematoma, osteogenic sarcoma, and fibrosarcoma, but may be due to a metastasis.
4. Are the lesions usually painful? Painful lesions in children are more likely to be due to fracture, osteomyelitis, hematoma, Ewing's tumors, scurvy, syphilis, battered baby syndrome, and rickets. Painful lesions in adults may be due to a giant cell tumor, metastasis, osteomyelitis, fracture, hematomas, osteogenic sarcoma, fibrosarcomas, and multiple myeloma.

DIAGNOSTIC WORKUP

Routine diagnostic studies include a CBC, sedimentation rate, urinalysis, chemistry panel, arthritis panel, serum protein electrophoresis, and plain films of the involved bones. A skeletal survey may be necessary. Bone scans are often useful. A search for a primary tumor may require chest x-ray, upper GI series, barium enema, intravenous pyelogram, mammography, prostatic examination, prostatic specific antigen titer, thyroid scans, lymph node biopsy, and bone marrow examinations.

CT scans of the area may help differentiate the mass or swelling. Needle biopsy or exploratory surgery and bone biopsy may be necessary before deciding what surgical approach should be undertaken.

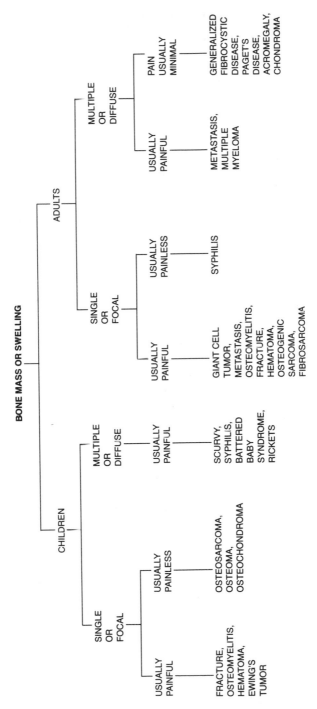

BONE MASS OR SWELLING

CHILDREN

SINGLE OR FOCAL

- USUALLY PAINFUL — FRACTURE, OSTEOMYELITIS, HEMATOMA, EWING'S TUMOR
- USUALLY PAINLESS — OSTEOSARCOMA, OSTEOMA, OSTEOCHONDROMA

MULTIPLE OR DIFFUSE

- USUALLY PAINFUL — SCURVY, SYPHILIS, BATTERED BABY SYNDROME, RICKETS

ADULTS

SINGLE OR FOCAL

- USUALLY PAINFUL — GIANT CELL TUMOR, METASTASIS, OSTEOMYELITIS, FRACTURE, HEMATOMA, OSTEOGENIC SARCOMA, FIBROSARCOMA
- USUALLY PAINLESS — SYPHILIS

MULTIPLE OR DIFFUSE

- USUALLY PAINFUL — METASTASIS, MULTIPLE MYELOMA
- PAIN USUALLY MINIMAL — GENERALIZED FIBROCYSTIC DISEASE, PAGET'S DISEASE, ACROMEGALY, CHONDROMA

Bone Mass or Swelling   67

BORBORYGMI

Ask the following questions:

1. Is there abdominal distention? If there is abdominal distention, an intestinal obstruction should be considered.
2. Is there obvious diarrhea? If there is diarrhea, one should look for malabsorption syndrome, lactase deficiency and carcinoid syndrome. Other causes of chronic diarrhea are discussed on page 137.
3. Is there flushing of the face? If there is significant flushing of the face along with the diarrhea, then carcinoid syndrome is the most likely possibility.

DIAGNOSTIC WORKUP

If there is significant distention of the abdomen, a flat plate of the abdomen with lateral decubiti should be done to rule out intestinal obstruction. A stool for occult blood culture, quantitative fat and ovum, and parasites should be done. If there is flushing, a urine for 5-hydroxyindoleacetic acid (5-HIAA) should be done to rule out carcinoid syndrome. After these tests are done, further workup can proceed. An upper GI series with an esophagram, a small bowel series, and a barium enema would be next in line. If all these studies are negative, perhaps referral to a gastroenterologist or psychiatrist would be indicated. Endoscopy is rarely necessary.

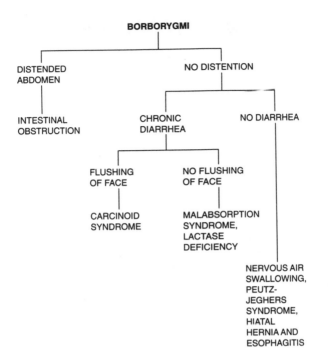

BORBORYGMI

- DISTENDED ABDOMEN
  - INTESTINAL OBSTRUCTION
- NO DISTENTION
  - CHRONIC DIARRHEA
    - FLUSHING OF FACE
      - CARCINOID SYNDROME
    - NO FLUSHING OF FACE
      - MALABSORPTION SYNDROME, LACTASE DEFICIENCY
  - NO DIARRHEA
    - NERVOUS AIR SWALLOWING, PEUTZ-JEGHERS SYNDROME, HIATAL HERNIA AND ESOPHAGITIS

BRADYCARDIA

Ask the following questions:

1. Is there fever? If there is fever, one should look for yellow fever, diphtheria, cerebral abscess, or meningitis. Perhaps the fever is related to increased intracranial pressure from apoplexy.
2. Are there episodes of syncope? The addition of syncope should make one think of a sick sinus syndrome, complete heart block, vasovagal syncope, or carotid sinus syncope.
3. Is there a heart murmur present? Heart murmurs are found in complete heart block, but they are also a sign of aortic stenosis, which can cause bradycardia.
4. Is there a history of drug ingestion? Several drugs can induce bradycardia, the most notable being digitalis, but propranolol, quinidine, and various cholinergic drugs may induce bradycardia. Opium poisoning may cause bradycardia.
5. Is there nonpitting edema? Obviously, this is a sign of myxedema and should be looked for in any patient presenting with bradycardia.
6. Is there chest pain? An acute myocardial infarction may present with bradycardia, although it is more typical for tachycardia to be associated with this condition. Heart disease can cause a second- and third-degree block, which may result in bradycardia, but also various other types of arrhythmia that cause the slowing of the pulse.

DIAGNOSTIC WORKUP

If there is fever without any definite focal signs, then a CBC, sedimentation rate, blood culture, chemistry panel, febrile agglutinins, and tests for other antibodies may be done. If there is fever with nuchal rigidity, a spinal tap should be done, preferably after a CT scan. An EKG will need to be done on all patients and if this shows simple sinus brady-cardia and there is no history of drug ingestion, a thyroid profile should be done. If there is chest pain, serial EKGs and cardiac enzymes should be done. If there is a heart murmur, echocardiography would be an important ancillary study. If the EKG shows various types of arrhythmia, a cardiologist should be consulted for further evaluation.

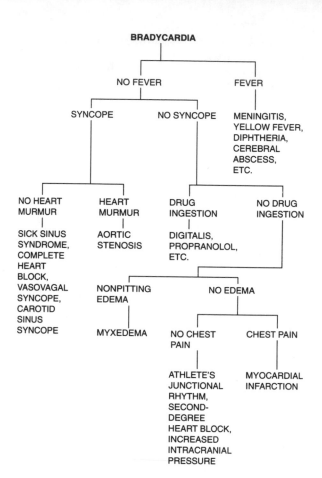

BREAST DISCHARGE

Ask the following questions:

1. Is the discharge unilateral or bilateral? If it is unilateral and watery or bloody, one should look for a neoplasm in the breast. If it is bilateral and milky, one should look for the various conditions that cause hyperprolactinemia or pregnancy.
2. Is the discharge bloody? A unilateral bloody discharge is most suggestive of carcinoma of the breast. Other types of lesions of the breast such as Paget's disease, papillary cystadenoma, and epithelioma of the nipple are causes of a bloody discharge also.
3. Is there a focal mass in the breast? A bloody discharge with a focal mass makes a neoplasm almost certain. If there is a focal mass, fever, and a nonbloody discharge, one should consider abscess.
4. Is there fever? Fever or chills along with a purulent discharge from the breast is most likely acute mastitis or an abscess.

DIAGNOSTIC WORKUP

If there is a bloody discharge, one should not hesitate to refer the patient to a general surgeon. He will probably order mammography and perform a biopsy. The type of biopsy may be either a fine needle aspiration or fine needle biopsy or excisional biopsy, but he can decide which is appropriate for any given patient.

If the discharge is bilateral and milky, a serum prolactin should be ordered. If the prolactin is high, referral to an endocrinologist is probably the best step to take next. He will probably order a CT scan of the brain and pituitary and do further workup studies based on his examination.

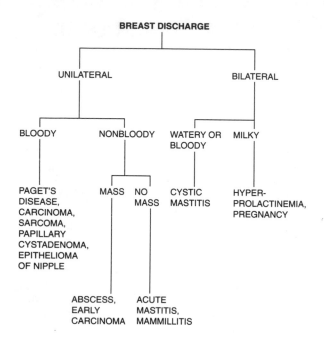

BREAST DISCHARGE

UNILATERAL

- **BLOODY**
  - PAGET'S DISEASE, CARCINOMA, SARCOMA, PAPILLARY CYSTADENOMA, EPITHELIOMA OF NIPPLE
- **NONBLOODY**
  - **MASS**
    - ABSCESS, EARLY CARCINOMA
  - **NO MASS**
    - ACUTE MASTITIS, MAMMILLITIS

BILATERAL

- **WATERY OR BLOODY**
  - CYSTIC MASTITIS
- **MILKY**
  - HYPER-PROLACTINEMIA, PREGNANCY

BREAST MASS

Ask the following questions:

1. Is the mass tender? A tender mass is most likely due to an infectious process such as mastitis or an abscess. However, chronic cystic mastitis may present with a tender mass. Also, advanced carcinoma of the breast usually produces a tender mass.
2. Is there a discharge? A bloody discharge from the breast means that the mass is most likely due to a malignant process. If there is a purulent discharge, abscess or mastitis must be considered. A watery discharge is often associated with chronic cystic mastitis and this occasionally may become bloody.
3. Does it transilluminate? Cysts of the breasts and galactoceles customarily transilluminate. A mass that does not transilluminate is probably a benign or malignant tumor.
4. Is there a deformity of the breast associated with the mass? An orange peel appearance of the skin over a tumor certainly suggests that it is a carcinoma. Retraction of the skin or the nipple suggests carcinoma. Also, in carcinoma there may be necrosis and ulceration of the tissues overlying the tumor.
5. Is there fever? Fever would suggest an acute mastitis or abscess.

DIAGNOSTIC WORKUP

A breast mass is a clear indication for a referral to a general surgeon. He will probably perform mammography and a biopsy before proceeding with surgery.

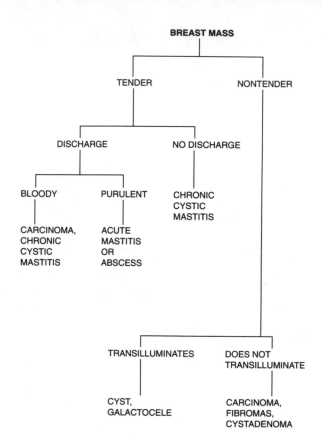

BREAST MASS

TENDER

NONTENDER

DISCHARGE

NO DISCHARGE

BLOODY

PURULENT

CHRONIC
CYSTIC
MASTITIS

CARCINOMA,
CHRONIC
CYSTIC
MASTITIS

ACUTE
MASTITIS
OR
ABSCESS

TRANSILLUMINATES

**DOES NOT
TRANSILLUMINATE**

CYST,
GALACTOCELE

CARCINOMA,
FIBROMAS,
CYSTADENOMA

BREAST PAIN

Ask the following questions:

1. Is it unilateral or bilateral? Unilateral breast pain should make one think of an infectious process or advanced carcinoma. Bilateral breast pain should make one think of pregnancy. This may be a normal pregnancy or an ectopic pregnancy.
2. Is there an associated mass? A tender breast mass is most likely a mastitis or abscess, but advanced carcinoma can also produce a tender breast mass. If there are tender masses in both breasts, then chronic cystic mastitis should be considered.
3. Is there a discharge? A bloody discharge associated with a tender breast should make one think of a carcinoma.
4. Is there fever? Fever associated with a tender breast or tender breast mass is most likely acute mastitis or abscess.

DIAGNOSTIC WORKUP

If there is a fever and discharge, then a culture and sensitivity of the discharge should be done before beginning antibiotics. When there is a localized tender mass, referral to a general surgeon should be made. Patients with bilateral breast pain without any masses identified should have a pregnancy test. If this is negative and the pain is associated with the menstrual cycle, they should be treated as having premenstrual tension. If there is persistent bilateral breast pain in a young unmarried female, perhaps a psychiatrist should be consulted.

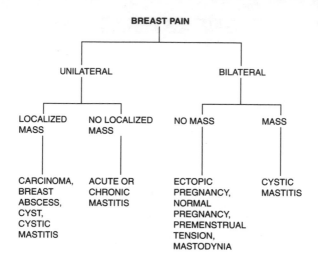

CARDIAC ARRHYTHMIA

Ask the following questions:

1. Is it acute or chronic? An acute cardiac arrhythmia should make one consider a myocardial infarction first.
2. Is the heart rate slow, normal, or fast? A rapid cardiac arrhythmia may be associated with hyperthyroidism, congestive heart failure, or drug toxicity. A slow cardiac arrhythmia is more likely to be associated with heart block and syncope. A myocardial infarction may produce either the rapid or slow cardiac arrhythmia.
3. Is the rhythm regular or irregular? A tachycardia with a regular rhythm is more likely to be a supraventricular tachycardia or ventricular tachycardia. A tachycardia with an irregular rhythm is more likely to be atrial fibrillation, but atrial flutter can also cause a rapid irregular rhythm. Irregular premature contractions and ventricular premature contractions may be associated with rapid, slow, or normal cardiac rates. A slow, fairly regular heart rate is associated with complete heart block.
4. Is there chest pain associated with the cardiac arrhythmia? Chest pain should make one think of myocardial infarction, pericarditis, or coronary insufficiency.
5. Is there fever? If there is fever, one should consider rheumatic fever, subacute bacterial endocarditis, and thyroid storm.
6. Is there a heart murmur associated with the arrhythmia? A heart murmur associated with arrhythmia should make one think of rheumatic fever or subacute bacterial endocarditis, myocardiopathy, or acute congestive heart failure.
7. Are there signs of congestive heart failure? Hepatomegaly, jugular vein distention, and pitting edema of the extremities would make one think that congestive heart failure was the cause of the arrhythmia.
8. Is there a thyroid enlargement? An enlarged thy-

roid gland would certainly make one think of thyrotoxicosis.

9. Is there hypertension? Hypertension is another important cause of cardiac arrhythmias that should not be forgotten.

DIAGNOSTIC WORKUP

All patients should have an EKG, chest x-ray, and a CBC to rule out anemia. A thyroid profile should be done to look for both hyperthyroidism and hypothyroidism. In acute arrhythmias, serial EKGs and tests for cardiac enzymes need to be done to exclude an acute myocardial infarction. Venous pressure and circulation time should be determined to rule out congestive heart failure; pulmonary function tests may be helpful, as they may rule out both congestive heart failure and emphysema. Echocardiograms should be done to rule out valvular disease and cardiomyopathy. If there are paroxysmal arrhythmias, Holter monitoring needs to be done. Patients on digitalis, quinidine, or other cardiac drugs should have blood levels of these drugs measured to determine if their levels are toxic. If there is a fever, blood culture should be done to rule out bacterial endocarditis. Referral to a cardiologist can be made at any point in the diagnostic workup.

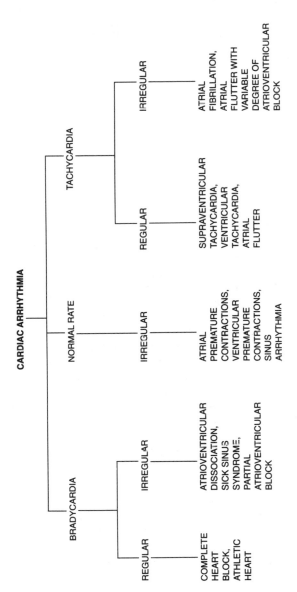

CARDIAC ARRHYTHMIA

BRADYCARDIA

REGULAR

COMPLETE
HEART
BLOCK,
ATHLETIC
HEART

IRREGULAR

ATRIOVENTRICULAR
DISSOCIATION,
SICK SINUS
SYNDROME,
PARTIAL
ATRIOVENTRICULAR
BLOCK

NORMAL RATE

IRREGULAR

ATRIAL
PREMATURE
CONTRACTIONS,
VENTRICULAR
PREMATURE
CONTRACTIONS,
SINUS
ARRHYTHMIA

TACHYCARDIA

REGULAR

SUPRAVENTRICULAR
TACHYCARDIA,
VENTRICULAR
TACHYCARDIA,
ATRIAL
FLUTTER

IRREGULAR

ATRIAL
FIBRILLATION,
ATRIAL
FLUTTER WITH
VARIABLE
DEGREE OF
ATRIOVENTRICULAR
BLOCK

CARDIAC MURMURS

Ask the following questions:

1. Could the murmur be extracardiac in origin? Extracardiac murmurs include the pericardial friction rub and cardiorespiratory murmurs.

2. Is the murmur continuous? A continuous murmur is most often due to a patent ductus arteriosus or combined valvular stenosis and insufficiency. However, arteriovenous aneurysms and ruptured aneurysm of the sinus of Valsalva must also be considered.

3. Is the murmur systolic or diastolic? Diastolic murmurs include aortic regurgitation and mitral stenosis, and are always organic. Many systolic murmurs are functional in nature.

4. Is there associated cardiomegaly? An enlarged heart associated with the murmur makes it more likely that it is pathologic. One would consider mitral regurgitation, aortic regurgitation, and aortic stenosis and various forms of congenital heart disease.

5. Is there hepatomegaly? Hepatomegaly associated with the murmur would make one think of congestive heart failure or tricuspid regurgitation and tricuspid stenosis.

6. Is there associated fever? Cardiac murmurs occurring with fever suggest acute rheumatic fever and subacute bacterial endocarditis.

7. Is there dyspnea? Dyspnea associated with a cardiac murmur suggests congestive heart failure.

8. Is there chest pain? If there is chest pain associated with a cardiac murmur, one must consider pericarditis and myocardial infarction.

9. Is there an enlarged thyroid or intention tremor? These findings suggest hyperthyroidism.

10. Is there cyanosis or clubbing? These findings suggest congenital heart disease.

DIAGNOSTIC WORKUP

If the murmur is believed to be organic, the most cost-effective approach would be to consult a cardiologist at the outset. If the astute clinician wishes to pursue the diagnostic workup on his own, it is suggested that a CBC, a sedimentation rate, a chemistry panel, a VDRL test, and a thyroid profile should be done for the initial blood work. In addition, a chest x-ray including obliques phonocardiograms, and EKG should be performed. These findings may provide a diagnosis. If there is fever, a streptozyme test, antistreptolysin-O (ASO) titer, and serial blood culture should be performed. If congestive heart failure is suspected, venous pressure and circulation time should be determined. Pulmonary function studies are also helpful. Echocardiography will be extremely helpful in diagnosing the various forms of valvular disease and will also help in identifying a pericardial effusion or the various cardiomyopathies. Cardiac catheterization and angiography and angiocardiography will identify the various congenital heart lesions and valvular disease. These studies, however, are most important when surgery is being considered.

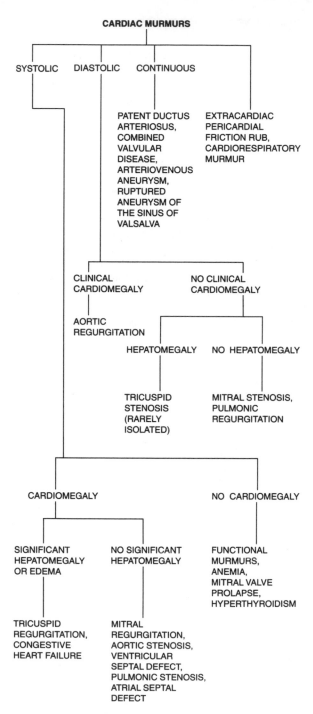

CARDIAC MURMURS

SYSTOLIC   DIASTOLIC   CONTINUOUS

PATENT DUCTUS
ARTERIOSUS,
COMBINED
VALVULAR
DISEASE,
ARTERIOVENOUS
ANEURYSM,
RUPTURED
ANEURYSM OF
THE SINUS OF
VALSALVA

EXTRACARDIAC
PERICARDIAL
FRICTION RUB,
CARDIORESPIRATORY
MURMUR

CLINICAL
CARDIOMEGALY

NO CLINICAL
CARDIOMEGALY

AORTIC
REGURGITATION

HEPATOMEGALY

NO HEPATOMEGALY

TRICUSPID
STENOSIS
(RARELY
ISOLATED)

MITRAL STENOSIS,
PULMONIC
REGURGITATION

CARDIOMEGALY

NO CARDIOMEGALY

SIGNIFICANT
HEPATOMEGALY
OR EDEMA

NO SIGNIFICANT
HEPATOMEGALY

FUNCTIONAL
MURMURS,
ANEMIA,
MITRAL VALVE
PROLAPSE,
HYPERTHYROIDISM

TRICUSPID
REGURGITATION,
CONGESTIVE
HEART FAILURE

MITRAL
REGURGITATION,
AORTIC STENOSIS,
VENTRICULAR
SEPTAL DEFECT,
PULMONIC STENOSIS,
ATRIAL SEPTAL
DEFECT

84   Cardiac Murmurs

CARDIOMEGALY

Ask the following questions:

1. Is there a murmur? Cardiomegaly with cardiac murmurs suggests valvular disease, but it also suggests congestive heart failure and advanced myocardiopathies. One should also be sure that the murmur is not a pericardial friction rub.
2. Is there fever? Fever with cardiomegaly should suggest rheumatic heart disease and bacterial endocarditis. However, it may also suggest an acute myocarditis or acute pericarditis.
3. Is there chest pain? Cardiomegaly with chest pain would certainly suggest a myocardial infarction, but it also may suggest an acute pericarditis.
4. Is there hepatomegaly? Cardiomegaly and hepatomegaly suggest congestive heart failure. It also may suggest one of the systemic diseases that causes a myocardiopathy such as amyloidosis.
5. Is there edema? The presence of peripheral edema would suggest congestive heart failure and if it is nonpitting it would suggest myxedema.
6. Is there hypertension? Cardiomegaly with hypertension would suggest that the cardiomegaly is due to left ventricular enlargement from the chronic hypertension.
7. Is there cyanosis? Cardiomegaly with cyanosis, particularly if there is an associated murmur, suggests congenital heart disease of the cyanotic type.

DIAGNOSTIC WORKUP

A CBC, sedimentation rate, ANA, chemistry panel, VDRL test, thyroid profile, EKG, and chest x-ray should be done on all patients. An echocardiogram will be helpful in diagnosing valvular disease, myocardiopathies, and pericardial effusion. If congestive heart failure is suspected, venous pressure and circulation time can be measured, and one should do pulmonary function studies. If there is fever, then one would want to do a streptozyme test, ASO titer, and serial blood cultures. If there is hypertension, a hypertensive workup may be indicated (see page 303). Patients with cyanosis need a workup for congenital heart disease, which will probably include cardiac catheterization and angiocardiography.

Most prudent physicians will refer the patient with cardiomegaly to a cardiologist before pursuing this extensive diagnostic workup.

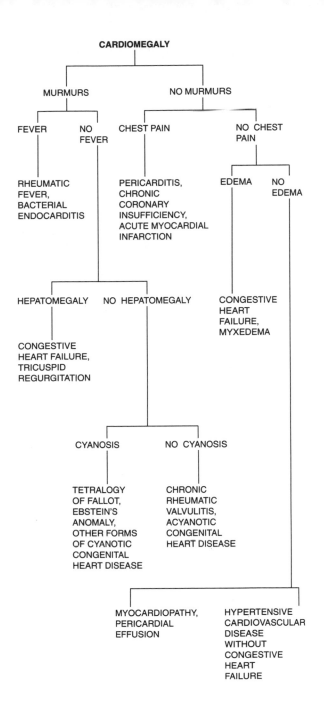

CHEST DEFORMITY

Many deformities of the chest may be observed on inspection of the patient and provide a clue to lung or systemic disease. Scoliosis may be a clue to syringomyelia, old poliomyelitis, muscular dystrophy, and Friedreich's ataxia. The "rachitic rosary" seen in rickets is due to swelling of the costochondral junctions. Expansion of one side of the chest may be seen in acute pneumothorax. A barrel chest is typical of emphysema. Emphysema may produce a localized swelling of the chest. An aortic aneurysm may cause a pulsatile swelling of the upper anterior chest. Hodgkin's disease, carcinoma of the lung, tuberculosis, actinomycosis, and various benign tumors of the lung will cause localized swellings in the chest.

DIAGNOSTIC WORKUP

Plain films of the chest, thoracic spine, and ribs will usually be diagnostic of chest deformities. Sputum culture and sensitivity, pleural fluid analysis, and culture and CT scans will be helpful in confusing cases. Referral to a pulmonologist will also help clear up the confusion.

CHEST PAIN

Ask the following questions:

1. Is the chest pain acute or chronic? If it is acute, one must consider acute myocardial infarction, pulmonary embolism, pneumothorax, pericarditis, and fractures. If the chest pain is chronic, one must consider chronic coronary insufficiency, esophagitis, hiatal hernia, and various chest wall conditions.

2. Is the pain constant or intermittent? Constant pain suggests acute myocardial infarction, pulmonary infarction, dissecting aneurysm, and pneumonia. Intermittent pain would suggest coronary insufficiency, Tietze's disease, and DaCosta's syndrome.

3. Is there associated significant hypertension? Significant hypertension would make one think of dissecting aneurysm, but it is also found occasionally in acute myocardial infarction.

4. Is the pain relieved by antacids? Relief by antacids should prompt one to consider esophagitis and hiatal hernia.

5. Is the pain precipitated or increased by breathing? The pain of pleurisy, costochondritis, rib fractures, and pneumothorax is precipitated or increased by breathing.

6. Is there associated hemoptysis? Hemoptysis should make one consider a pulmonary embolism.

7. Is there fever and purulent sputum? Fever and purulent sputum should make one consider pneumonia.

8. Is there dyspnea? Dyspnea should make one consider pneumothorax, pulmonary embolism, and pneumonia, as well as congestive heart failure secondary to acute myocardial infarction.

9. Is it aggravated by movement? Aggravation of the chest pain by movement should suggest pericarditis. Remember, myocardial infarctions may also have extension into the pericardium and must be considered at times.

10. Is it relieved by nitroglycerin? Relief by nitroglycerin should suggest a coronary insufficiency, but esophagospasm may be relieved by nitroglycerin also.

DIAGNOSTIC WORKUP

All patients should have a CBC, sedimentation rate, chemistry panel, VDRL test, chest x-ray, and EKG. If there is sputum, a smear and culture should be done as soon as possible.

If a myocardial infarction is suspected, then serial EKGs and tests for the CK-MB isoenzyme of creatine kinase should be done if the initial EKG and enzymes do not show any significant changes. Thallium-201 scintigraphy is useful in diagnosing both myocardial infarction and coronary insufficiency. Exercise Tolerance Tests may help diagnose coronary insufficiency.

If a pulmonary embolism is suspected, arterial blood gases and a ventilation-perfusion scan should be done. Pulmonary angiography may need to be done if these are negative and the pulmonary embolism is still strongly suspected.

If esophageal disease is suspected, an upper GI series with esophagram should be done; this can be followed with esophagoscopy and gastroscopy if needed.

If pericarditis is suspected, echocardiography and possibly a CT scan of the chest and pericardium may be necessary. Coronary angiography may be necessary to diagnose coronary insufficiency. Echocardiography is also helpful in diagnosing mitral valve prolapse and the various myocardiopathies. 24 hour Holter monitoring is useful in diagnosing many causes of intermittent chest pain.

Referral to a cardiologist or pulmonologist may be appropriate at any point in this workup.

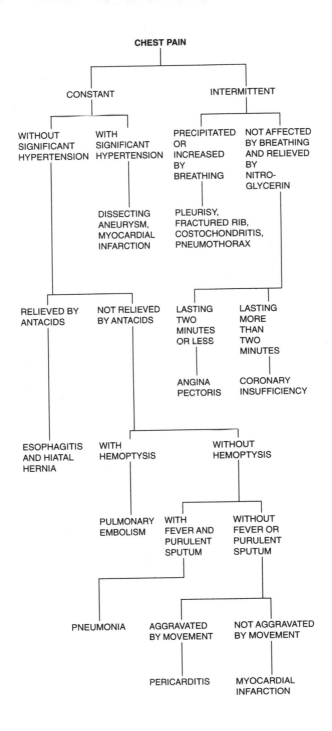

CHEST TENDERNESS

Ask the following questions:

1. Is there a history of trauma? Fractured or bruised ribs head the list of traumatic conditions that can cause chest tenderness. Intercostal myositis and burns may cause tenderness.
2. Are there significant signs of systemic diseases? Signs of petechiae or ecchymoses elsewhere may suggest blood dyscrasia. Splenomegaly and hepatomegaly may also suggest a systemic disease. Evidence of arthritic changes of the joints may suggest ankylosing spondylitis.
3. Is there a rash in the area of the tenderness? A rash in the area of tenderness suggests herpes zoster. At times only a few vesicles or bullae may be present and it is easy to miss this diagnosis in the early stages.
4. Are there abnormalities on auscultation and percussion of the lung? The pleura and pericardium may elicit a friction rub which will indicate pericarditis or pleurisy. Flatness or dullness to percussion may indicate pleural effusion, lobar pneumonia, or empyema. There may be a murmur beneath the area of tenderness and aortic aneurysm.

DIAGNOSTIC WORKUP

In any case of unexplained tenderness of the chest, x-rays of the chest and the ribs will be extremely useful in the diagnosis. If a systemic disease is suspected, a CBC and sedimentation rate, chemistry panel, and arthritis profile should be done. If cardiac disease is suspected, serial EKGs and serial cardiac enzymes may be necessary. A bone scan may diagnose subtle fractures or metastatic neoplasm of the ribs. A CT scan may be helpful in mediastinal tumors. Trigger point injections may help diagnose costochondritis.

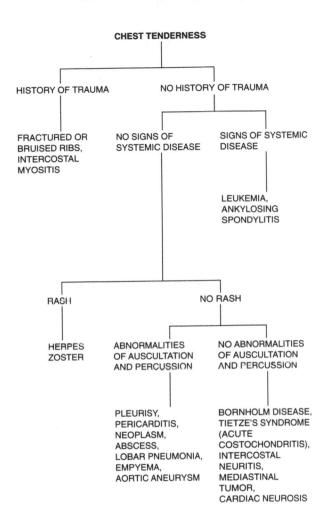

CHEST TENDERNESS

HISTORY OF TRAUMA

NO HISTORY OF TRAUMA

FRACTURED OR
BRUISED RIBS,
INTERCOSTAL
MYOSITIS

NO SIGNS OF
SYSTEMIC DISEASE

SIGNS OF SYSTEMIC
DISEASE

LEUKEMIA,
ANKYLOSING
SPONDYLITIS

RASH

NO RASH

HERPES
ZOSTER

ABNORMALITIES
OF AUSCULTATION
AND PERCUSSION

NO ABNORMALITIES
OF AUSCULTATION
AND PERCUSSION

PLEURISY,
PERICARDITIS,
NEOPLASM,
ABSCESS,
LOBAR PNEUMONIA,
EMPYEMA,
AORTIC ANEURYSM

BORNHOLM DISEASE,
TIETZE'S SYNDROME
(ACUTE
COSTOCHONDRITIS),
INTERCOSTAL
NEURITIS,
MEDIASTINAL
TUMOR,
CARDIAC NEUROSIS

CHILLS

Ask the following questions:

1. Is there a heart murmur? The presence of a heart murmur would suggest bacterial endocarditis.
2. Is there jaundice? The presence of jaundice should suggest ascending cholangitis and cholecystitis.
3. Is there frequency or burning of urination? The presence of frequency or burning of urination should suggest pyelonephritis, perinephric abscess, and prostatic abscess.
4. Is there hepatomegaly? The presence of an enlarged liver usually without jaundice is indicative of amebic abscess. The liver may be palpable, but not significantly enlarged in subdiaphragmatic abscess.
5. Are there neurologic signs? Neurologic findings would indicate a brain abscess, sinus thrombosis, various forms of encephalitis and epidural abscess. Don't forget that an epidural abscess of the spine may have its onset with chills. This type of abscess should be looked for in diabetics.
6. Is there cough or rales? The presence of cough or rales should prompt a search for a lung abscess, lobar pneumonia, bronchiectasis, and tuberculosis.
7. Is there bone pain or a bone mass? These findings are typical of osteomyelitis.
8. Are there no focal signs of infection? Without focal signs of infection, one should suspect septicemia, malaria, acute hemolytic anemias, relapsing fever, subdiaphragmatic abscess, and dental abscesses. However, chills may occur at the onset of any acute infection.

DIAGNOSTIC WORKUP

This is identical to the diagnostic workup for acute fever on page 218.

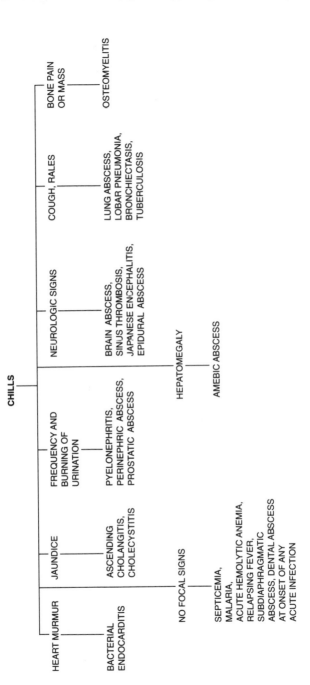

CHILLS

- HEART MURMUR
  - BACTERIAL ENDOCARDITIS
- JAUNDICE
  - ASCENDING CHOLANGITIS, CHOLECYSTITIS
- FREQUENCY AND BURNING OF URINATION
  - PYELONEPHRITIS, PERINEPHRIC ABSCESS, PROSTATIC ABSCESS
- NEUROLOGIC SIGNS
  - BRAIN ABSCESS, SINUS THROMBOSIS, JAPANESE ENCEPHALITIS, EPIDURAL ABSCESS
- COUGH, RALES
  - LUNG ABSCESS, LOBAR PNEUMONIA, BRONCHIECTASIS, TUBERCULOSIS
- BONE PAIN OR MASS
  - OSTEOMYELITIS
- HEPATOMEGALY
  - AMEBIC ABSCESS
- NO FOCAL SIGNS
  - SEPTICEMIA, MALARIA, ACUTE HEMOLYTIC ANEMIA, RELAPSING FEVER, SUBDIAPHRAGMATIC ABSCESS, DENTAL ABSCESS AT ONSET OF ANY ACUTE INFECTION

CHOREIFORM MOVEMENTS

Ask the following questions:

1. What is the patient's age? Children are likely to develop Sydenham's chorea, Tourette's syndrome, or Wilson's disease. Huntington's chorea and senile chorea usually occur in adults.
2. Is there associated fever or joint pains? The presence of fever or joint pains would make one think of Sydenham's chorea, encephalitis lethargica, or systemic lupus erythematosus.
3. Is there a family history? A family history will be found in patients with Huntington's chorea, Tourette's syndrome, and Wilson's disease.
4. Is there a history of drug ingestion? Several drugs can lead to choreiform movements, including the phenothiazines, levodopa, anticonvulsants, and birth control pills.

DIAGNOSTIC WORKUP

A sedimentation rate, antistreptolysin-O (ASO) titer, streptozyme test, and EKG will help diagnose Sydenham's chorea. Serum copper and ceruloplasmin will help diagnose Wilson's disease. An antinuclear antibody (ANA) assay may be done in cases suspected of having lupus erythematosus. If these tests are unrewarding, a neurologist should be consulted.

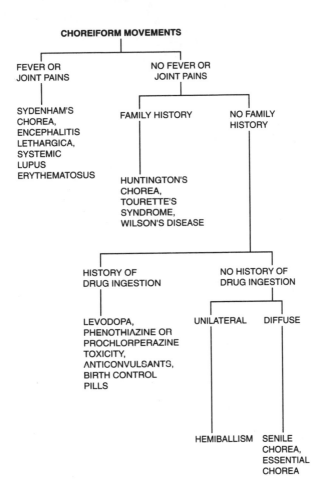

CLUBBING OF
THE FINGERS

Ask the following questions:

1. Is there cyanosis? Cyanosis should make one think of cyanotic congenital heart disease and pulmonary arteriovenous aneurysms.
2. Is there a cough or dyspnea? A cough or shortness of breath should make one think of a pulmonary condition such as bronchiectasis, chronic interstitial fibrosis, asbestosis, emphysema, or carcinoma of the lung. Lung abscesses and tuberculosis must also be considered, although they are less frequent.
3. Is there a fever? A fever along with the clubbing should make one think of empyema, lung abscess, tuberculosis, or subacute bacterial endocarditis.

DIAGNOSTIC WORKUP

An EKG and chest x-ray will identify the most common causes of clubbing. A CBC, sedimentation rate, and chemistry panel should also be done routinely. If there is fever, a sputum smear, culture and sensitivity, and blood culture should be done. An upper GI series, esophagram, and a barium enema will identify most gastrointestinal disorders. Cyanotic congenital heart disease will require further workup, including a cardiology consultation, cardiac catheterization, and angiocardiography. A thoracentesis may be necessary to diagnose empyema. Bronchoscopy may be necessary to diagnose carcinoma of the lung. A bronchogram may be necessary to diagnose bronchiectasis.

If a more extensive workup is necessary, a referral to a pulmonologist or cardiologist should be considered.

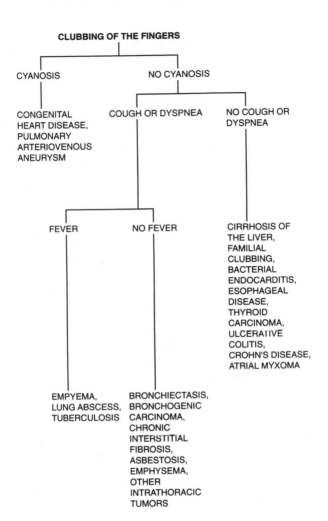

CLUBBING OF THE FINGERS

CYANOSIS

CONGENITAL
HEART DISEASE,
PULMONARY
ARTERIOVENOUS
ANEURYSM

NO CYANOSIS

COUGH OR DYSPNEA

NO COUGH OR
DYSPNEA

FEVER

NO FEVER

CIRRHOSIS OF
THE LIVER,
FAMILIAL
CLUBBING,
BACTERIAL
ENDOCARDITIS,
ESOPHAGEAL
DISEASE,
THYROID
CARCINOMA,
ULCERATIVE
COLITIS,
CROHN'S DISEASE,
ATRIAL MYXOMA

EMPYEMA,
LUNG ABSCESS,
TUBERCULOSIS

BRONCHIECTASIS,
BRONCHOGENIC
CARCINOMA,
CHRONIC
INTERSTITIAL
FIBROSIS,
ASBESTOSIS,
EMPHYSEMA,
OTHER
INTRATHORACIC
TUMORS

COMA

Ask the following questions:

1. Is there a history of drug or alcohol ingestion? This is a very important question to ask, as many cases of coma are due to acute alcohol intoxication, delirium tremens, opium poisoning, barbiturate poisoning, and other toxic cerebral depressants.
2. Is there a history of trauma? Most of the time it will be obvious that the patient has suffered a blow to the head. However, there are many times when one must get a hold of the family or other people who witnessed the onset of the coma to determine if there was trauma.
3. Are there focal neurological signs? Focal neurologic signs would make one think of a stroke, brain abscess, brain tumor, or epidural or subdural hematoma.
4. Is there papilledema? Papilledema certainly would indicate a possible space-occupying lesion such as a brain tumor, brain abscess, or subdural hematoma.
5. Is there a sweet odor to the breath? A sweet odor to the breath should make one think of a diabetic coma or alcoholism.
6. Is there fever? If there is fever, one should be thinking of meningitis, subarachnoid hemorrhage, or acute encephalitis. However, aspiration pneumonia, urinary tract infection, or septicemia may explain the fever.
7. Is there nuchal rigidity? The presence of nuchal rigidity suggests a meningitis or subarachnoid hemorrhage.
8. Are there sibilant or crepitant rales on examination of the lung? Sibilant rales would suggest the possibility that pulmonary emphysema is responsible for the coma, while crepitant rales would suggest that there is congestive heart failure or possibly pneumonia.

DIAGNOSTIC WORKUP

When one encounters a patient with coma, the first thing to do is to establish an airway. Next, the blood pressure is taken. If there are any signs of shock, an intravenous access is established and the shock is treated appropriately. Blood should then be drawn for a CBC, sedimentation rate, chemistry panel, electrolytes, blood ammonia level, and blood alcohol levels. Before removing the syringe, 50 cc of 50% dextrose is given unless the patient is suspected of having hyperosmolar nonketotic diabetic coma. A urinalysis and urine drug screen must be done also. Arterial blood gas analysis should be done. If the situation is urgent or emergent, a CT scan is done before the results of the laboratory tests are available. If the laboratory tests are inconclusive, a CT scan must be done anyway.

If all of the above studies are negative, a spinal tap is done for cell count, protein, glucose, VDRL test, smear, and culture and sensitivity. This is especially true when there is fever or nuchal rigidity.

If the diagnosis is still in doubt, blood tests for other toxic materials such as the lead level, and blood cultures and EEG are done. A neurologist or neurosurgeon is usually consulted as soon as one is available.

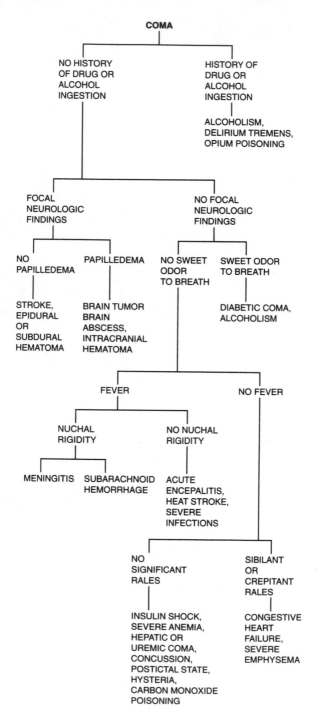

COMA

NO HISTORY OF DRUG OR ALCOHOL INGESTION

HISTORY OF DRUG OR ALCOHOL INGESTION

ALCOHOLISM, DELIRIUM TREMENS, OPIUM POISONING

FOCAL NEUROLOGIC FINDINGS

NO FOCAL NEUROLOGIC FINDINGS

NO PAPILLEDEMA

STROKE, EPIDURAL OR SUBDURAL HEMATOMA

PAPILLEDEMA

BRAIN TUMOR BRAIN ABSCESS, INTRACRANIAL HEMATOMA

NO SWEET ODOR TO BREATH

SWEET ODOR TO BREATH

DIABETIC COMA, ALCOHOLISM

FEVER

NO FEVER

NUCHAL RIGIDITY

MENINGITIS   SUBARACHNOID HEMORRHAGE

NO NUCHAL RIGIDITY

ACUTE ENCEPALITIS, HEAT STROKE, SEVERE INFECTIONS

NO SIGNIFICANT RALES

INSULIN SHOCK, SEVERE ANEMIA, HEPATIC OR UREMIC COMA, CONCUSSION, POSTICTAL STATE, HYSTERIA, CARBON MONOXIDE POISONING

SIBILANT OR CREPITANT RALES

CONGESTIVE HEART FAILURE, SEVERE EMPHYSEMA

CONSTIPATION

Ask the following questions:

1. Is the constipation acute or chronic? If the constipation is acute and there is abdominal pain or vomiting, one must consider the possibility of intestinal obstruction. An examination may disclose an empty rectum, in which case it is more likely complete intestinal obstruction; or there may be some feces in the rectum, in which case there may be incomplete intestinal obstruction. If the constipation is a chronic problem, one should investigate the patient's diet and emotional status and toilet habits over the life span.
2. What kind of a diet is the patient on? Many patients today eat on the run, and they eat mostly fast foods which are devoid of fiber. Frequently they don't take the time to go to the bathroom. Some patients are on special diets to lose weight or have a fear of gaining weight; therefore, they don't eat well at all. If what the patient labels as constipation is simply infrequent bowel movements, but the bowel movements are normal in consistency, this is not really true constipation.
3. Does the patient take drugs of any kind? The first drug that one wants to question the patient about is the chronic use of laxatives. Americans have the misconception that they must have a bowel movement every day and, therefore, they get in the habit of using something to stimulate the bowels, which can lead them to believe they have chronic constipation. Chronic narcotic use can lead to constipation, as can the use of antispasmodics for ulcer or urinary incontinence.
4. Associated symptoms: We have already mentioned that abdominal pain and vomiting may be a sign of acute intestinal obstruction and occasionally this is a sign of a chronic intestinal obstruction. If there is alternating diarrhea and constipation, one must consider the possibility of irritable bowel syndrome or a colon carcinoma. Blood in the stool along with painful defecation

may indicate hemorrhoids and anal fissure. A person who is suffering from these conditions may delay moving his bowels for fear of the pain that accompanies this situation, and the hard stool which caused the hemorrhoids and anal fissure in the first place perpetuates the condition because it contributes to the constipation. If blood is found in the stool, well mixed with the stool, and defecation is basically painless, then colon carcinoma and diverticulitis must be considered. Blood and mucus in the stool would indicate an irritable bowel syndrome.

5. What are the findings on physical examination? The finding of an empty rectum indicates an intestinal obstruction. A finding of an abdominal mass or a rectal mass certainly would indicate carcinoma of the colon. Vaginal examination may disclose hemorrhoids or anal fissure as causing the chronic constipation and allow one to test the stool for occult blood.

DIAGNOSTIC WORKUP

If the constipation is acute, a flat plate of the abdomen and a CBC would be in order to determine if the patient has intestinal obstruction. The workup of chronic constipation should include stool for occult blood, sigmoidoscopy, barium enema, or a colonoscopy. A chemistry panel and other diagnostic studies may be necessary to rule out systemic causes of constipation such as diabetes, hypothyroidism, and various conditions associated with hypercalcemia. If diagnostic tests yield no positive findings, referral to a psychiatrist or a gynecologist may be in order.

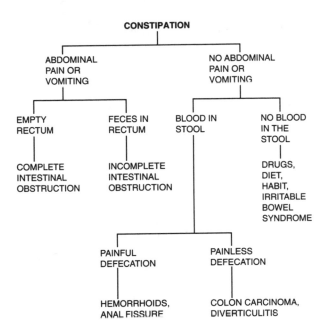

CONVULSIONS

Ask the following questions:

1. Are the episodes of loss of consciousness really seizures? Real seizures, especially grand mal, present with incontinence and/or tongue biting. Hysterical seizures with actual tonic or clonic movements may occur, but there is no tongue biting or incontinence. Syncope usually is not accompanied by convulsive movements, but it occasionally can be after the drop in blood pressure or anoxia to the brain has continued for a period of time. If there are no convulsive movements to the blackouts, then the possibility of syncope must be considered (page 549). In addition, cerebrovascular accidents, narcolepsy, and breath-holding attacks must be considered when there are no definite convulsive movements.
2. Is there a history of drug or alcohol abuse? Alcohol withdrawal seizures and seizures due to cocaine abuse are becoming more and more common. Patients frequently lie about their use of illicit drugs or alcohol. In young adults and teenagers a urine drug screen should be done.
3. Is there fever? Fever should make one think of meningitis or encephalitis or if it has been extended over a longer period of time, a cerebral abscess. In children one should consider the possibility of febrile convulsions.
4. What type of seizure disorder is it? If there are convulsions, are they focal or jacksonian type? That would certainly suggest a space-occupying lesion as opposed to a generalized convulsion. Loss of awareness with no actual collapse for one minute or less is suggestive of a petit mal type seizure. In these seizures the patient just simply stares. Longer attacks of loss of awareness are more likely to be due to complex partial seizures and occasionally an observer will note unusual behavior during these episodes. The patient may note unusual odors.
5. Are there focal neurologic signs and pa-

pilledema? These findings are more typical of a space-occupying lesion such as a cerebral tumor, cerebral abscess, or a subdural hematoma.

DIAGNOSTIC WORKUP

All patients deserve a CBC, urinalysis, sedimentation rate, ANA, VDRL test, and chemistry panel. In older patients a chest x-ray should be done to look for the possibility of a primary lung tumor. A urine drug screen is useful especially in young adults. All patients also need a wake-and-sleep EEG. There is some argument over whether a CT scan or MRI should be done on all patients with definite convulsions. The author believes that a CT scan should be done on all patients, even without focal neurologic signs or papilledema. Isotope brain scans, arteriography, and pneumoencephalography are no longer indicated unless something is found on the CT scan that needs further clarification. A spinal tap should also be done when there is fever or when central nervous system lues or multiple sclerosis are suspected. Visual evoked potentials (VEPs) and brain stem evoked potentials (BSEPs) may also help diagnose multiple sclerosis. It should be noted that seizures occur in 7% of cases with multiple sclerosis.

A consultation with a neurologic specialist can be done at any point in this workup. Certainly, it would be very important to have it done early if there are focal neurologic signs or papilledema.

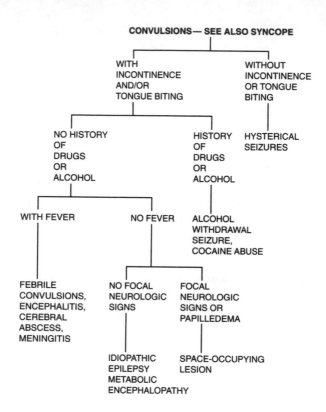

CONVULSIONS— SEE ALSO SYNCOPE

WITH INCONTINENCE AND/OR TONGUE BITING

WITHOUT INCONTINENCE OR TONGUE BITING

NO HISTORY OF DRUGS OR ALCOHOL

HISTORY OF DRUGS OR ALCOHOL

HYSTERICAL SEIZURES

WITH FEVER

NO FEVER

ALCOHOL WITHDRAWAL SEIZURE, COCAINE ABUSE

FEBRILE CONVULSIONS, ENCEPHALITIS, CEREBRAL ABSCESS, MENINGITIS

NO FOCAL NEUROLOGIC SIGNS

FOCAL NEUROLOGIC SIGNS OR PAPILLEDEMA

IDIOPATHIC EPILEPSY METABOLIC ENCEPHALOPATHY

SPACE-OCCUPYING LESION

COUGH

Ask the following questions:

1. Is it acute or chronic? Acute onset of a cough would suggest an acute upper respiratory infection, viral pneumonia, or bronchopneumonia. A chronic cough is more suggestive of pneumoconiosis, chronic bronchitis, emphysema, bronchiectasis, tuberculosis, carcinoma of the lung, or bronchial asthma.
2. Is there exposure to toxic fumes? The most common toxic fume is cigarette smoke. However, if one asks the patient's occupation one might find that he is a miner and therefore pneumoconiosis comes to mind. One might find that he is an aircraft maker or shipbuilder, in which case berylliosis and asbestosis would come to mind, or that he is a farmer and, therefore, farmer's lung would come to mind.
3. Is there significant sputum production? If so, what is the nature of the sputum? Purulent sputum would suggest a pneumonia, abscess, tuberculosis, or bronchiectasis; bloody sputum would suggest carcinoma of the lung, tuberculosis, and bronchiectasis; mucoid sputum would suggest asthma. If the sputum is foamy, one would consider congestive heart failure, mitral stenosis, and inhalation of poison gas.
4. Is there fever? If there is fever associated with the cough, obviously one would suspect an infectious process to be present. This could be viral or bacterial. Most likely the patient has bronchopneumonia, but the possibility of an abscess or pulmonary infarct would still have to be entertained.
5. What other symptoms and signs are associated with the cough? The first thing to be considered would be dyspnea. In acute cases dyspnea would be a sign of congestive heart failure, pulmonary embolism and, of course, advancing pneumonia. In chronic cases dyspnea would be a sign of emphysema, chronic pulmonary fibrosis, and

chronic congestive heart failure. Wheezing would be a sign of asthma or congestive heart failure, but of course it is also found in pulmonary emphysema. Cardiomegaly would suggest congestive heart failure and if there is an associated murmur, then that makes congestive heart failure even more likely. If there is hepatosplenomegaly, one would suspect a systemic disease involving the lungs such as periarteritis nodosa or other collagen diseases.

DIAGNOSTIC WORKUP

All patients require a CBC and differential count, a sedimentation rate, and a chemistry panel. A sputum for routine smear and culture should be done and in chronic cases a sputum for acid-fast bacillus culture and smear must be done. One should keep a high index of suspicion for mycoplasma pneumoniae and Legionaire's disease. Also, sputum for fungi culture should be done on chronic cases.

Asthma can be further elucidated and confirmed by doing a sputum for eosinophils. Carcinoma of the lung can be confirmed with a sputum for Papanicolaou's smear. If there is fever, blood cultures may be useful and febrile agglutinins should also be done. An x-ray of the chest, with anteroposterior, lateral, and apical lordotic views should be done and when there is a tumor suspected tomography should be done or a CT scan. In cases of chronic cough, skin testing for coccidioidomycosis, cystoplasmosis, tuberculosis, and blastomycosis should be done. A Kveim test to rule out sarcoidosis may be necessary. When these tests fail to make a diagnosis, bronchoscopy and possibly bronchograms to look for a bronchiectasis should be done. Lung biopsy may be necessary also. Pulmonary function tests should be done in suspected cases of emphysema and asthma. Allergy skin testing is extremely valuable in cases of asthma. Look for alpha 1-antitrypsin deficiency in difficult cases. If congestive heart failure is suspected, an arm-to-tongue circulation time would be valuable.

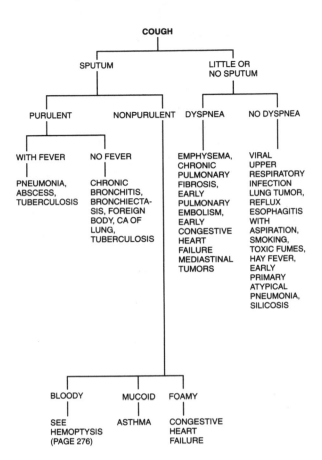

COUGH

SPUTUM

PURULENT

WITH FEVER

PNEUMONIA,
ABSCESS,
TUBERCULOSIS

NO FEVER

CHRONIC
BRONCHITIS,
BRONCHIECTA-
SIS, FOREIGN
BODY, CA OF
LUNG,
TUBERCULOSIS

NONPURULENT

LITTLE OR
NO SPUTUM

DYSPNEA

EMPHYSEMA,
CHRONIC
PULMONARY
FIBROSIS,
EARLY
PULMONARY
EMBOLISM,
EARLY
CONGESTIVE
HEART
FAILURE
MEDIASTINAL
TUMORS

NO DYSPNEA

VIRAL
UPPER
RESPIRATORY
INFECTION
LUNG TUMOR,
REFLUX
ESOPHAGITIS
WITH
ASPIRATION,
SMOKING,
TOXIC FUMES,
HAY FEVER,
EARLY
PRIMARY
ATYPICAL
PNEUMONIA,
SILICOSIS

BLOODY

SEE
HEMOPTYSIS
(PAGE 276)

MUCOID

ASTHMA

FOAMY

CONGESTIVE
HEART
FAILURE

CRAMPS, MENSTRUAL

There are usually physiologic cramps occurring during menstruation and not associated with pathology of the female reproductive organs. If there is associated menorrhagia, then the differential diagnosis of this symptom should be consulted (page 362).

Menstrual cramps occur more frequently in the virginal uterus, but may establish themselves after the first pregnancy. All women have experienced menstrual cramps at some time in their life. These cramps may be the first sign of endometriosis, pelvic inflammatory disease, or ectopic pregnancy.

CRAMPS, MUSCULAR

Ask the following questions:

1. Is there a history of drug ingestion? Many drugs produce muscular cramps. The most notable are the diuretics.
2. Are there absent or diminished peripheral pulses? Absent or diminished peripheral pulses suggest the cramps are due to ischemia from peripheral arteriosclerosis or arterial embolism.
3. Are the femoral pulses diminished? Diminished femoral pulses suggest a Leriche syndrome or saddle embolism of the terminal aorta.
4. Is there hypertension? Hypertension suggests aldosteronism and chronic glomerulonephritis.
5. Are the cramps limited to one extremity? Limitation of the cramps to one extremity suggests an occupational neurosis (professional cramps).
6. Is there a positive Chvostek's and/or Trousseau's sign? These are signs of tetany, as might be associated with hypoparathyroidism, uremia, alkalosis, and other causes.
7. Is there fever? Fever is associated with dehydration, heat stroke, and many infectious diseases that cause cramps.

DIAGNOSTIC WORKUP

All patients should have a CBC, sedimentation rate, chemistry panel, electrolytes, and urinalysis. If there is associated diminished or absent peripheral pulses, then Doppler studies and arteriography should be done. If the cramps are acute in onset, time should not be wasted in performing these studies. If there is associated hypertension, then a 24-hr urine aldosterone and plasma renin studies should be done. If there are positive Trousseau's and/or Chvostek's signs, a thorough investigation for hypoparathyroidism should be done. A single serum calcium and phosphorus and alkaline phosphatase is not enough, but repeated studies should be done. In addition, 24-hr urine collection for calcium and serum parathyroid hormones should be done. An endocrinologist should probably be consulted if there is any doubt about the existence of hypoparathyroidism or any of the other causes of hypocalcemia.

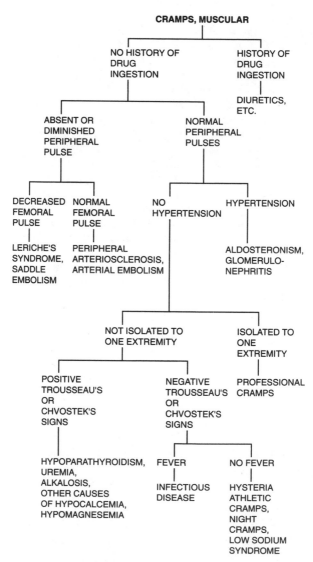

CREPITUS

The most classical example of crepitus is subcutaneous emphysema following a chest injury, especially a fractured rib. This may also occur around a tracheotomy site. Crepitus is felt over arthritic joints, especially when there is synovitis. In tenosynovitis of the wrist there is often a marked crepitus over the flexor tendons. A grating sound or crepitus may be felt over fractured bones if an effort is made to move the two portions of fractured bones. Palpation of a malignant bone tumor will elicit crepitus if the bone cortex has been penetrated. In patients with gas gangrene, crepitus may be felt over the infected area due to subcutaneous gas.

DIAGNOSTIC WORKUP

This will depend on the type of crepitus felt. Plain films will verify the presence of gas, fractures, and tumors. Undoubtedly, other symptoms and signs will be present to key the rest of the diagnostic workup using the pages in this book.

CYANOSIS

Ask the following questions:

1. Is there a history of drug ingestion? Potassium chlorate, sulfanilamide, and coal tar products are only a few of the drugs that may cause methemoglobinemia and sulfhemoglobinemia.
2. Is the cyanosis limited to one extremity? If the cyanosis is limited to one extremity, one should suspect an arterial embolism or phlebothrombosis.
3. Is the cyanosis limited to the extremities or is it generalized? Cyanosis that is limited to the extremities only, suggests Raynaud's disease, Raynaud's phenomena, shock, and acrocyanosis.
4. Is there associated dyspnea? If there is significant dyspnea, one should consider a pulmonary or cardiac origin for the cyanosis such as cyanotic congenital heart disease, pulmonary emphysema, pulmonary fibrosis, or pulmonary embolism.
5. Is the patient a child or an adult? Certain causes of cyanosis are limited to children, such as laryngismus stridulus, laryngotracheitis, and acute subglottic laryngitis.
6. Is there a heart murmur or cardiomegaly? A heart murmur or cardiomegaly suggests rheumatic carditis, congenital heart disease, or congestive heart failure.

DIAGNOSTIC WORKUP

Arterial blood gases, EKG, chest x-ray, and pulmonary function studies will diagnose most cases that are due to pulmonary or cardiac causes. If there is a history of drug ingestion, the blood should be drawn for methemoglobin and sulfhemoglobin testing. If a pulmonary embolism is suspected, a ventilation-perfusion scan and pulmonary arteriography may need to be done. If a peripheral embolism is suspected, angiography of the vessel involved will be diagnostic. Sputum or nose and throat cultures will be useful in diagnosing the infectious diseases associated with cyanosis.

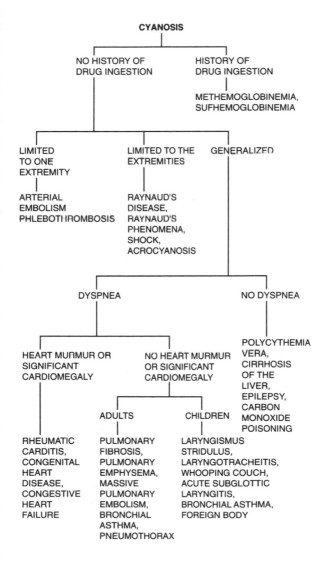

DEAFNESS

Ask the following questions:

1. Is it unilateral or bilateral? Unilateral deafness may be due to local conditions such as wax, a foreign body, otitis media, or ruptured drum or it may be due to neurologic conditions such as Ménière's disease, acoustic neuroma, or multiple sclerosis. Bilateral deafness is more likely due to otosclerosis, acoustic trauma, presbyacusis, or drug toxicity.
2. Are there abnormalities on otoscopic examination of the ear? It is very important to do a thorough examination of the ear, as one may find wax, foreign body, otitis media, cholesteatoma, or ruptured drum.
3. Is there associated vertigo? The presence of vertigo should make one think of Ménière's disease or some neurologic condition such as acoustic neuroma, multiple sclerosis, or basilar artery insufficiency.
4. What are the results of the Rinne test? Normally, the Rinne test should show a 2 to 1 ratio of air to bone hearing. In otosclerosis, the ratio approaches 1 to 1, but in sensory neural deafness the ratio is preserved at 2 to 1. In unilateral deafness, the Weber test is helpful. This will lateralize to the affected ear if the problem is a conductive deafness and it will lateralize to the good ear if the problem is a sensory neural deafness.

DIAGNOSTIC WORKUP

Audiometry and caloric testing or electronystagmography should be done in almost all cases where the ear examination is normal. It is probably wise to consult an otolaryngologist at this point. Tympanography will be helpful in diagnosing subtle cases of serous otitis media. X-rays of the mastoids, petrous bones, and internal auditory canal should be done for chronic otitis media, cholesteatoma, and acoustic neuroma. If an acoustic neuroma is suspected, however, a CT scan of the brain must be done. If basilar artery insufficiency is suspected, four-vessel cerebral angiography should be done. If multiple sclerosis is suspected, then MRI of the brain, brain stem evoked potentials, and visual evoked potential studies along with a spinal tap for spinal fluid analysis may be done.

Rather than perform these tests, the most cost-effective approach would be to refer the patient to a neurologist if other focal neurologic findings are evident.

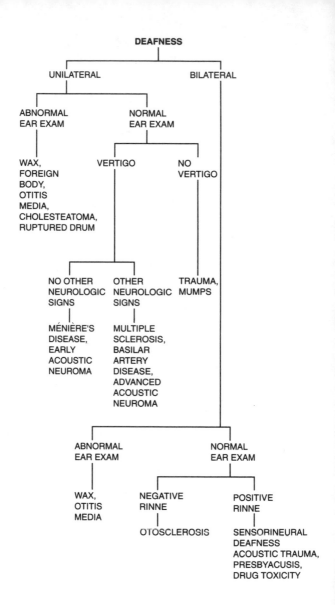

DELAYED PUBERTY

Ask the following questions:

1. Is there a positive drug history? Boys and girls may take anabolic steroids or androgens and thyroid hormones. These hormones may cause a delay in puberty.
2. Is there a significant weight loss? Significant weight loss would suggest anorexia nervosa, hyperthyroidism, celiac disease, cystic fibrosis, and uncontrolled diabetes among other conditions.
3. Is there a short stature? The presence of a short stature would suggest pituitary tumors, hypothalamic syndromes, gonadal dysgenesis, adrenal tumors, hyperplasia, hypothyroidism, and ovarian tumors.
4. Is there a hemianoptic field defect? The presence of a hemianoptic field defect would suggest a pituitary tumor. The presence of a normal or tall stature would suggest constitutional delayed puberty among other more rare conditions.

DIAGNOSTIC WORKUP

Before proceeding with an expensive diagnostic workup, it is perhaps best to consult an endocrinologist. If one is not available, routine tests would be a CBC, chemistry panel, and thyroid profile. Blood tests for a serum follicle-stimulating hormone (FSH), luteinizing hormone (LH), and testosterone or estradiol may be done, although urine gonadotrophins may be a cheaper screening test.

Pelvic ultrasound and CT scans of the abdomen and pelvis will help identify ovarian and adrenal tumors and abnormal configuration of the uterus. CT scans of the brain will help identify pituitary tumors. If all these studies are negative, a psychiatrist may need to be consulted. Remember, the family may be in more need of the psychiatrist than the child.

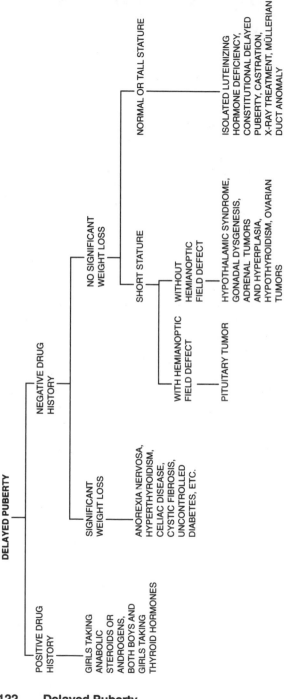

DELAYED PUBERTY

- POSITIVE DRUG HISTORY
  - GIRLS TAKING ANABOLIC STEROIDS OR ANDROGENS, BOTH BOYS AND GIRLS TAKING THYROID HORMONES

- NEGATIVE DRUG HISTORY
  - SIGNIFICANT WEIGHT LOSS
    - ANOREXIA NERVOSA, HYPERTHYROIDISM, CELIAC DISEASE, CYSTIC FIBROSIS, UNCONTROLLED DIABETES, ETC.
  - NO SIGNIFICANT WEIGHT LOSS
    - SHORT STATURE
      - WITH HEMIANOPTIC FIELD DEFECT
        - PITUITARY TUMOR
      - WITHOUT HEMIANOPTIC FIELD DEFECT
        - HYPOTHALAMIC SYNDROME, GONADAL DYSGENESIS, ADRENAL TUMORS AND HYPERPLASIA, HYPOTHYROIDISM, OVARIAN TUMORS
    - NORMAL OR TALL STATURE
      - ISOLATED LUTEINIZING HORMONE DEFICIENCY, CONSTITUTIONAL DELAYED PUBERTY, CASTRATION, X-RAY TREATMENT, MÜLLERIAN DUCT ANOMALY

DELIRIUM

Ask the following questions:

1. Is there associated fever? Delirium with fever may simply indicate a self-limited infectious process, but it should bring to mind encephalitis and meningitis as well as cerebral abscess and cerebral hemorrhage.
2. Is there a history of trauma? A history of head trauma would make one suspect a subdural or epidural hematoma.
3. Is there a history of drug or alcohol ingestion? This is probably the most important single question to ask in the average case coming into the emergency room these days without a good history. Very often the problem is alcoholism or various popular drugs such as cocaine, lysergic acid diethylamide (LSD), and phencyclidine (PCP).
4. Are there focal neurologic signs? Focal neurologic signs along with the delirium would make one think of subdural or epidural hematoma, cerebral abscess, or cerebral hemorrhage. Remember a cerebral thrombosis or embolism may present with delirium also.
5. Is there nuchal rigidity? If there is nuchal rigidity, the patient may have meningitis or subarachnoid hemorrhage.
6. Is there a sweet odor to the breath? A sweet odor to the breath should make one think of diabetic coma or alcoholism.
7. What is the response to intravenous thiamine? If the patient responds to intravenous thiamine, the diagnosis is usually Wernicke's encephalopathy or Korsakoff's syndrome.
8. Intermittent delirium should suggest psychomotor epilepsy.

DIAGNOSTIC WORKUP

Routine laboratory tests include a CBC, sedimentation rate, ANA, chemistry panel including electrolytes and blood urea nitrogen (BUN) and VDRL tests, a blood alcohol level, urinalysis, and urine drug screen. A CT scan of the brain is usually indicated also. Acute delirium may be an indication to administer I.V. glucose and thiamine. If there is fever, then blood cultures and a spinal tap for analysis and culture need to be done. Arterial blood gases and carboxyhemoglobin should be determined. Generally, a neurologist or neurosurgeon should be consulted early.

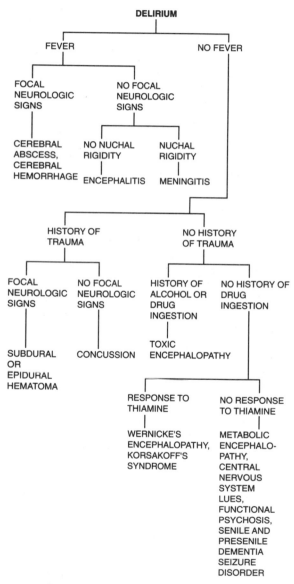

DELUSIONS

Ask the following questions:

1. Is there a history of drug or alcohol ingestion? Many drugs may be associated with delusions, especially cocaine, PCP, and LSD. The confabulations of Korsakoff's psychosis may be confused with delusions.
2. Is there impairment of memory? If there is impairment of memory, an organic psychosis should be suspected, such as senile and presenile dementia or general paresis. When there is no impairment of memory, the problem is probably a psychiatric disorder such as schizophrenia or manic-depressive psychosis.

DIAGNOSTIC WORKUP

If there is a history of alcohol or drug ingestion, then a blood alcohol level and urine for drug screen should be done. A CT scan, EEG, and spinal fluid analysis will often need to be done before referring a patient to a psychiatrist for further evaluation.

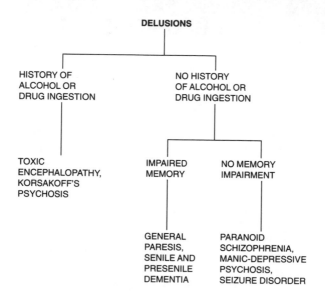

DEMENTIA

Ask the following questions:

1. Is there a history of drug or alcohol ingestion? Chronic barbiturate intoxication, ergotism, and other psychotropic or antidepressant drugs may cause dementia. Alcoholism may cause dementia in the form of Korsakoff's psychosis or Wernicke's encephalopathy.
2. Is there headache, papilledema, or focal neurologic signs? The most important condition to rule out in this category would be a space-occupying lesion, but normal pressure hydrocephalus, cerebral arteriosclerosis, acute cerebrovascular accident, and general paresis may present with focal neurologic signs.
3. Is there a response to niacin, thiamine, vitamin B_{12}, or thyroid? Response to these drugs would indicate that the patient has pellagra, Korsakoff's psychosis, pernicious anemia, or myxedema. However, laboratory tests should be done before administering the medications. Laboratory tests include serum B_{12} and folic acid and a thyroid profile. Unfortunately, most laboratories do not have a test for niacin or thiamine.
4. Is there insight? In patients with cerebral arteriosclerosis, the patient notices that his memory is slipping. This is also true of AIDS.
5. Are there extrapyramidal tract signs? Extrapyramidal tract signs should suggest Huntington's chorea or Parkinson's disease.
6. Are there pyramidal tract signs or myoclonus? Pyramidal tract signs are seen in general paresis and Jakob-Creutzfeldt syndrome, but also myoclonus is seen in Jakob-Creutzfeldt syndrome.

DIAGNOSTIC WORKUP

Routine laboratory tests include a CBC, sedimentation rate, chemistry panel, VDRL, HIV antibody titer, ANA, blood alcohol level, urine drug screens, thyroid profile, serum B_{12}, and folic acid. A CT scan should probably be done in all cases. An EEG may be helpful in demonstrating drug intoxication. A spinal tap may need to be done to diagnose central nervous system lues. The best test for that is the fluorescent treponema antibody absorption test (FTA-ABS). MRI may be useful in distinguishing Alzheimer's disease from cerebral arteriosclerosis, as in the cerebral arteriosclerosis small infarcts may be demonstrated. A radioiodinated serum albumin (RISA) cisternography study is useful to diagnose normal pressure hydrocephalus. Arterial blood gases should be drawn. Psychiatric testing will help differentiate organic brain syndrome from other psychiatric disorders and malingering. A neurologist or psychiatrist should be consulted before ordering expensive diagnostic tests.

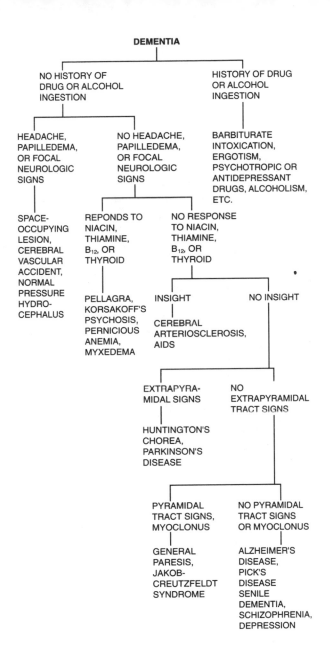

DEMENTIA

NO HISTORY OF DRUG OR ALCOHOL INGESTION

HISTORY OF DRUG OR ALCOHOL INGESTION

HEADACHE, PAPILLEDEMA, OR FOCAL NEUROLOGIC SIGNS

NO HEADACHE, PAPILLEDEMA, OR FOCAL NEUROLOGIC SIGNS

BARBITURATE INTOXICATION, ERGOTISM, PSYCHOTROPIC OR ANTIDEPRESSANT DRUGS, ALCOHOLISM, ETC.

SPACE-OCCUPYING LESION, CEREBRAL VASCULAR ACCIDENT, NORMAL PRESSURE HYDRO-CEPHALUS

REPONDS TO NIACIN, THIAMINE, B₁₂, OR THYROID

NO RESPONSE TO NIACIN, THIAMINE, B₁₂, OR THYROID

PELLAGRA, KORSAKOFF'S PSYCHOSIS, PERNICIOUS ANEMIA, MYXEDEMA

INSIGHT

NO INSIGHT

CEREBRAL ARTERIOSCLEROSIS, AIDS

EXTRAPYRA-MIDAL SIGNS

NO EXTRAPYRAMIDAL TRACT SIGNS

HUNTINGTON'S CHOREA, PARKINSON'S DISEASE

PYRAMIDAL TRACT SIGNS, MYOCLONUS

NO PYRAMIDAL TRACT SIGNS OR MYOCLONUS

GENERAL PARESIS, JAKOB-CREUTZFELDT SYNDROME

ALZHEIMER'S DISEASE, PICK'S DISEASE SENILE DEMENTIA, SCHIZOPHRENIA, DEPRESSION

Dementia 129

DEPRESSION

Ask the following questions:

1. Is there associated headache, papilledema, dementia, or focal neurologic signs? These findings would suggest a space-occupying lesion. This is something the clinician does not want to miss.
2. Are there endocrine changes? A number of endocrinologic diseases may present with depression, including Cushing's disease, myxedema, hyperthyroidism, and menopause.
3. Is there marked loss of appetite, weight, and libido? Endogenous depression, unipolar depression, and the depressive phase of manic-depressive psychosis may present with these findings. On the other hand, neurotic depressive reaction usually is not associated with significant loss of appetite, weight, or libido.

DIAGNOSTIC WORKUP

Routine laboratory studies include a CBC, sedimentation rate, chemistry panel, VDRL test, and thyroid profile. If Cushing's syndrome is suspected, a serum cortisol and cortisol suppression test should be done. If menopause is suspected, order a serum FSH and estradiol level. A trial of estrogen therapy may be warranted. A CT scan of the brain should probably be done in all cases to exclude a brain tumor, especially if there is no response to treatment! A referral to a psychiatrist should also be considered early if the depression is severe or if there is suicidal ideation.

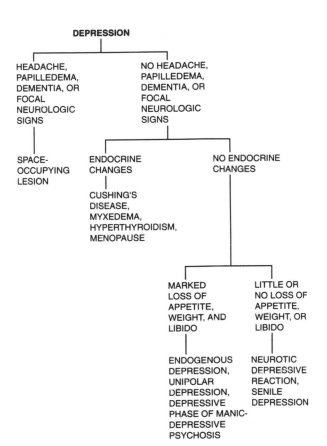

DIAPHORESIS

Ask the following questions:

1. Is there a history of drug or alcohol ingestion? Many drugs can cause diaphoresis, but caffeine and nicotine head the list. Alcohol can be associated with significant diaphoresis also.
2. Is there associated fever? Obviously, infectious disease is a very important cause of diaphoresis, particularly when the fever breaks. Look for tuberculosis, malaria, acute rheumatic fever, and bacterial endocarditis. Thyroid storm can be associated with fever also.
3. Is there associated chest pain or hypotension? Chest pain with diaphoresis would make one think of an acute myocardial infarction, but this combination is also found in coronary insufficiency. Shock, whatever the cause, produces significant diaphoresis.
4. Is there associated weight loss, hypertension, or both? Weight loss and hypertension should make one think of hyperthyroidism and pheochromocytoma.
5. Is there associated weight gain? The triad of obesity, diaphoresis, and increased appetite is typical of an insulinoma. Diabetics taking excessive insulin will also sweat.
6. Is there a rash? Several skin diseases may cause hyperhidrosis.

DIAGNOSTIC WORKUP

Routine diagnostic studies include a CBC, sedimentation rate, chemistry panel, electrolytes, thyroid profile, blood alcohol level, EKG, and chest x-ray. Serial EKGs and cardiac enzymes should be done if a myocardial infarction is suspected. A 24-hr urine collection for catecholamine can be done if a pheochromocytoma is suspected. A glucose tolerance test 36–72 hr. fast, and insulin tolerance test may be done for an insulinoma. If infectious disease is strongly suspected, a workup for fever of unknown origin can be done (see page 218).

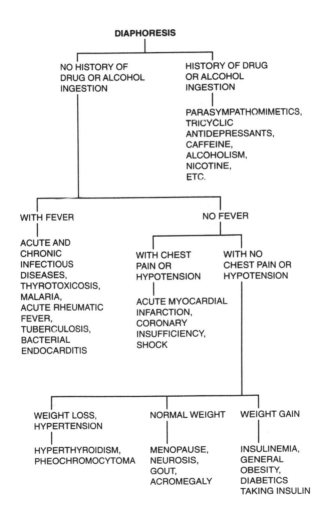

DIAPHORESIS

NO HISTORY OF DRUG OR ALCOHOL INGESTION

HISTORY OF DRUG OR ALCOHOL INGESTION

PARASYMPATHOMIMETICS, TRICYCLIC ANTIDEPRESSANTS, CAFFEINE, ALCOHOLISM, NICOTINE, ETC.

WITH FEVER

ACUTE AND CHRONIC INFECTIOUS DISEASES, THYROTOXICOSIS, MALARIA, ACUTE RHEUMATIC FEVER, TUBERCULOSIS, BACTERIAL ENDOCARDITIS

NO FEVER

WITH CHEST PAIN OR HYPOTENSION

WITH NO CHEST PAIN OR HYPOTENSION

ACUTE MYOCARDIAL INFARCTION, CORONARY INSUFFICIENCY, SHOCK

WEIGHT LOSS, HYPERTENSION

HYPERTHYROIDISM, PHEOCHROMOCYTOMA

NORMAL WEIGHT

MENOPAUSE, NEUROSIS, GOUT, ACROMEGALY

WEIGHT GAIN

INSULINEMIA, GENERAL OBESITY, DIABETICS TAKING INSULIN

DIARRHEA, ACUTE

Ask the following questions:

1. Is there blood in the stool? From the algorithm, blood in the stool should indicate to you that there is *Salmonella, Shigella, Campylobacter jejuni*, ulcerative colitis, and amebic dysentery. Without blood in the stool, it is more likely that the acute diarrhea is due to a staphylococcal toxin, giardiasis, traveler's diarrhea, a virus or contaminated food.

2. Is there a fever? Fever, especially with an elevated white count and blood in the stool, would suggest *Salmonella, Shigella, Campylobacter jejuni*, or ulcerative colitis in its acute stage. The absence of fever would suggest amebic dysentery or giardiasis, although there may be fever in amebic dysentery in the severe cases. Even traveler's diarrhea and toxic staphylococcal gastroenteritis do not usually give more than a low-grade temperature at best. Pseudomembranous colitis may result in a significant elevation of the temperature once the patient becomes severely dehydrated.

3. Is there severe vomiting? Severe vomiting is seen in toxic staphylococcal gastroenteritis! This follows 2 to 4 hr after eating food poisoned with the toxin. Traveler's diarrhea and viral gastroenteritis may also cause severe vomiting, as may food that is contaminated. On the other hand, there is little or no vomiting in giardiasis and pseudomembranous colitis.

4. Did several members of the family experience acute diarrhea also? This is a key question because it indicates whether there is a possibility of toxic staphylococcal gastroenteritis or the possibility of a contagious condition such as infection with *Salmonella, Shigella*, or *Campylobacter*. If only one member of the family was suffering from diarrhea and everybody is eating the same food, then it is less likely to be a contagious condition and one must consider ulcera-

tive colitis, pseudomembranous colitis, and conditions listed under chronic diarrhea.
5. Was there recent foreign travel? Recent foreign travel would suggest the possibility of traveler's diarrhea, cholera, shigellosis, salmonellosis, and giardiasis.
6. Is there neurologic symptomatology? This should point one in the direction of botulism and generally a little epidemiologic research will disclose that other people in the community have been suffering from the same condition.

DIAGNOSTIC WORKUP

The first thing to do is a stool for occult blood. This will help distinguish those patients who are having obvious infectious disease of the large intestine or maybe even the small intestine. It will also make one suspicious of ulcerative colitis. All patients need a stool culture and stool for ova and parasites. A stool for *Giardia* antigen can also be done. Serologic studies will not be of much help in the acute condition, but they may help later on in cases of salmonellosis and amebiasis. The clinician himself should do a smear for leukocytes and examine a wet saline preparation of the stool. If the diarrhea persists or if there is blood, then sigmoidoscopy or colonoscopy should be performed. It is always important to examine the rectum for hemorrhoids and anal fissures that may be causing the positive stool for occult blood. When the diarrhea persists and becomes chronic, the diagnostic workup should include the studies that are listed under chronic diarrhea (page 138).

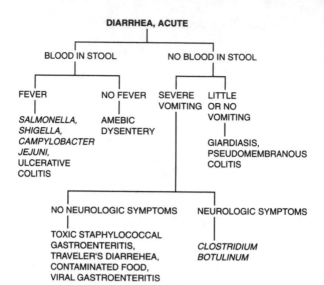

DIARRHEA, CHRONIC

Ask the following questions:

1. Is there a positive drug or alcohol history? It is well known that alcohol can cause diarrhea, as do drugs in common use such as digitalis, diuretics, beta-blockers, aspirin, colchicine, and other nonsteroidal anti-inflammatory drugs. Perhaps there is overuse of laxatives. Remember, patients may lie about the use of laxatives.
2. Is there blood in the stool? Blood in the stool certainly is significant for ulcerative colitis, carcinoma, and diverticulitis, but it is also found in amebiasis and the Zollinger-Ellison syndrome.
3. Is there a lot of mucus in the stool? Mucus is often found in ulcerative colitis, Crohn's disease, and irritable bowel syndrome.
4. Is there evidence of steatorrhea? Large volumes of stools that are partially formed or formed and float in the commode suggest steatorrhea. Stool analysis can be done, as will be discussed later.
5. Is there an abdominal mass? A mass in the right lower quadrant would suggest carcinoma or diverticulitis. Tenderness in the left lower quadrant with or without a significant mass would be suggestive of ulcerative colitis, diverticulitis, and irritable bowel syndrome. A mass in the area of the ascending or descending colon or the transverse colon should be looked for also, as these would suggest carcinoma.
6. Are there signs of systemic disease? Many systemic diseases may cause diarrhea. Among them are thyrotoxicosis, in which case one would be looking for a thyroid tumor and a tremor and tachycardia; carcinoid syndrome, which would cause considerable flushing; Addison's disease, which would cause hyperpigmentation of the skin; and pellagra, which may cause dermatitis and dementia.
7. Does significant diarrhea persist on fasting? Diarrhea that persists after fasting suggests a secretory diarrhea from a polypeptide-secreting tu-

mor, such as villous adenoma, a gastrinoma, or a carcinoid tumor.

DIAGNOSTIC WORKUP

Most patients will be diagnosed by a stool culture, stool for occult blood, and stool for ovum and parasites, along with a sigmoidoscopy and barium enema. Giardiasis may be best diagnosed by the finding of *Giardia* antigen in the stool. If a systemic disease is suspected, CBC, sedimentation rate, chemistry panel, and thyroid profile should be done. A urine test for 5-hydroxyindoleacetic acid (5-HIAA) will uncover a carcinoid syndrome. A serum gastrin will usually reveal a gastrinoma. If these tests do not provide a diagnosis, the most cost-effective approach at this point is to refer the patient to a gastroenterologist.

If a gastroenterologist is not available, the clinician may proceed with a quantitative 24-hr stool analysis for fat. If there is 10 gm or more of fat in the stool in a day, then steatorrhea can be diagnosed and one can proceed with the workup of steatorrhea (page 539). If there is less than 7 gm of fat per day in the stool, the stool volume after fasting should be done. If it is large and we have ruled out surreptitious laxative abuse, a polypeptide-secreting tumor should be considered. Here again, it would be best to refer the patient to a gastroenterologist. If the volume after a fast is small, the problem is most likely lactose or other food intolerance or an irritable bowel syndrome. Occasionally, the problem is dysfunction of the anal sphincter. Once again, a GI specialist is probably best consulted for workup of a dysfunctional anal sphincter.

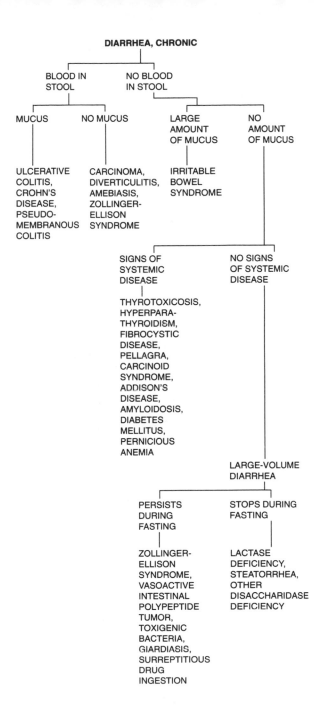

DIARRHEA, CHRONIC

BLOOD IN STOOL

NO BLOOD IN STOOL

MUCUS

NO MUCUS

LARGE AMOUNT OF MUCUS

NO AMOUNT OF MUCUS

ULCERATIVE COLITIS, CROHN'S DISEASE, PSEUDO-MEMBRANOUS COLITIS

CARCINOMA, DIVERTICULITIS, AMEBIASIS, ZOLLINGER-ELLISON SYNDROME

IRRITABLE BOWEL SYNDROME

SIGNS OF SYSTEMIC DISEASE

NO SIGNS OF SYSTEMIC DISEASE

THYROTOXICOSIS, HYPERPARA-THYROIDISM, FIBROCYSTIC DISEASE, PELLAGRA, CARCINOID SYNDROME, ADDISON'S DISEASE, AMYLOIDOSIS, DIABETES MELLITUS, PERNICIOUS ANEMIA

LARGE-VOLUME DIARRHEA

PERSISTS DURING FASTING

STOPS DURING FASTING

ZOLLINGER-ELLISON SYNDROME, VASOACTIVE INTESTINAL POLYPEPTIDE TUMOR, TOXIGENIC BACTERIA, GIARDIASIS, SURREPTITIOUS DRUG INGESTION

LACTASE DEFICIENCY, STEATORRHEA, OTHER DISACCHARIDASE DEFICIENCY

DIFFICULTY URINATING

Ask the following questions:

1. Is there pain on urination? The presence of pain on urination should suggest cystitis, urethritis, urethral caruncle, vesicular calculus, urethral stricture, and acute prostatitis.
2. Are there focal neurologic signs? The presence of focal neurologic signs should suggest multiple sclerosis, poliomyelitis, cauda equina tumor, acute spinal cord injury, tabes dorsalis, and diabetic neuropathy.
3. Is the prostate enlarged? The presence of an enlarged prostate would suggest benign prostatic hypertrophy or an advanced malignancy. A small nodular prostate may suggest an early carcinoma of the prostate. Chronic prostatitis would present with a normal sized or small sized prostate which is firm.

DIAGNOSTIC WORKUP

Routine laboratory tests include a CBC, sedimentation rate, urinalysis, VDRL test, urine culture, colony count, and sensitivity. If there is a urethral discharge, a Gram stain and culture for gonococcus should be done. If this is negative, a culture for chlamydia should be done. The patient should be catheterized for residual urine. Alternatively, ultrasonography may be done to demonstrate residual urine. If there is a significant amount of residual urine, referral to a urologist for cystoscopy and cystometric testing is done.

If there are focal neurologic signs, a neurologist is consulted. An enlarged prostate or a prostate that is nodular should be an indication for a consultation with a urologist and ordering a prostate-specific antigen titer.

DIFFICULTY URINATING

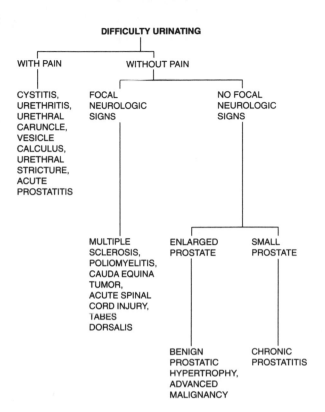

WITH PAIN

WITHOUT PAIN

CYSTITIS,
URETHRITIS,
URETHRAL
CARUNCLE,
VESICLE
CALCULUS,
URETHRAL
STRICTURE,
ACUTE
PROSTATITIS

FOCAL
NEUROLOGIC
SIGNS

NO FOCAL
NEUROLOGIC
SIGNS

MULTIPLE
SCLEROSIS,
POLIOMYELITIS,
CAUDA EQUINA
TUMOR,
ACUTE SPINAL
CORD INJURY,
TABES
DORSALIS

ENLARGED
PROSTATE

SMALL
PROSTATE

BENIGN
PROSTATIC
HYPERTROPHY,
ADVANCED
MALIGNANCY

CHRONIC
PROSTATITIS

DIPLOPIA

Ask the following questions:

1. Is it unilateral? Diplopia that is unilateral is rare, but can be encountered in ectopia lentis as associated with Marfan's disease, as well as in congenital double pupil, cataracts, and corneal opacities.
2. Is it intermittent? Intermittent diplopia would make one think of myasthenia gravis, but remember, Eaton-Lambert syndrome can do the same thing.
3. Is there associated proptosis? If there is associated proptosis, one should consider hyperthyroidism or pituitary exophthalmos, especially if it is bilateral. However, when it is associated with chemosis and ecchymosis, one should consider an infectious process.
4. Is there chemosis, ecchymosis, or periorbital edema? These findings should make one think immediately of cavernous sinus thrombosis, but an arteriovenous aneurysm can produce unilateral chemosis, ecchymosis, and exophthalmos.
5. Are there associated long tract neurologic signs? The findings of associated pyramidal tract or other long tract signs would make one think of a brain stem infarct or a brain stem tumor. Advanced intercranial pressure will put pressure on the sixth nerve and cause diplopia. Multiple sclerosis may cause long tract signs along with extraocular muscle palsies.
6. Is there fever or chills? Findings of fever and chills and diplopia should make one think of an orbital abscess, a brain abscess, or a cavernous sinus thrombosis. There is also the possibility of diphtheria.

DIAGNOSTIC WORKUP

An expensive diagnostic workup may be avoided by referring the patient to an ophthalmologist or a neurologist at the outset. If the diplopia is intermittent, a Tensilon test would be indicated. If there are fever and chills, one should do a CBC, sedimentation rate, and possibly blood cultures, a skull x-ray, and x-rays of the sinuses. However, under these circumstances, it will usually be necessary to perform a CT scan of the brain, sinuses, and orbits. If there is chemosis or ecchymosis, immediate admission to the hospital and administration of antibiotics after blood culture has been drawn are indicated. Magnetic resonance imaging of the brain may be necessary to diagnose multiple sclerosis and some of the brain stem infarcts.

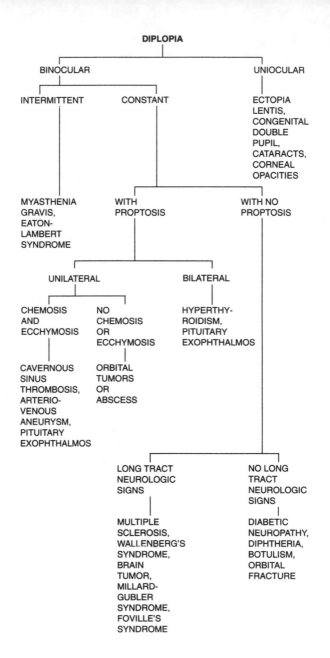

DIPLOPIA

BINOCULAR
- INTERMITTENT
  - MYASTHENIA GRAVIS, EATON-LAMBERT SYNDROME
- CONSTANT
  - WITH PROPTOSIS
    - UNILATERAL
      - CHEMOSIS AND ECCHYMOSIS
        - CAVERNOUS SINUS THROMBOSIS, ARTERIO-VENOUS ANEURYSM, PITUITARY EXOPHTHALMOS
      - NO CHEMOSIS OR ECCHYMOSIS
        - ORBITAL TUMORS OR ABSCESS
    - BILATERAL
      - HYPERTHY-ROIDISM, PITUITARY EXOPHTHALMOS
  - WITH NO PROPTOSIS
    - LONG TRACT NEUROLOGIC SIGNS
      - MULTIPLE SCLEROSIS, WALLENBERG'S SYNDROME, BRAIN TUMOR, MILLARD-GUBLER SYNDROME, FOVILLE'S SYNDROME
    - NO LONG TRACT NEUROLOGIC SIGNS
      - DIABETIC NEUROPATHY, DIPHTHERIA, BOTULISM, ORBITAL FRACTURE

UNIOCULAR
- ECTOPIA LENTIS, CONGENITAL DOUBLE PUPIL, CATARACTS, CORNEAL OPACITIES

DIZZINESS

Ask the following questions:

1. Is it true vertigo? True vertigo is characterized by the fact that the subject feels he or his environment is turning. One other form of true vertigo is lateral pulsion, where the subject feels as if he or she is moving to the left or right or may be moving forward or backward. True vertigo is a sign of neurologic or otologic disease, whereas dizziness that is not true vertigo is more likely a sign of cardiovascular disease.

2. Is there associated tinnitus or deafness? The presence of tinnitus or deafness, especially if the ear examination is negative, is a sign of a more serious otologic or neurologic condition. Such disorders as cholesteatoma, acoustic neuroma, and Ménière's disease must be considered.

3. Are there other neurologic findings? The finding of abnormalities of other cranial nerves or the long tracts such as the pyramidal tracts would suggest multiple sclerosis, an advanced brain stem tumor, acoustic neuroma, or basilar artery insufficiency.

4. Are there findings on otoscopic examination? A normal neurologic examination with an abnormal ear exam would suggest otitis media, cholesteatoma, or petrositis.

5. Is there tachypnea during the attack? If there is hyperventilation during the attack, then hyperventilation syndrome should be considered.

6. Is there a history of trauma? A history of trauma would suggest a postconcussion syndrome.

7. Are there abnormalities of the blood pressure? If the dizziness is really lightheadedness, hypertension may be present, but hypertension may also cause true vertigo. Hypotension is more likely to cause lightheadedness, which is not true vertigo. Be sure to take the blood pressures while the patient is lying down and again after rapidly arising to the standing position.

8. Are there abnormal cardiac findings? A thorough

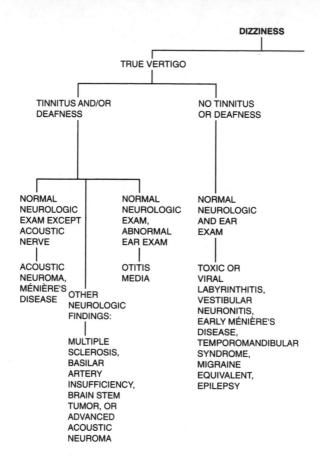

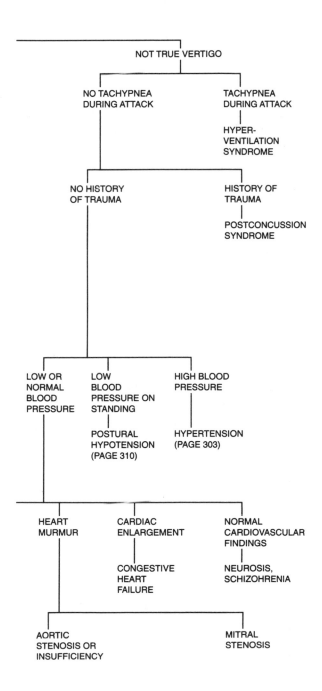

cardiovascular examination should be done. Irregularities of the heart beat, heart murmurs, or cardiac enlargement will suggest cardiac arrhythmia, aortic stenosis and insufficiency, mitral stenosis, prolapse of the mitral valve, and congestive heart failure.

9. Is there pallor? Moderate to severe anemia will cause lightheadedness and dizziness, but usually not true vertigo.

DIAGNOSTIC WORKUP

If there is true vertigo, then an audiogram and a caloric test or electronystagmography should be done. If these are abnormal, an x-ray of the mastoids, petrous bones, and internal auditory canals should be done. A CT scan of the brain should be done, especially if the findings are only unilateral. If the CT scan of the brain is negative, a spinal fluid examination can be done to exclude such disorders as central nervous system lues and multiple sclerosis. If there are long tract signs and the CT scan is negative, an MRI of the brain needs to be done to distinguish multiple sclerosis. Brain stem evoked potentials, visual evoked potentials, and somatosensory evoked potentials will also be helpful in making the diagnosis of multiple sclerosis, along with the spinal fluid analysis mentioned above. A wake-and-sleep EEG needs to be done to exclude temporal lobe epilepsy. If migraine or migraine equivalents are suspected, perhaps a trial of beta-blockers would help make this diagnosis.

If the dizziness is not true vertigo, a CBC and chemistry panel should be done at the outset. Additional studies in the form of 24-hr blood pressure monitoring, Holter monitoring, and echocardiography all have a valuable place in the diagnostic workup of dizziness without true vertigo. However, a referral to a cardiologist is wise before undertaking these expensive studies. If all studies are negative, perhaps a psychiatrist should be consulted.

DROP ATTACKS

Ask the following questions:

1. Is there loss of consciousness? If there is loss of consciousness, the differential diagnosis for syncope should be considered (page 549).
2. Are there other neurologic signs and symptoms? Focal neurologic signs and symptoms should make one think of basilar artery insufficiency, cerebral arteriosclerosis, Ménière's disease, and cerebellar atrophy. A brain tumor should also be considered if there are focal signs.
3. Is there hypotension, cardiomegaly, or a heart murmur? These findings should make one think of orthostatic hypotension, aortic stenosis and insufficiency, and cardiac arrhythmia.

DIAGNOSTIC WORKUP

Basic studies for the workup of drop attacks are CBC, sedimentation rate, chemistry panel, VDRL test, chest x-ray, and EKG. These will help identify anemia, hypoglycemia, and cardiovascular diseases. An electroencephalogram (EEG) should also be done to rule out epilepsy. If there are focal neurologic signs, a CT scan or MRI should be done. Remember, the MRI is double the cost and the diagnostic yield is only slightly higher. A neurologist should be consulted to help decide which study is appropriate. A 5-hr glucose tolerance test can be done to help diagnose hypoglycemia. Four-vessel angiography is necessary to diagnose vertebral basilar disease. Holter monitoring will be useful to diagnose complete heart block and other cardiac arrhythmias. If the chest x-ray or EKG has revealed possible cardiac findings, a referral to a cardiologist would be wise.

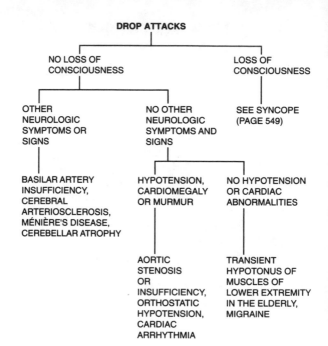

DROP ATTACKS

NO LOSS OF CONSCIOUSNESS

LOSS OF CONSCIOUSNESS

OTHER NEUROLOGIC SYMPTOMS OR SIGNS

NO OTHER NEUROLOGIC SYMPTOMS AND SIGNS

SEE SYNCOPE (PAGE 549)

BASILAR ARTERY INSUFFICIENCY, CEREBRAL ARTERIOSCLEROSIS, MÉNIÈRE'S DISEASE, CEREBELLAR ATROPHY

HYPOTENSION, CARDIOMEGALY OR MURMUR

NO HYPOTENSION OR CARDIAC ABNORMALITIES

AORTIC STENOSIS OR INSUFFICIENCY, ORTHOSTATIC HYPOTENSION, CARDIAC ARRHYTHMIA

TRANSIENT HYPOTONUS OF MUSCLES OF LOWER EXTREMITY IN THE ELDERLY, MIGRAINE

DWARFISM

Ask the following questions:

1. Is there disproportion of the trunk and extremities? These findings would suggest achondroplasia.
2. Is there obesity? The finding of obesity would suggest Fröhlich's syndrome, Laurence-Moon-Bardet-Biedl syndrome, and Brissaud's infantilism.
3. Is there appearance of wasting and/or malnutrition? The presence of wasting or other signs of malnutrition suggests chronic nephritis, congenital heart disease, progeria, malnutrition, and rickets.
4. Is there an unusual appearance to the skull or face? These findings suggest mongolism, cretinism, microcephaly, hydrocephalus, and cleidocranial dysostosis, among other conditions.
5. Are there abnormal secondary sex characteristics? The development of secondary sex characteristics is impaired in Turner's syndrome and pituitary dwarfism.

DIAGNOSTIC WORKUP

Routine studies should include a CBC, sedimentation rate, urinalysis, chemistry panel, thyroid profile, VDRL test, quantitative stool fat, a sweat test, and x-rays of the skull and long bones.

If Turner's syndrome is suspected, a buccal smear for sex chromogen may be done. If pituitary dwarfism is suspected, a CT scan of the skull may be helpful. Additional endocrine tests include a serum growth hormone level before and after exercise, a resting somatomedin-C level, and an overnight dexamethasone suppression test. In patients suspected of having rickets and hypoparathyroidism, 24-hr urine calciums may be done. However, it is best to consult a pediatrician, endocrinologist, or orthopedic surgeon before proceeding with very expensive diagnostic tests.

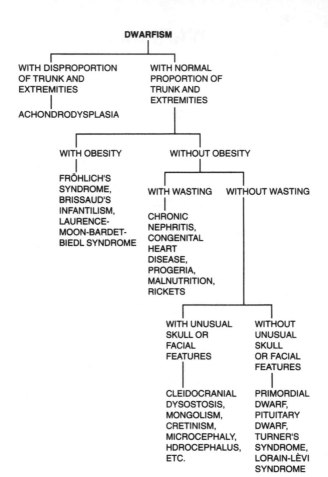

DWARFISM

WITH DISPROPORTION OF TRUNK AND EXTREMITIES
— ACHONDRODYSPLASIA

WITH NORMAL PROPORTION OF TRUNK AND EXTREMITIES

WITH OBESITY
— FRÖHLICH'S SYNDROME, BRISSAUD'S INFANTILISM, LAURENCE-MOON-BARDET-BIEDL SYNDROME

WITHOUT OBESITY

WITH WASTING
— CHRONIC NEPHRITIS, CONGENITAL HEART DISEASE, PROGERIA, MALNUTRITION, RICKETS

WITHOUT WASTING

WITH UNUSUAL SKULL OR FACIAL FEATURES
— CLEIDOCRANIAL DYSOSTOSIS, MONGOLISM, CRETINISM, MICROCEPHALY, HDROCEPHALUS, ETC.

WITHOUT UNUSUAL SKULL OR FACIAL FEATURES
— PRIMORDIAL DWARF, PITUITARY DWARF, TURNER'S SYNDROME, LORAIN-LÈVI SYNDROME

DYSARTHRIA

Ask the following questions:

1. Is it intermittent? Intermittent dysarthria should make one think of myasthenia gravis, epilepsy, and transient ischemic attacks.
2. Is there associated ataxia or nystagmus? The findings of nystagmus or ataxia should make one think of a cerebellar disorder such as multiple sclerosis, drug intoxication, or cerebellar ataxia.
3. Is there a history of drug or alcohol ingestion? Alcohol and phenytoin (Dilantin®) are just two of the toxic substances that may affect speech.
4. Is there tremor or rigidity? If there is tremor or rigidity, one should suspect Parkinson's disease, hepatolenticular degeneration, and phenothiazine toxicity.

DIAGNOSTIC WORKUP

The yield for diagnoses of dysarthria is high for a blood alcohol level and urine drug screen. If the dysarthria is intermittent, an EEG and Tensilon test should be done. If transient ischemic attacks are suspected, a carotid scan should be done, but the only way to completely exclude this possibility is by doing four-vessel cerebral angiography. A CT scan or MRI should be done in all cases of persistent dysarthria. A neurologist can help decide which study would be most appropriate. If Wilson's disease is suspected, a test for serum iron and ceruloplasmin should be done. A spinal tap may help diagnose multiple sclerosis and intracranial hemorrhage.

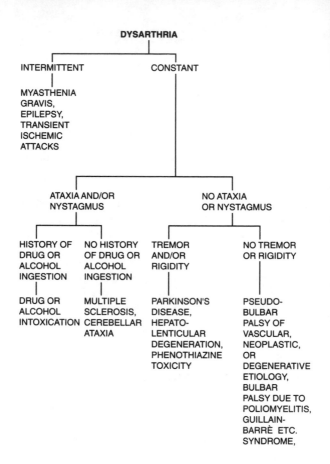

DYSARTHRIA

INTERMITTENT

MYASTHENIA
GRAVIS,
EPILEPSY,
TRANSIENT
ISCHEMIC
ATTACKS

CONSTANT

ATAXIA AND/OR
NYSTAGMUS

HISTORY OF
DRUG OR
ALCOHOL
INGESTION

DRUG OR
ALCOHOL
INTOXICATION

NO HISTORY
OF DRUG OR
ALCOHOL
INGESTION

MULTIPLE
SCLEROSIS,
CEREBELLAR
ATAXIA

NO ATAXIA
OR NYSTAGMUS

TREMOR
AND/OR
RIGIDITY

PARKINSON'S
DISEASE,
HEPATO-
LENTICULAR
DEGENERATION,
PHENOTHIAZINE
TOXICITY

NO TREMOR
OR RIGIDITY

PSEUDO-
BULBAR
PALSY OF
VASCULAR,
NEOPLASTIC,
OR
DEGENERATIVE
ETIOLOGY,
BULBAR
PALSY DUE TO
POLIOMYELITIS,
GUILLAIN-
BARRÈ ETC.
SYNDROME,

DYSMENORRHEA

Ask the following questions:

1. Are there abnormalities on pelvic examination? A tubo-ovarian mass on pelvic examination should suggest salpingo-oophoritis, endometriosis with a chocolate cyst, or ectopic pregnancy. Perhaps the uterus is abnormal, in which case one should suspect fibroids, endometrial carcinoma, uterine pregnancy, retroverted uterus, endometrial cast, or cervical polyp. A normal examination should suggest ovarian dysfunction, endocrine imbalance, and psychogenic causes.
2. What is the age of the patient? If the patient is young, she probably has a virginal uterus and may be considered to have primary dysmenorrhea. These cases are usually due to uterine hypoplasia, congenital malformations, ovarian dysfunction, or psychogenic causes.

DIAGNOSTIC WORKUP

Routine studies should include a CBC, sedimentation rate, chemistry panel, and thyroid profile. If there is vaginal discharge, a smear and culture should be done for gonorrhea and chlamydia. If there is a tubo-ovarian mass or enlarged uterus, abdominal ultrasound may help in differentiating the cause. A pregnancy test should be done. If a ruptured ectopic pregnancy is expected, a peritoneal tap or culdocentesis may help if abdominal ultrasound is not conclusive. Laparoscopy may also be helpful in the diagnosis. A fern test and basal body temperature may help diagnose endometriosis. An exploratory laparotomy may be the only way to make a diagnosis in cases of a pelvic mass. If the pelvic examination is perfectly normal, sometimes a course of progesterone hormones is useful in alleviating the problem. A dilation and curettage may also be done to address the problem. Referral to a gynecologist is usually made before doing expensive diagnostic tests.

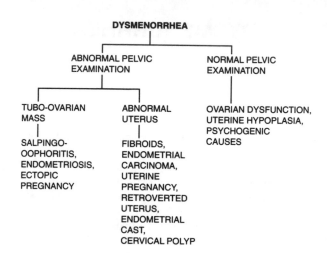

DYSMENORRHEA

ABNORMAL PELVIC EXAMINATION

NORMAL PELVIC EXAMINATION

TUBO-OVARIAN MASS

SALPINGO-OOPHORITIS, ENDOMETRIOSIS, ECTOPIC PREGNANCY

ABNORMAL UTERUS

FIBROIDS, ENDOMETRIAL CARCINOMA, UTERINE PREGNANCY, RETROVERTED UTERUS, ENDOMETRIAL CAST, CERVICAL POLYP

OVARIAN DYSFUNCTION, UTERINE HYPOPLASIA, PSYCHOGENIC CAUSES

DYSPAREUNIA

Ask the following questions:

1. Are there abnormalities on the pelvic examination? Abnormalities on pelvic examination include an ovarian mass, salpingo-oophoritis, a retroverted uterus, endometriosis, bartholinitis, and urethritis.
2. Does the history indicate that the difficulty is on penetration? Difficulties on penetration usually point to a vulval or vaginal origin for the problem. In that case, bartholinitis, vulvitis, vulval dystrophy, cystitis, urethritis, and urethral caruncle should be suspected.
3. Is the urinalysis abnormal? An abnormal urinalysis may indicate cystitis or a bladder calculus.
4. Are there abnormalities on rectal examination? Hemorrhoids, anal fissures, and impacted feces may cause dyspareunia.
5. Is the pelvic examination totally normal? If this is true, one would consider functional dyspareunia or it may be that the patient does not have dyspareunia at all and simply has no sexual desire or dislikes the sexual act.

DIAGNOSTIC WORKUP

Routine studies include a CBC, a sedimentation rate, a urinalysis, a urine culture and sensitivity, and a vaginal smear and culture. A Pap smear should also be done. If pregnancy is suspected, a pregnancy test should be done. If there is a pelvic mass, pelvic ultrasound may be helpful. A referral to a gynecologist is usually made before ordering this study, however. If vulval dystrophy is suspected, a vaginal biopsy may be useful. If the vaginal examination is normal, perhaps a psychiatrist should be consulted.

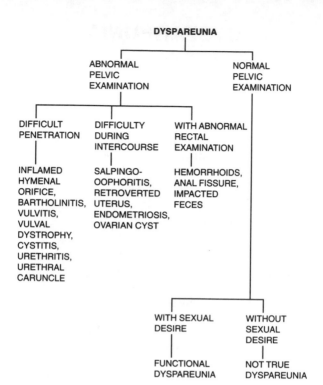

DYSPAREUNIA

- ABNORMAL PELVIC EXAMINATION
  - DIFFICULT PENETRATION
    - INFLAMED HYMENAL ORIFICE, BARTHOLINITIS, VULVITIS, VULVAL DYSTROPHY, CYSTITIS, URETHRITIS, URETHRAL CARUNCLE
  - DIFFICULTY DURING INTERCOURSE
    - SALPINGO-OOPHORITIS, RETROVERTED UTERUS, ENDOMETRIOSIS, OVARIAN CYST
  - WITH ABNORMAL RECTAL EXAMINATION
    - HEMORRHOIDS, ANAL FISSURE, IMPACTED FECES
- NORMAL PELVIC EXAMINATION
  - WITH SEXUAL DESIRE
    - FUNCTIONAL DYSPAREUNIA
  - WITHOUT SEXUAL DESIRE
    - NOT TRUE DYSPAREUNIA

DYSPHAGIA

Ask the following questions:

1. Are there abnormalities on oropharyngeal examination? If that is true, then of course the cause may be local. This is particularly true if there are painful ulcerations of the mouth, glossitis, or tonsillitis. There may be neoplasms in the oropharynx or larynx that may be either obstructing swallowing or causing pain on swallowing.

2. Is the dysphagia constant or intermittent? Intermittent dysphagia would make one think of myasthenia gravis and if there are other neurologic findings to suggest that, then it would be the most likely working diagnosis. Without neurologic findings, a Schatzki ring may be present.

3. Does the patient have difficulty swallowing both liquids and solids or only solids? If the patient has difficulty with both liquids and solids, a diagnosis of achalasia, scleroderma, or diffuse esophageal spasm should be entertained. Patients who have difficulty swallowing solids only usually should be considered to have esophageal carcinoma until proven otherwise.

4. Is heartburn present? If there is heartburn as well as dysphagia, a diagnosis of reflux esophagitis with or without hiatal hernia should be entertained. Many conditions including achalasia, diffuse esophageal spasm, and even advanced esophageal carcinoma may be associated with pain on swallowing or chest pain.

5. Is the patient male or female? Dysphagia in a male is suggestive of esophageal carcinoma and that would be especially true with a history of significant smoking and drinking. Dysphagia in a female would suggest esophageal web, as in Plummer-Vinson syndrome.

6. Is there significant weight loss? Significant weight loss is very often associated with esophageal carcinoma, but not until it is advanced a significant degree. One often forgets that weight loss is also associated with achalasia.

7. Is there a history of syphilis? Obviously, this would suggest an aortic aneurysm and in considering aortic aneurysm, one should also consider other mediastinal masses that might be associated with this condition.

8. Are there dermatologic signs and symptoms? This would bring up the possibility of scleroderma.

DIAGNOSTIC WORKUP

In a patient with definite dysphagia, it is wise to consult a gastroenterologist at the outset! The most useful diagnostic test (and most inexpensive) is the barium swallow and an upper GI series might as well be done as well. The barium swallow will often display fairly definitive features of carcinoma of the esophagus, achalasia, hiatal hernia, and esophagitis. The barium swallow, however, must be frequently followed by esophagoscopy to obtain a more definitive diagnosis and a tissue biopsy, particularly in the case of carcinoma of the esophagus. If both of these tests are negative, the possibility of myasthenia gravis should be considered and a Tensilon test should be done. Esophageal manometry may detect achalasia or diffuse esophageal spasm. When a mediastinal mass is suspected, a CT scan of the mediastinum should be done. When all testing is negative, hysteria should be considered.

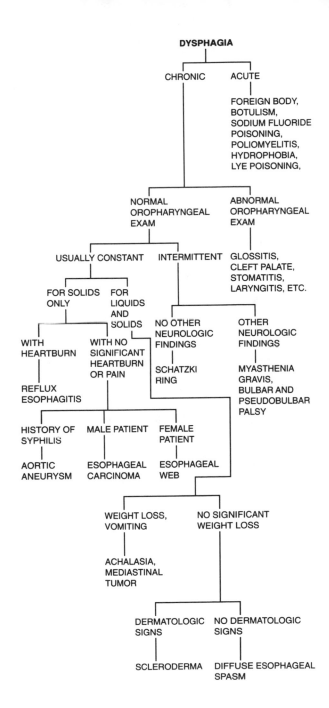

DYSPNEA

Ask the following questions:

1. Is the dyspnea acute? If the dyspnea is acute onset, one should then ask is there a drug history, particularly a history of mainlining narcotics. If so, then adult respiratory distress syndrome should be considered. Furthermore, is there an embolic source for a possible pulmonary embolism? If the onset is gradual, one should move on to consider chronic diseases such as congestive heart failure and pulmonary emphysema and fibrosis.
2. Is there fever or purulent sputum? Obviously, fever and purulent sputum should make one think of pneumonia.
3. What kind of rales are there? If there are crepitant rales, one should consider congestive heart failure. If there are sibilant and sonorous rales or wheezing, one should consider bronchial asthma or pulmonary emphysema.
4. Is there hepatomegaly? Hepatomegaly would be a sign of congestive heart failure. However, in the acute stages it may not manifest immediately. Hepatomegaly may also be an indication of other systemic diseases that are associated with either lung disease or heart disease. The collagen diseases in particular come to mind.

DIAGNOSTIC WORKUP

The basic workup of acute onset dyspnea should include a CBC to exclude anemia, a chest x-ray and arterial blood gases to exclude pneumothorax, pneumonia, and other pulmonic diseases, and an EKG and serial cardiac enzymes to exclude myocardial infarction and some of the causes of congestive heart failure. A sputum smear and culture should always be done when there is adequate sputum. Eosinophils should be looked for. It is important to make sure that you have an adequate specimen and, therefore, leukocytes should be reported on the smear.

If there is chest pain accompanied by hemoptysis, then arterial blood gases and a ventilation-perfusion scan should be done to rule out pulmonary embolism. Even without chest pain and hemoptysis, a pulmonary embolism may need to be excluded. If the ventilation-perfusion scan is inconclusive, a pulmonary angiography may still need to be done in difficult cases. If routine smears and cultures are negative, cultures for acid-fast bacilli and fungi may need to be done, especially when there is continuing purulent sputum. The clinician should also consider doing skin testing for these diseases.

If congestive heart failure is suspected, an arm-to-tongue circulation time and pulmonary function testing should also be done. A therapeutic trial of a diuretic may be valuable. When there is significant wheezing, a trial of sublingual isoproterenol hydrochloride (Isuprel®) or epinephrine 0.3 cc subcutaneously may clear up the confusion.

In chronic dyspnea the chest x-ray and EKG should be complemented by pulmonary function testing, exercise testing, and arterial blood gases. Pulmonary function testing will be very useful in diagnosing asthma and distinguishing pulmonary emphysema from pulmonary fibrosis. The advice of a pulmonologist should be sought when extensive pulmonary function testing such as compliance and diffusing capacity need to be determined. Bronchoscopy may need to be done to exclude a foreign body, neoplasm, or bronchiectasis. Cardiac catheterization and pulmonary angiography may be needed to identify chronic recurrent pulmonary embolism, intracardiac shunts and pulmonary hypertension.

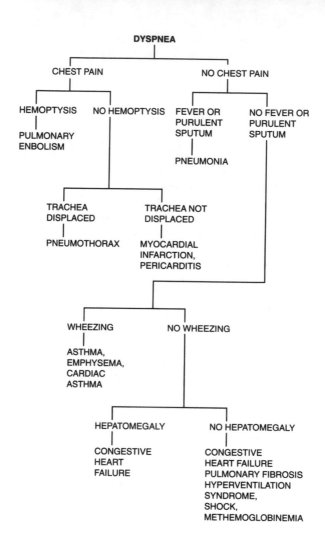

DYSPNEA

CHEST PAIN

HEMOPTYSIS

PULMONARY
ENBOLISM

NO HEMOPTYSIS

TRACHEA
DISPLACED

PNEUMOTHORAX

TRACHEA NOT
DISPLACED

MYOCARDIAL
INFARCTION,
PERICARDITIS

NO CHEST PAIN

FEVER OR
PURULENT
SPUTUM

PNEUMONIA

NO FEVER OR
PURULENT
SPUTUM

WHEEZING

ASTHMA,
EMPHYSEMA,
CARDIAC
ASTHMA

NO WHEEZING

HEPATOMEGALY

CONGESTIVE
HEART
FAILURE

NO HEPATOMEGALY

CONGESTIVE
HEART FAILURE
PULMONARY FIBROSIS
HYPERVENTILATION
SYNDROME,
SHOCK,
METHEMOGLOBINEMIA

DYSURIA

Ask the following questions:

1. Is there fever? A significant fever would suggest either pyelonephritis, particularly in females, or acute prostatitis in males.
2. Is the urine grossly bloody or are there a significant number of red cells on microscopic examination? Grossly bloody urine in a young female should suggest acute cystitis, particularly if she has just returned from a honeymoon. In older patients it may indicate bladder carcinoma, but generally these patients have blood in their urine before they develop dysuria. Really significant blood in the urine may also indicate schistosomiasis or tuberculous cystitis. Dysuria and hematuria can occur in renal or vesicular calculi as well.
3. Is there a urethral or vaginal discharge? If either of these signs is present, one must consider that the patient may have gonorrhea until proven otherwise. Repeated negative smears and cultures for gonococcus should suggest that the patient may have female urethral syndrome or nonspecific urethritis due to chlamydia.
4. Are there systemic symptoms? If there are systemic symptoms, one must consider the possibility of Reiter's syndrome or collagen disease. One should not forget that systemic symptoms of arthritis and rash may also be present in gonorrhea.
5. Is the pain very severe? Severe pain, particularly a need to stay close to the restroom so one can empty one's bladder, may indicate tabes dorsalis, although this condition is rarely seen today.

DIAGNOSTIC WORKUP

Obviously, a urinalysis and urine culture, sensitivity, and colony count must be done in all cases. I also recommend a urethral smear and a vaginal smear and culture if sufficient material can be obtained. Even 4 white cells per high-powered field on a urethral smear probably indicates urethritis. Cultures for both gonorrhea and chlamydia should be done. In persistent cases of dysuria, an intravenous pyelogram and a cystoscopy must be done. Cultures for anaerobic bacilli and tuberculosis may be necessary in persistent pyuria. It should go without saying that a rectal and vaginal examination should be done in all cases. However, this is frequently neglected.

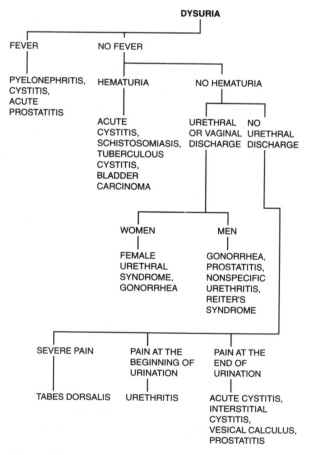

EARACHE

Ask the following questions:

1. Are there abnormalities on the ear examination? The ear examination may reveal severe otitis externa, an epithelioma of the pinna, a foreign body, or impacted wax. It may also show inflammation and bulging of the ear drum. A vesicular rash of the drum and external auditory canal may indicate herpes zoster.
2. Is there pain on moving the pinna? Pain on moving the ear suggests otitis externa, foreign body, impacted wax, or keratosis obturans.
3. Is there hearing loss? Hearing loss with an abnormal drum would suggest serous or bacterial otitis media. It may also suggest a cholesteatoma. Hearing loss with a normal ear exam suggests aerootitis.
4. Could the pain be a referred pain? Dental caries, dental abscesses, impacted teeth, tonsillitis, and temporomandibular joint syndrome may refer pain to the ear.

DIAGNOSTIC WORKUP

If there is an exudate, a culture and sensitivity should be ordered. Perhaps a throat culture should be done also. X-rays of the mastoids and petrous bones should be done if the exudate is believed to be from a deeper source. Perhaps a CT scan is also needed. If there is hearing loss, an audiogram needs to be done and a tympanogram will be useful in diagnosing serous otitis media. A trial of carbamazepine (Tegretol®) or phenytoin (Dilantin®) may be useful in diagnosing glossopharyngeal neuralgia or tic douloureux. If the discharge is thought to be cerebrospinal fluid, a CT scan and RISA study should be done.

Referral to an ear, nose and throat specialist or neurologist should be considered before ordering expensive diagnostic tests.

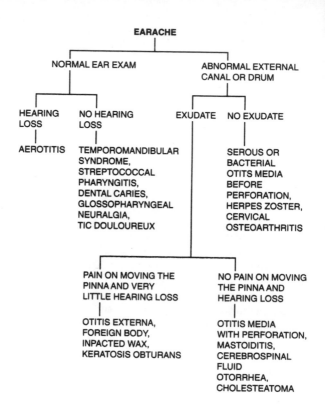

EARACHE

- **NORMAL EAR EXAM**
  - **HEARING LOSS**
    - AEROTITIS
  - **NO HEARING LOSS**
    - TEMPOROMANDIBULAR SYNDROME, STREPTOCOCCAL PHARYNGITIS, DENTAL CARIES, GLOSSOPHARYNGEAL NEURALGIA, TIC DOULOUREUX
- **ABNORMAL EXTERNAL CANAL OR DRUM**
  - **EXUDATE**
    - **PAIN ON MOVING THE PINNA AND VERY LITTLE HEARING LOSS**
      - OTITIS EXTERNA, FOREIGN BODY, INPACTED WAX, KERATOSIS OBTURANS
    - **NO PAIN ON MOVING THE PINNA AND HEARING LOSS**
      - OTITIS MEDIA WITH PERFORATION, MASTOIDITIS, CEREBROSPINAL FLUID OTORRHEA, CHOLESTEATOMA
  - **NO EXUDATE**
    - SEROUS OR BACTERIAL OTITS MEDIA BEFORE PERFORATION, HERPES ZOSTER, CERVICAL OSTEOARTHRITIS

EAR DISCHARGE

Ask the following questions:

1. Is it acute? Acute ear discharge suggests acute otitis media with rupture or an otitis externa, especially if it is painful. A chronic discharge would suggest cholesteatoma, chronic otitis media, and possibly cerebrospinal fluid.
2. Is it painful? A painful ear with a discharge is most likely acute otitis media with rupture. It may, however, be due to otitis externa, a foreign body, or serous otitis media.
3. Is there associated fever? An ear discharge with fever suggests otitis media, mastoiditis, and petrositis.
4. What is the character of the discharge? A mucopurulent discharge suggests chronic otitis media and mastoiditis, while a fetid discharge with whitish debris suggests a cholesteatoma. If the discharge is clear, a cerebrospinal fluid otorrhea should be suspected.

DIAGNOSTIC WORKUP

The most important test to do is a smear, culture and sensitivity of the discharge. If there is fever, a CBC, sedimentation rate, and chemistry panel should be done. The ears should be examined after thorough irrigation. X-rays of the mastoids and petrous bones should be done if a deep source for the discharge is suspected. Audiograms are helpful if there is hearing loss. If the discharge is thought to be cerebrospinal fluid, a RISA study and CT scan of the brain may need to be done. An ear, nose and throat specialist should be consulted before ordering expensive diagnostic tests.

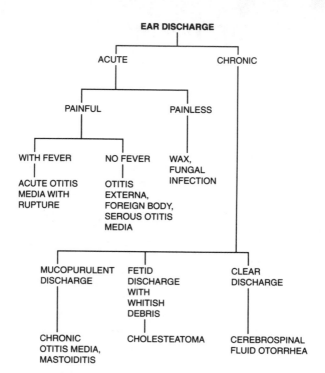

EAR DISCHARGE

- ACUTE
  - PAINFUL
    - WITH FEVER
      - ACUTE OTITIS MEDIA WITH RUPTURE
    - NO FEVER
      - OTITIS EXTERNA, FOREIGN BODY, SEROUS OTITIS MEDIA
  - PAINLESS
    - WAX, FUNGAL INFECTION
- CHRONIC
  - MUCOPURULENT DISCHARGE
    - CHRONIC OTITIS MEDIA, MASTOIDITIS
  - FETID DISCHARGE WITH WHITISH DEBRIS
    - CHOLESTEATOMA
  - CLEAR DISCHARGE
    - CEREBROSPINAL FLUID OTORRHEA

EDEMA, GENERALIZED

Ask the following questions:

1. Does the edema pit on pressure? Edema that pits on pressure is more likely to be due to heart, liver, or kidney disease. Edema that does not pit on pressure is more likely due to myxedema or lymphedema.
2. Is there hepatomegaly? If there is hepatomegaly, one should consider liver disease such as cirrhosis or cardiac disease.
3. Is there ascites? If there is ascites along with hepatomegaly, cirrhosis of the liver is the most likely cause of the edema. However, one should not forget constrictive pericarditis. If there is no ascites along with the hepatomegaly then congestive heart failure should be considered.
4. Is there jugular vein distention? Jugular vein distention certainly would be most suggestive of congestive heart failure, but other causes of jugular vein distention include superior vena cava syndrome due to a mediastinal mass such as carcinoma of the lung and constrictive pericarditis. Right heart failure secondary to pulmonary emphysema and fibrosis can also cause jugular vein distention.
5. Is there an abnormal urinary sediment? If there is an abnormal urinary sediment, consider nephritis, whether it might be due to chronic glomerulonephritis or whether it is secondary to diabetes mellitus or a collagen disease.
6. Is the patient taking any drugs that could cause the edema? Among the drugs that should be considered are corticosteroids, progesterone, estrogen, anti-inflammatory drugs like naproxen (Naprosyn®) and ibuprofen (Motrin®), antihypertensive drugs like methyldopa (Aldomet®) and clonidine hydrochloride, calcium channel blockers, beta-adrenergic blockers, and antidepressants.

DIAGNOSTIC WORKUP

A CBC should be done to rule out significant anemia that may be the cause of the edema. If there is anemia, we need to determine its source. Liver function tests are done to rule out liver disease, and serum protein electrophoresis and tests for blood urea nitrogen (BUN) and creatinine should be done to exclude renal disease. The urinalysis is very important both for the routine studies and also to examine the urinary sediment for diseases such as chronic glomerulonephritis and collagen disease. If there is significant loss of protein in the urine, we should be considering nephrosis. An EKG, chest x-ray, and venous pressure and circulation time will be extremely helpful in diagnosing congestive heart failure, but pulmonary function tests can be done as the vital capacity is significantly reduced in this disease. A thyroid profile should be done to diagnose myxedema. A CT scan of the chest will help diagnose constrictive pericarditis. Occasionally, the edema is due to an abdominal tumor. A CT scan of the abdomen and pelvis will be helpful in those cases. Contrast lymphangiography may be necessary to diagnose lymphedema.

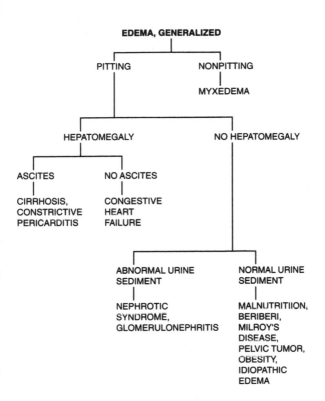

EDEMA, GENERALIZED

PITTING

NONPITTING

MYXEDEMA

HEPATOMEGALY

NO HEPATOMEGALY

ASCITES

CIRRHOSIS, CONSTRICTIVE PERICARDITIS

NO ASCITES

CONGESTIVE HEART FAILURE

ABNORMAL URINE SEDIMENT

NEPHROTIC SYNDROME, GLOMERULONEPHRITIS

NORMAL URINE SEDIMENT

MALNUTRITIION, BERIBERI, MILROY'S DISEASE, PELVIC TUMOR, OBESITY, IDIOPATHIC EDEMA

EDEMA, LOCALIZED

Ask the following questions:

1. Is the edema acute or chronic? Acute edema, if it is localized, should always bring to mind a deep vein thrombophlebitis. It also should bring to mind acute lymphangitis, particularly if there is erythema in the area. Finally, it should also make one think of trauma or a focal infection such as cellulitis. Chronic localized edema, on the other hand, is more likely related to varicose veins or lymphedema.
2. Is the edema pitting or nonpitting? If the edema pits, it is more likely related to inflammation or venous incompetence. If it is nonpitting, it is more likely due to obstruction of the lymphatics, i.e., lymphedema.
3. Is there erythema, a rash, or focal tenderness, or all three? Erythema and focal tenderness would suggest cellulitis, lymphangitis, thrombophlebitis, angioneurotic edema, insect bite, or snake bite. It also would suggest a sprain or contusion. Focal tenderness alone with pitting edema and no significant erythema or rash would suggest a deep vein thrombophlebitis. When there is no erythema or tenderness in a case of pitting edema of a localized nature, one should consider varicose veins or, in the lower extremities, a popliteal cyst that might be obstructing the veins on a chronic basis.
4. If the edema is of the lower extremities, is there a positive Homans' sign? A positive Homans' sign should always be looked for because this would suggest a deep vein thrombophlebitis. Action must be taken immediately in such cases.

DIAGNOSTIC WORKUP

A venous ultrasound study, impedance plethysmography, and contrast venography are very useful in the diagnosis of deep vein thrombophlebitis. Patients with suspected cellulitis or osteomyelitis should have a CBC, sedimentation rate, and cultures of the blood or any fluid that is available from the site of the lesion, either direct or by aspiration. X-rays and CT scans of the involved area are useful as well. Bone scans are often of value in diagnosing osteomyelitis and fractures. Lymphangiography will be helpful in the diagnosis of carcinomatosis or lymphedema from other causes. A CT scan of the abdomen or pelvis may also demonstrate the malignant lymph nodes. A thyroid profile will diagnose cases of pretibial myxedema due to thyrotoxicosis. Patients with upper extremity edema should have a chest x-ray and CT scan of the mediastinum to determine the causes of superior vena cava syndrome.

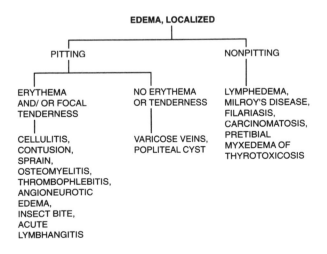

EDEMA, LOCALIZED

PITTING — NONPITTING

ERYTHEMA AND/ OR FOCAL TENDERNESS — NO ERYTHEMA OR TENDERNESS — LYMPHEDEMA, MILROY'S DISEASE, FILARIASIS, CARCINOMATOSIS, PRETIBIAL MYXEDEMA OF THYROTOXICOSIS

CELLULITIS, CONTUSION, SPRAIN, OSTEOMYELITIS, THROMBOPHLEBITIS, ANGIONEUROTIC EDEMA, INSECT BITE, ACUTE LYMBHANGITIS — VARICOSE VEINS, POPLITEAL CYST

ENOPHTHALMOS

If the condition is unilateral, it is almost always due to paralysis of the cervical sympathetic ganglion and part of Horner's syndrome. Horner's syndrome includes enophthalmos, partial ptosis, constricted pupil, absence of sweating, and the presence of blushing on the side of the sympathetic paralysis. The various causes of Horner's syndrome can be found on page 292. Prolonged endophthalmitis may cause unilateral enophthalmos due to shrinkage of the eyeball.

Bilateral enophthalmos may be due to starvation or cachexia (in which case the cause should be obvious) or congenital.

ENURESIS

Ask the following questions:

1. Is the bed-wetting frequent or only occasional? If the bed-wetting is frequent, that should signify pathology in the urogenital tract or endocrine system. If it is infrequent, one should consider epilepsy.
2. Are there abnormalities found on the urogenital examination? There are many causes of enuresis that can be found on a simple examination such as phimosis, balanitis, meatal stricture, vulvitis, or intestinal worms.
3. Are there abnormalities on the urinalysis? Urinalysis alone is usually not adequate and a urine culture should be done to rule out cystitis and pyelonephritis. The simple examination of the urine sediment for bacteria is also helpful. Sugar in the urine may indicate diabetes mellitus, but it may also indicate Fanconi's syndrome.
4. Is there polyuria? Polyuria might indicate diabetes insipidus, diabetes mellitus, hyperthyroidism, and hypoparathyroidism.
5. Are there abnormalities on the neurologic examination? Here one would be looking for cerebral palsy and congenital anomalies of the spinal cord.

Finally, if the neurologic examination, urogenital examination, and urinalysis are normal, perhaps the patient has a simple neurosis or situational maladjustment.

DIAGNOSTIC WORKUP

Patients who are suspected of having a urological condition as the cause of their enuresis should have a urinalysis, intravenous pyelogram, and voiding cystogram along with a urine culture and colony count. Referral to a urologist for cystometric testing may be required. If there is polyuria, then a glucose tolerance test, a thyroid profile, and tests for calcium phosphorus, alkaline phosphatase, and parathyroid hormone level should be done. If epilepsy is suspected, an EEG should be ordered. If the neurologic examination is abnormal, referral to a neurologic specialist would be in order. If all the studies and examinations are within normal limits, a referral to a psychiatrist or psychologist may be in order. However, the child may have simple enuresis in which case all that is required is to reassure the parents that the child will grow out of it by puberty.

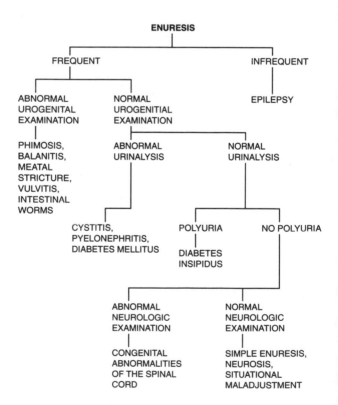

EPIPHORA

Ask the following questions:

1. Is the epiphora unilateral or bilateral? If it is bilateral, it is most likely due to emotional weeping or to the effects of drugs such as bromides, arsenic, and mercury.
2. Is the eye examination normal? If the eye examination is abnormal, there are most likely obvious findings of conjunctivitis, foreign bodies, corneal ulcer, or other problems. A foreign body may be difficult to find, as may a corneal ulcer, and referral to an ophthalmologist would be in order. In any event, the conjunctiva will be red and inflamed. In addition, there may be lid problems, particularly in the elderly and these may constitute ectropion or entropion. There is also the possibility of Bell's palsy causing incomplete closure of the eye and therefore the eye will be chronically inflamed from constant exposure to air.

    If the eye examination is normal, one must consider the possibility of obstruction of the nasolacrimal duct due to either trauma, congenital causes, a calculus, neoplasm, or dacryocystitis. Crocodile tears may occur when, due to aberrant nerve regeneration following facial paralysis, the lacrimal gland is stimulated to produce excessive tears while eating.

DIAGNOSTIC WORKUP

The first thing to do if the epiphora is bilateral is to determine if the patient has been on any particular drugs or has emotional problems. If the eye examination is abnormal or there are problems with the lids, referral to an ophthalmologist is in order. Even if the eye examination is normal, the referral to an ophthalmologist would be necessary to determine if obstruction of the nasolacrimal duct is the problem.

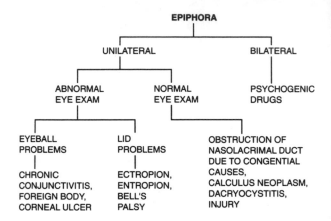

EPIPHORA

UNILATERAL — BILATERAL

UNILATERAL:
- ABNORMAL EYE EXAM
- NORMAL EYE EXAM

BILATERAL:
- PSYCHOGENIC DRUGS

ABNORMAL EYE EXAM:
- EYEBALL PROBLEMS
- LID PROBLEMS

EYEBALL PROBLEMS:
CHRONIC CONJUNCTIVITIS, FOREIGN BODY, CORNEAL ULCER

LID PROBLEMS:
ECTROPION, ENTROPION, BELL'S PALSY

NORMAL EYE EXAM:
OBSTRUCTION OF NASOLACRIMAL DUCT DUE TO CONGENTIAL CAUSES, CALCULUS NEOPLASM, DACRYOCYSTITIS, INJURY

EPISTAXIS

Ask the following questions:

1. Is there hypertension? The patient with hypertension could have either essential or symptomatic hypertension. Be sure to recheck the blood pressure, as other health professionals may miss the auscultatory gap. Next, treat the hypertension and investigate the patient for symptomatic hypertension later (page 303).
2. Is the bleeding from Little's area or is it further up the nasal passageway? Ninety percent of epistaxis results from bleeding in Little's area, and this area is most easily controlled. Bleeding from this area is usually not a serious problem. However, when the bleeding is from the posterior nasal areas, one must always consider the possibility of carcinoma.
3. Is there a history or clinical signs of a coagulation disorder? There may be a history of hemophilia or leukemia. There may be splenomegaly. There may be bleeding sites elsewhere to indicate that there is a systemic disorder associated with the epistaxis. One can easily perform a Rumpel-Leede test to determine if there is a platelet deficiency or dysfunction.

DIAGNOSTIC WORKUP

The diagnostic workup of epistaxis should include a coagulation profile with prothrombin time, partial thromboplastin time (PTT), bleeding time, platelet count, Rumpel-Leede test, and CBC. If these tests suggest a coagulation disorder, referral to a hematologist can be done for further diagnostic workup.

A nasal smear should be done for eosinophils to determine if the patient has chronic allergic rhinitis.

When a carcinoma of the nasal pharynx or sinuses is suspected, x-rays of the paranasal sinuses can be done, as well as nasopharyngoscopy. A CT scan of the sinuses is also of value in difficult diagnostic problems.

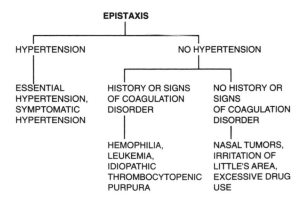

EUPHORIA

Ask the following questions:

1. Is there a history of drug ingestion? The patient will frequently not tell the truth about drug ingestion, but one should then ask family and friends about whether the patient uses any of the illicit drugs such as LSD, marijuana, or cocaine. Other drugs that are prescribed by physicians may cause euphoria such as corticosteroids and various narcotics.
2. Is the neurologic examination abnormal? The patient may demonstrate simply disorientation or disturbance in the thought process or excessive jocularity, as may be seen in witzelsucht. All these findings may suggest a frontal lobe tumor, a general paresis or other forms of dementia. When there are long tract signs such as posterior column or pyramidal tract involvement, one must consider the possibility of multiple sclerosis or a pontine glioma.
3. Is there significant incoherence, delusions, or hallucinations? These findings would most likely suggest schizophrenia.
4. Is the euphoria sustained for long periods or very short-lived? If the euphoria is intermittent and very brief, one should consider temporal lobe epilepsy. If it is more sustained, one would consider manic-depressive psychosis.

DIAGNOSTIC WORKUP

A drug screen should be axiomatic on all patients, as the patient may lie. If this is negative, one may proceed with the more expensive testing such as MRI or at least a CT scan to rule out a brain tumor. If these tests are negative and the problem persists, the patient should be referred to a psychiatrist.

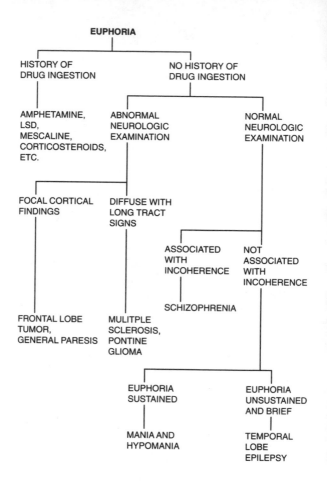

EXOPHTHALMOS

Ask the following questions:

1. Is it bilateral or unilateral? Bilateral exophthalmos would suggest hyperthyroidism. Unilateral exophthalmos suggests orbital tumor, abscess, or aneurysm.
2. If it is bilateral, are there signs of hyperthyroidism? If there are other indications of hyperthyroidism, Graves' disease would be the diagnosis.
3. If it is unilateral, does the eyeball pulsate? A pulsating eyeball would suggest an arteriovenous fistula and there should be a loud blowing murmur over the orbit.
4. Is there fever? Fever would suggest acute cellulitis, acute sinusitis, periostitis, or a cavernous sinus thrombosis.
5. Is there chemosis or ecchymosis? These signs are suggestive of a cavernous sinus thrombosis.

DIAGNOSTIC WORKUP

In cases of bilateral exophthalmos, particularly if there is no fever or chemosis or ecchymosis, a thyroid profile is the most valuable test. Other endocrine studies may be necessary once hyperthyroidism has been excluded. In cases of unilateral exophthalmos, plane films of the orbits and sinuses may be helpful, but a CT scan of the brain and sinuses is the most valuable diagnostic aid. Carotid angiography will need to be done to diagnose an arteriovenous fistula.

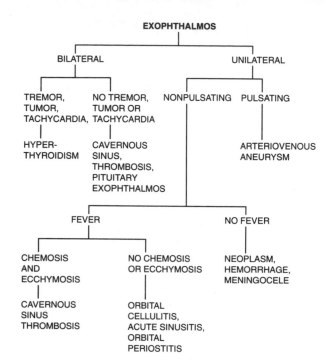

EXOPHTHALMOS

BILATERAL

- TREMOR, TUMOR, OR TACHYCARDIA,
  - HYPER-THYROIDISM
- NO TREMOR, TUMOR OR TACHYCARDIA
  - CAVERNOUS SINUS, THROMBOSIS, PITUITARY EXOPHTHALMOS

UNILATERAL

- NONPULSATING
- PULSATING
  - ARTERIOVENOUS ANEURYSM

FEVER

- CHEMOSIS AND ECCHYMOSIS
  - CAVERNOUS SINUS THROMBOSIS
- NO CHEMOSIS OR ECCHYMOSIS
  - ORBITAL CELLULITIS, ACUTE SINUSITIS, ORBITAL PERIOSTITIS

NO FEVER

- NEOPLASM, HEMORRHAGE, MENINGOCELE

EXTREMITY PAIN, LOWER EXTREMITY

Ask the following questions:

1. Is the extremity pain of acute or gradual onset? Acute onset would suggest arterial embolism, deep vein thrombophlebitis, and cellulitis. If there is a history of trauma, it would suggest a fracture, sprain, or torn ligament.
2. Is there limitation of motion of the joints? A positive Patrick's test would indicate hip pathology, including greater trochanter bursitis. A positive McMurray test would indicate a torn meniscus.
3. Are there positive neurologic findings? A positive femoral stretch test would suggest a herniated disk at L2–L3 or L3–L4, while a positive Lasègue's sign would indicate a herniated disk at L4–L5 or L5–S1. Combined motor and sensory deficits may indicate radiculopathy or neuropathy.
4. Is there a positive Homans' sign? This is a very important examination, as one would not want to miss a deep vein thrombophlebitis.
5. Is there diminished or absent peripheral pulses? Diminished or absent pulses would suggest arterial embolism, peripheral arteriosclerosis, or Leriche's syndrome (thrombosis of the terminal aorta).
6. Is there focal tenderness, swelling, or erythema of the extremity? This would suggest cellulitis, superficial thrombophlebitis, osteomyelitis, lymphangitis, and other types of infections. Tenderness without significant swelling or erythema would be suggestive of bursitis or deep vein thrombophlebitis.

DIAGNOSTIC WORKUP

If there is clear-cut joint pathology, an x-ray of the joints, arthritis profile, and synovial fluid analysis will usually provide a diagnosis. Magnetic resonance imaging is useful in the diagnosis of a torn meniscus. If a deep pain thrombophlebitis is suspected, venous Doppler ultrasound, impedance plethysmography, or a contrast venogram may be done. If an arterial embolism or chronic peripheral arterial disease is suspected, femoral angiography can be done. If a herniated disk or other pathology of the lumbar spine is suspected, plain films of the lumbar spine should be obtained. It might be wise at this point also to obtain a CBC, a sedimentation rate, and a chemistry panel to determine the alkaline phosphatase, calcium, and phosphorus. In older males, tests for acid phosphatase and prostate-specific antigen (PSA) should be done.

If these tests are unrevealing, it is wise to refer the patient to a neurologic specialist before any more expensive tests are ordered. He will probably order a CT scan of the lumbar spine and may do nerve conduction velocity studies, electromyographic examinations, or dermatomal somatosensory evoked potential studies as indicated. In difficult neurologic problems, a combined myelography and CT scan is preferred over MRI. Bone scans will help diagnose obscure fractures and osteomyelitis, both of the lumbar spine and the lower extremities.

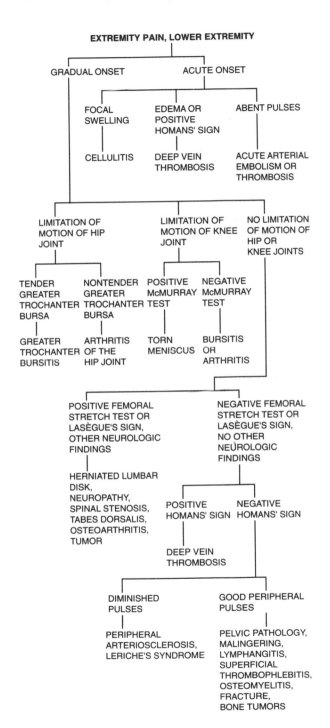

EXTREMITY PAIN, UPPER EXTREMITY

Ask the following questions:

1. Is there limitation of motion of the joints? Limitation of motion of a joint would suggest not only various types of arthritis, fracture, or torn ligaments, but also inflammation of surrounding structures such as the bursa or tendons. For example, limitation of motion of the shoulder would suggest impingement syndrome, frozen shoulder, rheumatoid or osteoarthritis, subacromial bursitis, and a torn rotator cuff.

2. Is the limitation of motion both active and passive or active only? If the limitation of motion is only active, one should suspect tendinitis or bursitis. If the limitation of motion is both active and passive, one should suspect the various forms of arthritis, as well as bone tumors, osteomyelitis, and adhesive capsulitis.

3. Is there weakness or paresthesia? Weakness and especially paresthesia suggest a neurologic origin for the pain and then one should be considering brachial plexus neuritis, carpal tunnel syndrome, ulnar entrapment, and radiculopathy.

4. Are there vasomotor or trophic changes? Vasomotor changes would suggest Raynaud's phenomena and sympathetic dystrophy. Trophic changes along with vasomotor changes would suggest a peripheral neuropathy also.

5. Are there positive neurologic signs in the lower extremities? Diffuse hypoactive reflexes with stocking deficits in the lower extremities would suggest a peripheral neuropathy, while hyperactive reflexes in the lower extremities would suggest a cervical cord tumor, cervical spondylosis, or multiple sclerosis.

6. Is there a positive Tinel's sign at the wrist or elbow? Tinel's sign at the wrist would suggest carpal tunnel syndrome, while Tinel's sign at the elbow would suggest ulnar entrapment if it is

over the ulnar nerve, or pronator syndrome if it is over the median nerve.

7. Are Adson's tests positive? Adson's tests are positive in thoracic outlet syndrome whether it is due to a cervical rib, scalenus-anticus syndrome, Wright syndrome (pectoralis minor syndrome), or a costoclavicular compression.

DIAGNOSTIC WORKUP

X-rays of the affected joints need to be done if there is tenderness or limitation of motion. Further workup of joint pain can be found on page 339. When there are abnormal neurologic findings, an x-ray of the cervical spine, nerve conduction velocity studies, and electromyographic examinations need to be done. Referral to a neurologist should be made for these tests. If there is a typical radicular pain and a herniated cervical disk is strongly suspected, then MRI of the cervical spine should done. This is an expensive test, but when there are obvious signs of radiculopathy, it is worthwhile. Perhaps dermatomal somatosensory studies should be done when there is confusion about whether a herniated disk is pathologic or not. If a vascular lesion is suspected angiography and venography should be ordered.

When there is intermittent pain, an exercise tolerance test should be done to exclude coronary insufficiency. A stellate ganglion block may be helpful in diagnosing reflex sympathetic dystrophy. Remember that other nerve blocks may be done and one should not hesitate to call an anesthesiologist for help in this area. Various forms of bursitis may be diagnosed by a therapeutic trial of lidocaine and corticosteroid injections.

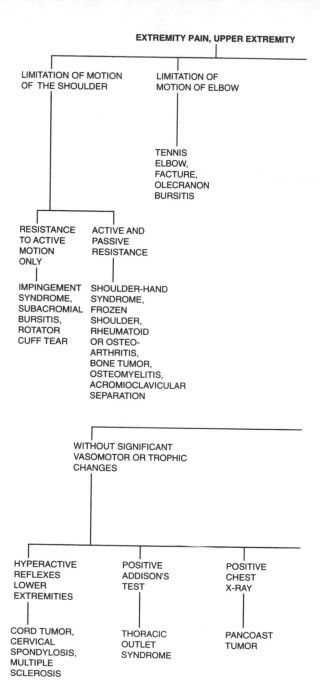

EXTREMITY PAIN, UPPER EXTREMITY

LIMITATION OF MOTION OF THE SHOULDER

LIMITATION OF MOTION OF ELBOW

TENNIS ELBOW, FACTURE, OLECRANON BURSITIS

RESISTANCE TO ACTIVE MOTION ONLY

ACTIVE AND PASSIVE RESISTANCE

IMPINGEMENT SYNDROME, SUBACROMIAL BURSITIS, ROTATOR CUFF TEAR

SHOULDER-HAND SYNDROME, FROZEN SHOULDER, RHEUMATOID OR OSTEO-ARTHRITIS, BONE TUMOR, OSTEOMYELITIS, ACROMIOCLAVICULAR SEPARATION

WITHOUT SIGNIFICANT VASOMOTOR OR TROPHIC CHANGES

HYPERACTIVE REFLEXES LOWER EXTREMITIES

POSITIVE ADDISON'S TEST

POSITIVE CHEST X-RAY

CORD TUMOR, CERVICAL SPONDYLOSIS, MULTIPLE SCLEROSIS

THORACIC OUTLET SYNDROME

PANCOAST TUMOR

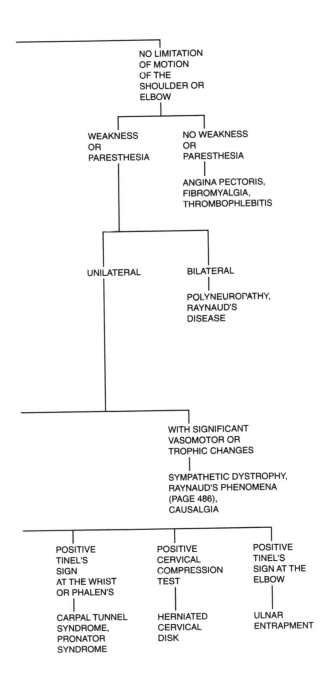

NO LIMITATION OF MOTION OF THE SHOULDER OR ELBOW

WEAKNESS OR PARESTHESIA

NO WEAKNESS OR PARESTHESIA

ANGINA PECTORIS, FIBROMYALGIA, THROMBOPHLEBITIS

UNILATERAL

BILATERAL

POLYNEUROPATHY, RAYNAUD'S DISEASE

WITH SIGNIFICANT VASOMOTOR OR TROPHIC CHANGES

SYMPATHETIC DYSTROPHY, RAYNAUD'S PHENOMENA (PAGE 486), CAUSALGIA

POSITIVE TINEL'S SIGN AT THE WRIST OR PHALEN'S

POSITIVE CERVICAL COMPRESSION TEST

POSITIVE TINEL'S SIGN AT THE ELBOW

CARPAL TUNNEL SYNDROME, PRONATOR SYNDROME

HERNIATED CERVICAL DISK

ULNAR ENTRAPMENT

EYE PAIN

Ask the following questions:

1. Is there redness of the eye? Redness of the eye suggests definite eye pathology. Without redness, one should suspect disease in the adjacent structures or retrobulbar neuritis.
2. If there is redness, is there periorbital edema as well? Periorbital edema should suggest a cavernous sinus thrombosis or herpes zoster.
3. If there is periorbital edema, is there a rash? A rash, particularly vesicular rash, would suggest herpes zoster.
4. In cases without redness of the eye, is there any abnormality on examination both with the naked eye and with the ophthalmoscope? A dilated pupil would certainly suggest glaucoma; ophthalmoscopic examination may show optic neuritis or retinal detachment. A visual field examination may detect optic neuritis, retrobulbar neuritis, and retinal artery occlusion. A visual acuity check may pick up a refractive error.
5. Finally, is there headache associated with the eye pain? This would be suggestive of migraine or cluster headache.

DIAGNOSTIC WORKUP

The primary care specialist may want to treat cases of obvious conjunctivitis without a culture and sensitivity. He may also use fluorescein dye to diagnose a foreign body. Most primary care physicians feel competent to use a tonometry to diagnose glaucoma. He may feel competent to use a slit lamp. However, when there is any doubt about the diagnosis, the most cost-effective approach is to refer the patient to an ophthalmologist.

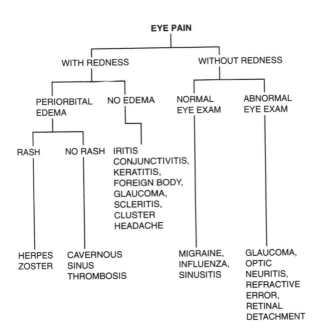

FACE PAIN

Ask the following questions:

1. Is the pain constant or intermittent? Intermittent pain would suggest trigeminal neuralgia, cluster headaches, or atypical migraine. Constant pain would suggest any local abnormalities in the structures underlying the face such as an abscessed sinus, an abscessed tooth, or a neoplasm in these areas.
2. Is the pain increased by chewing? Pain that is increased by chewing very often may be related to the temporomandibular joint syndrome, but it could be related to trigeminal neuralgia or dental caries.
3. Is there an associated nasal discharge? An associated bloody nasal discharge would make one think of a nasopharyngeal carcinoma, but a purulent discharge would make one think of acute or chronic sinusitis. A watery nasal discharge often accompanies cluster headaches or atypical migraine.
4. Are there abnormal neurologic findings? Face pain sometimes accompanies multiple sclerosis, acute Wallenberg's syndrome and advanced acoustic neuromas. The pain in the trigeminal distribution associated with multiple sclerosis often is intermittent and suggests trigeminal neuralgia.

DIAGNOSTIC WORKUP

The first thing to determine is whether there is an infectious or neoplastic process in the structures underlying the face. X-rays of the sinuses and teeth, and CT scans of the sinuses and brain may be necessary to further elucidate this. An x-ray of the temporomandibular joint may be helpful. Referral to a dentist to evaluate the patient's teeth or to an ear, nose and throat specialist to evaluate sinusitis may be necessary.

To rule out cluster headaches or atypical migraine, a histamine test may be done. It may be wise to see the patient during an attack so that superficial temporal artery compression can be done to rule out migraine and/or a shot of sumatriptan succinate can be given which should give immediate results in cluster headache and atypical migraine.

A trial of carbamazepine (Tegretol) can be given in cases of suspected trigeminal neuralgia, but referral to a neurosurgeon for an alcoholic injection of the maxillary or mandibular branches of trigeminal nerve will more likely make the diagnosis and solve the patient's problem.

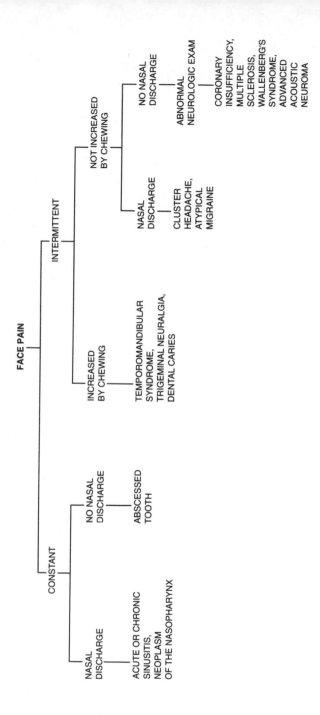

FACIAL FLUSHING

Ask the following questions:

1. Is the flushing constant or intermittent? Intermittent flushing suggests menopause, carcinoid syndrome, systemic mastocytosis, pheochromocytoma, and Zollinger-Ellison syndrome. Constant flushing might suggest alcoholism, polycythemia, or the malar flush of mitral stenosis.
2. Is there associated obesity? Associated obesity would certainly bring to mind Cushing's syndrome, but it may also be associated with alcoholism.
3. Is there associated rash on the face or elsewhere? A rash would most likely bring to mind rosacea if it is on the face, but if it is elsewhere one might consider systemic mastocytosis or dermatomyositis.
4. Are there associated systemic symptoms and signs? Diarrhea would suggest carcinoid or Zollinger-Ellison syndrome. A headache along with the flushing would suggest a systemic mastocytosis. Fainting might suggest pheochromocytoma or epilepsy.

DIAGNOSTIC WORKUP

Urinalysis for 5-hydroxyindoleacetic acid (5-HIAA) should be done if carcinoid syndrome is suspected. Urine samples may be taken for drug and alcohol screen in all cases where there is any doubt about drug or alcohol history. Tests for serum FSH and estradiol should be done in patients suspected of having menopause. A 24-hr urine collection for catecholamine should be done for patients suspected of having pheochromocytoma. Serum gastrin tests should be done for patients suspected of Zollinger-Ellison syndrome. In patients with systemic mastitis or dermatomyositis, a skin biopsy or muscle biopsy can be done. In patients with suspected Cushing's disease, a serum cortisol and cortisol suppression test can be done.

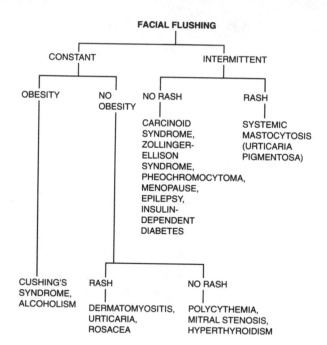

FACIAL FLUSHING

CONSTANT

OBESITY

CUSHING'S
SYNDROME,
ALCOHOLISM

NO
OBESITY

RASH

DERMATOMYOSITIS,
URTICARIA,
ROSACEA

NO RASH

POLYCYTHEMIA,
MITRAL STENOSIS,
HYPERTHYROIDISM

INTERMITTENT

NO RASH

CARCINOID
SYNDROME,
ZOLLINGER-
ELLISON
SYNDROME,
PHEOCHROMOCYTOMA,
MENOPAUSE,
EPILEPSY,
INSULIN-
DEPENDENT
DIABETES

RASH

SYSTEMIC
MASTOCYTOSIS
(URTICARIA
PIGMENTOSA)

FACIAL MASS

A facial mass may come from the skin, the subcutaneous tissue, the teeth, the sinuses, the bones, or the salivary glands. In the skin there may be moles, simple nevi, sebaceous cysts, papillomas, carcinoma, comedones, and urticaria. In the subcutaneous tissue there may be angioneurotic edema, trauma, and erysipelas and actinomycosis.

Swelling coming from the teeth includes dental abscess or dental cyst. The sinuses may become infected and cause swelling over the surface. The bones may develop an odontoma, a sarcoma, or a dermoid cyst. The bones may be fractured and there may be bruising with considerable swelling. If the bones of the sinuses are broken, there may be subcutaneous emphysema.

Mumps and uveoparotid fever may cause swelling of the salivary glands. Mixed tumors of the parotid gland cause unilateral swelling of the face. A stone may obstruct Stensen's or Wharton's ducts, causing intermittent swelling. Nonspecific inflammation of the parotid glands occurs in the elderly and malnourished individuals.

DIAGNOSTIC WORKUP

Most of the skin lesions will be obvious, but a skin biopsy can be performed when in doubt. Smears and cultures should be done when infection is suspected. A therapeutic trial of epinephrine or antihistamines can be tried in angioneurotic edema or urticaria. X-rays of the skull, jaw, and sinuses may be necessary. A CT scan may be needed to identify some fractures and sinus infections. Referral to an oral surgeon or otolaryngologist should be made early in confusing cases.

FACIAL PARALYSIS

Ask the following questions:

1. Is it unilateral or bilateral? Bilateral facial paralysis should make one think of a Guillain-Barré syndrome, especially when it is acute, and this will usually progress to weakness of all four extremities. In addition, congenital bilateral facial paralysis, myotonic dystrophy, and myasthenia gravis may present as bilateral facial paralysis. The majority of cases of unilateral facial paralysis are due to Bell's palsy.

2. Is it acute or gradual onset? If it is acute onset, Bell's palsy, diabetic neuropathy, and cerebral vascular accident must be considered. If it is a gradual onset, one must consider an acoustic neuroma, advancing petrositis, or a brain tumor or abscess.

3. Is there associated hemiplegia or hemiparesis? If there is associated hemiplegia or hemiparesis and it is acute onset, one should consider cerebral vascular accident or extradural or subdural hematoma. If the hemiparesis, however, is contralateral, one should consider a brain stem thrombosis or hemorrhage. There are two clinical syndromes that are due to basilar artery lesions: Foville's syndrome and Millard-Gubler syndrome. If the hemiparesis is gradual onset, one should consider brain tumor or abscess or degenerative disease.

4. Is there earache or hearing loss? Associated earache or hearing loss should make one think of acoustic neuroma, petrositis, mastoiditis, herpes zoster, and cholesteatoma.

DIAGNOSTIC WORKUP

First, one should do a complete examination of the ear, nose, and throat to determine if there is any rupture of the drum, discharge, evidence of otitis media, etc. Then x-rays of the mastoids and petrous bones should be done along with tomography. A CT scan of the brain with emphasis on the internal auditory foramina should be done if acoustic neuroma is suspected. Culture of the discharge from the ears and blood culture should be done if there are associated signs of an infectious process. Spinal fluid analysis should be done to look for Guillain-Barré syndrome. If myasthenia gravis is suspected, a Tensilon test may be done. Spinal fluid culture should be done in cases of brain abscess. Carotid scans and a workup for an embolic source should be done in cases of cerebral vascular accident. Of course, when there is a brain tumor or abscess or a cerebral vascular accident is suspected, CT scans of the brain should be done. If these are not helpful or are inconclusive, MRI of the brain can be done. Glucose tolerance testing should be done to rule out diabetic neuropathy. If lead poisoning is suspected, a blood level for lead should be done.

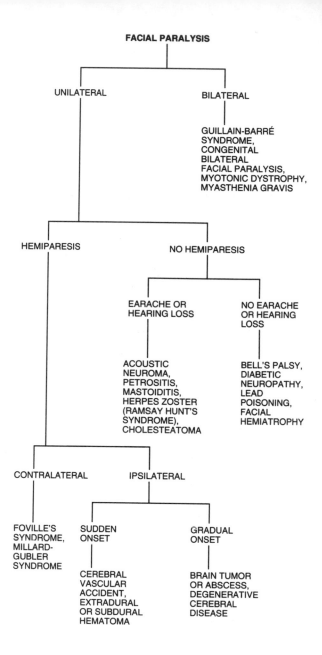

FACIAL PARALYSIS

UNILATERAL

BILATERAL

GUILLAIN-BARRÉ
SYNDROME,
CONGENITAL
BILATERAL
FACIAL PARALYSIS,
MYOTONIC DYSTROPHY,
MYASTHENIA GRAVIS

HEMIPARESIS

NO HEMIPARESIS

EARACHE OR
HEARING LOSS

NO EARACHE
OR HEARING
LOSS

ACOUSTIC
NEUROMA,
PETROSITIS,
MASTOIDITIS,
HERPES ZOSTER
(RAMSAY HUNT'S
SYNDROME),
CHOLESTEATOMA

BELL'S PALSY,
DIABETIC
NEUROPATHY,
LEAD
POISONING,
FACIAL
HEMIATROPHY

CONTRALATERAL

IPSILATERAL

FOVILLE'S
SYNDROME,
MILLARD-
GUBLER
SYNDROME

SUDDEN
ONSET

GRADUAL
ONSET

CEREBRAL
VASCULAR
ACCIDENT,
EXTRADURAL
OR SUBDURAL
HEMATOMA

BRAIN TUMOR
OR ABSCESS,
DEGENERATIVE
CEREBRAL
DISEASE

FACIAL SWELLING

Ask the following questions:

1. Is the facial swelling focal or diffuse? If it is focal, then one should consider a local condition in the structures underlying the face such as the salivary glands, the teeth, or the sinuses. Mumps is a common condition, of course, especially in children. If it is diffuse facial swelling, one should consider a systemic disease such as glomerulonephritis, myxedema, or Cushing's disease.

2. Is the swelling associated with generalized edema? If there is generalized edema, one must consider acute glomerulonephritis, nephrotic syndrome, congestive heart failure, or cirrhosis. If the generalized edema is nonpitting, one would consider myxedema and cretinism. If there is no generalized edema, one must consider conditions such as Cushing's syndrome, dermatomyositis, acromegaly, mongolism, and Paget's disease.

3. If the edema is generalized, is it pitting edema or nonpitting edema? Nonpitting edema would suggest myxedema and cretinism.

4. Is there associated flushing? With flushing one would consider Cushing's syndrome, dermatomyositis, and a superior vena cava syndrome. If there is no flushing, one should consider acromegaly, mongolism, or Paget's disease.

5. Is there associated fever? If there is associated fever, look for infections in the structures underlying the skin such as mumps, abscess of the salivary gland, an abscessed tooth, sinusitis, or syphilis.

DIAGNOSTIC WORKUP

Cases of focal swelling should have a routine CBC and sedimentation rate. X-rays of the sinuses and teeth should be done. If mumps is suspected, a mumps skin test or antibody titer may be done. If all these tests are negative and there is a focal swelling, referral to an oral surgeon may be wise at this point.

If the swelling is diffuse, the basic workup is a CBC, chemistry panel, and urinalysis. A streptozyme test or ASO titer can be done if glomerulonephritis is suspected, but a microscopic examination of the urine is extremely important in this condition. If congestive heart failure is suspected, a chest x-ray, EKG, arm-to-tongue circulation time and pulmonary function testing should be done. In cases of Cushing's disease, a serum cortisol and cortisol suppression test may be done. X-rays of the skull and long bones should be done in suspected cases of acromegaly or Paget's disease.

FACIAL SWELLING

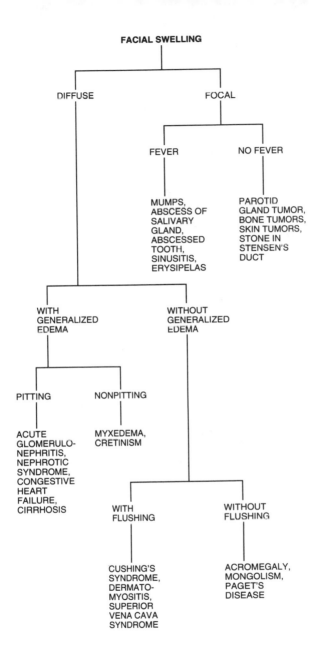

FACIES, ABNORMAL

Perhaps every clinician has at one time or another experienced the joy of seeing a patient's face and making the diagnosis. The round flushed face of Cushing's disease, the pop-eyes of hyperthyroidism or the expressionless face of Parkinson's disease quickly come to mind. There are many other abnormal facies you will want to remember. Let's enumerate them.

1. In glomerulonephritis the face is pale and puffy with edematous bags under the eyes.
2. In myxedema the facial features become coarse, consequently the nostrils are broad and the lips are thick. The face is expressionless and puffy.
3. In mongolism there is epicanthus and the face is Oriental in appearance with the tongue protruding.
4. In mental retardation the face is often dull and expressionless.
5. In tetanus we see the sarcastic smile of risus sardonicus.
6. In myasthenia gravis the face is also expressionless, but the variable degree of ptosis should be a warning.
7. In mitral stenosis the malar flush is very helpful in making the diagnosis.
8. The flushing of the face in alcoholism, carcinoid syndrome, and menopause is also helpful.
9. In acromegaly the features are coarse, but the brows are enlarged and the jaw protrudes. The spaces between the lower teeth widen.
10. In myotonic dystrophy the face is hatchet-shaped due to the facial wasting and weakness and there is bilateral partial ptosis.
11. In bulbar and pseudobulbar palsy regardless of the cause, the face is expressionless, the mouth remains open most of the time and there is drooling.
12. In Bell's palsy the mouth is drawn to the unaffected side during a smile and the nasolabial fold is flat. The eye does not close completely.

13. In Paget's disease the forehead protrudes and the face appears disproportionately small.
14. In scleroderma there is smoothing out of all the wrinkles of the face along with thinning of the skin, giving a waxy appearance.
15. In cachectic states the face begins to appear like a skull with skin over it.
16. In hypertelorism the eyes are wide apart.
17. In Wilson's disease the face looks like it is ready to crack a smile and the mouth is open with frequent drooling.
18. The cyanosis of congenital heart disease would hardly be missed.

There are many other rare faces that once seen won't be forgotten.

FAILURE TO THRIVE

Ask the following questions:

1. Is there a history of an abnormal gestation? There may be a history that the mother was a chronic alcoholic or ingested such drugs as phenytoin, trimethadione, or narcotics. The mother may have had toxoplasmosis, rubella, herpes simplex, or other diseases during her gestation.
2. Is the child's environment abnormal? Careful investigation may disclose that the child has been neglected or that there are economic circumstances to indicate that the child is not getting enough food. Investigation may also indicate that the child is not getting adequate love or practicing good hygiene.
3. Are there abnormalities found on the neurologic examination? Neurologic examination may reveal findings to suggest microcephaly, muscular atrophy, hydrocephalus, spastic diplegia, and other neurologic causes of mental retardation.
4. Are there endocrine abnormalities? Cretinism, pituitary tumors, and genital abnormalities may be suggested from the endocrine examination.
5. Are there findings to suggest a gastrointestinal disorder? Wasting and a distended abdomen may suggest a malabsorption syndrome. The history of frequent pneumonia may indicate fibrocystic disease. Cataracts may suggest galactosemia.

DIAGNOSTIC WORKUP

The routine diagnostic workup should include a CBC, sedimentation rate, urinalysis, urine culture, chemistry panel, thyroid profile, sweat test, stool for quantitative fat, chest x-ray, and an EKG. Bone age x-rays are often helpful in indicating a growth delay.

If there are focal neurologic signs or a pituitary tumor is suspected, a CT scan of the brain may be necessary. Additional endocrinologic tests include serum growth hormone level before and after exercise, somatomedin-C level, and overnight dexamethasone suppression test. However, an endocrinologist, pediatrician, or orthopedic surgeon should be consulted before ordering expensive diagnostic tests.

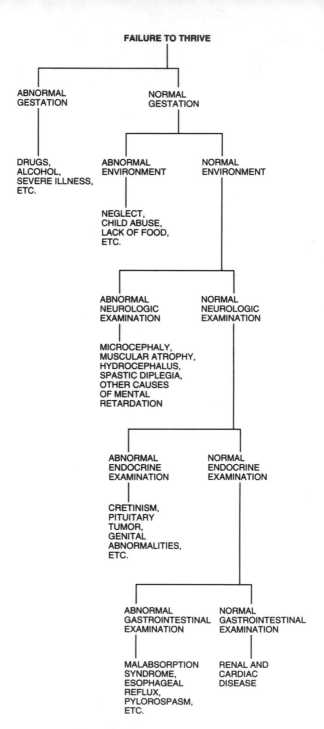

FAILURE TO THRIVE

- **ABNORMAL GESTATION**
  - DRUGS, ALCOHOL, SEVERE ILLNESS, ETC.
- **NORMAL GESTATION**
  - **ABNORMAL ENVIRONMENT**
    - NEGLECT, CHILD ABUSE, LACK OF FOOD, ETC.
  - **NORMAL ENVIRONMENT**
    - **ABNORMAL NEUROLOGIC EXAMINATION**
      - MICROCEPHALY, MUSCULAR ATROPHY, HYDROCEPHALUS, SPASTIC DIPLEGIA, OTHER CAUSES OF MENTAL RETARDATION
    - **NORMAL NEUROLOGIC EXAMINATION**
      - **ABNORMAL ENDOCRINE EXAMINATION**
        - CRETINISM, PITUITARY TUMOR, GENITAL ABNORMALITIES, ETC.
      - **NORMAL ENDOCRINE EXAMINATION**
        - **ABNORMAL GASTROINTESTINAL EXAMINATION**
          - MALABSORPTION SYNDROME, ESOPHAGEAL REFLUX, PYLOROSPASM, ETC.
        - **NORMAL GASTROINTESTINAL EXAMINATION**
          - RENAL AND CARDIAC DISEASE

FATIGUE

Ask the following questions:

1. Is there weight loss? If there is weight loss, one must consider a neoplasm, endocrine disorders such as hyperthyroidism or diabetes mellitus, malnutrition or malabsorption, and chronic infectious diseases such as tuberculosis or subacute bacterial endocarditis.
2. Is there fever? If there is fever, one should consider an infectious disease such as tuberculosis, subacute bacterial endocarditis, toxoplasmosis, infectious mononucleosis, or brucellosis.
3. Is there pallor? If there is pallor, the most likely cause is a type of anemia such as that associated with malabsorption syndrome or iron deficiency anemia, pernicious anemia, or anemia blood loss.
4. Is the fatigue intermittent or constant? Intermittent fatigue would make one suspect myasthenia gravis. Constant fatigue would be related to any of the conditions we have already discussed. Constant fatigue, however, with no weight loss would make one consider a psychiatric disorder.
5. Is there a positive drug or alcohol history? Alcoholism, cocaine abuse, and chronic aspirin ingestion are just a few of the disorders that can be associated with chronic fatigue. Don't forget caffeine abuse!
6. Are there associated neurologic findings? Many neurologic disorders are associated with fatigue and they include muscular dystrophy, amyotrophic lateral sclerosis, and Parkinson's disease.
7. Is there polyuria? Polyuria would make one think of hyperthyroidism, diabetes mellitus, hyperparathyroidism, and chronic renal failure.

DIAGNOSTIC WORKUP

All patients should have routine laboratory studies including CBC, sedimentation rate, chemistry panel, VDRL test, and a urinalysis including analysis for myoglobin. A thyroid profile should be done to rule out hyperthyroidism. Further endocrine workup including serum cortisol will help differentiate Addison's disease and hypopituitarism. Since fatigue is associated with aldosteronism, a 24-hr urine aldosterone determination should be done.

Tests for chronic infectious disease such as febrile agglutinins, brucellin antibody titer, heterophile antibody titer or monospot test, sputum for acid-fast bacilli, and various skin tests for tuberculosis and fungi can be done. Serial blood cultures also would be of value if there is significant fever. Tests for chronic organ failure such as BUN, creatinine, serum electrolytes, and liver function tests should be done. A workup of anemia including a workup of malabsorption syndrome may be necessary. Consequently, stools for fat content as well as D-xylose absorption testing may be done.

A search for neoplasm will include chest x-rays, x-rays of the skull and long bones, a bone scan, an upper GI series, and small bowel follow-through as well as a barium enema and intravenous pyelogram. A muscle biopsy will help differentiate certain collagen diseases, muscular dystrophy, and trichinosis. An ANA test and serum complement to screen for collagen disease should be done. A Tensilon test may be necessary to differentiate myasthenia gravis. If a neurologic disease is suspected, referral to a neurologist would be in order. Consider electromyography also.

If all the tests prove negative, referral to a psychiatrist would be appropriate. On the other hand, it may be appropriate to refer the patient to a psychiatrist earlier in the course of the workup.

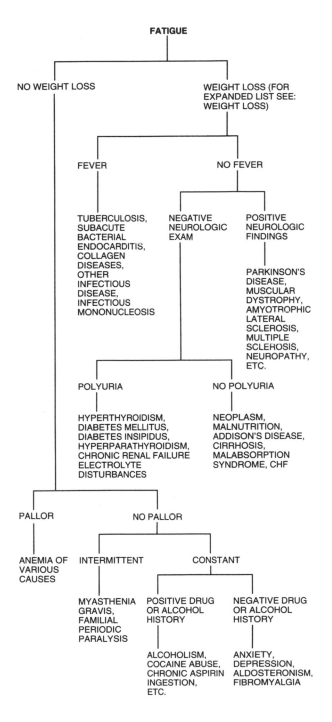

FATIGUE

NO WEIGHT LOSS

WEIGHT LOSS (FOR
EXPANDED LIST SEE:
WEIGHT LOSS)

FEVER

NO FEVER

TUBERCULOSIS,
SUBACUTE
BACTERIAL
ENDOCARDITIS,
COLLAGEN
DISEASES,
OTHER
INFECTIOUS
DISEASE,
INFECTIOUS
MONONUCLEOSIS

NEGATIVE
NEUROLOGIC
EXAM

POSITIVE
NEUROLOGIC
FINDINGS

PARKINSON'S
DISEASE,
MUSCULAR
DYSTROPHY,
AMYOTROPHIC
LATERAL
SCLEROSIS,
MULTIPLE
SCLEROSIS,
NEUROPATHY,
ETC.

POLYURIA

NO POLYURIA

HYPERTHYROIDISM,
DIABETES MELLITUS,
DIABETES INSIPIDUS,
HYPERPARATHYROIDISM,
CHRONIC RENAL FAILURE
ELECTROLYTE
DISTURBANCES

NEOPLASM,
MALNUTRITION,
ADDISON'S DISEASE,
CIRRHOSIS,
MALABSORPTION
SYNDROME, CHF

PALLOR

NO PALLOR

ANEMIA OF
VARIOUS
CAUSES

INTERMITTENT

CONSTANT

MYASTHENIA
GRAVIS,
FAMILIAL
PERIODIC
PARALYSIS

POSITIVE DRUG
OR ALCOHOL
HISTORY

NEGATIVE DRUG
OR ALCOHOL
HISTORY

ALCOHOLISM,
COCAINE ABUSE,
CHRONIC ASPIRIN
INGESTION,
ETC.

ANXIETY,
DEPRESSION,
ALDOSTERONISM,
FIBROMYALGIA

Fatigue   215

FEMORAL MASS
OR SWELLING

Ask the following questions:

1. Is it reducible? If the mass is reducible, it is most likely a femoral hernia or saphenous varix.
2. Is there an associated kyphotic curvature of the spine? The findings of a kyphotic curvature of the spine suggest a psoas abscess, which is usually tuberculous.
3. Is the mass firm and ovoid? A firm ovoid mass suggests an enlarged lymph node or an ectopic testis.
4. Is there resonance or bowel sounds over the mass? These findings suggest a femoral hernia.
5. Is the corresponding half of the scrotum empty? These findings suggest an ectopic testis.

DIAGNOSTIC WORKUP

A reducible mass would suggest a femoral hernia, but an upper GI series with a small bowel follow-through would confirm this diagnosis. Of course, if it is felt that the femoral hernia is irreducible, this study would not be done and exploratory surgery would be indicated. If the mass is suspected to be a lymph node, a biopsy should be done. If the mass is suspected to be an abscess, an incision and drainage should be done. If tuberculosis is suspected, a tuberculin test as well as an acid-fast bacillus smear and culture should be done. If the mass is suspected to be a saphenous varix, venography will confirm the diagnosis. Exploratory surgery of the groin will clarify the diagnosis in confusing cases.

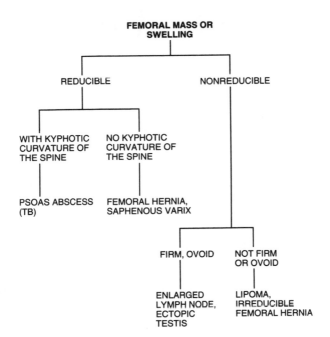

FEVER, ACUTE

Ask the following questions:

1. Is there a history of drug ingestion or injection? This will help diagnosis drug reactions and serum sickness, which are common and easily discovered in the history.
2. Is there a rash? The presence of a rash should make one think of a drug reaction, meningococcemia, the various exanthems, and subacute bacterial endocarditis.
3. Is there localized pain? If there is a sore throat, obviously streptococcal pharyngitis or a viral upper respiratory infection is likely. If there is headache, meningitis or encephalitis must be considered. If there is chest pain, one should consider a pulmonary infarct, myocardial infarction, or Bornholm disease. If there is abdominal pain, one would consider pyelonephritis, cholecystitis, and appendicitis among the various conditions. If there is joint pain, one should consider rheumatic fever, rheumatoid arthritis, or septic arthritis.
4. Is there a focal discharge? A productive cough would make one consider pneumonia. A rectal discharge would make one consider a perirectal abscess. A urethral discharge should make one think of gonorrhea.
5. Are there other localizing signs? Frequency of urination should make one think of pyelonephritis. A productive cough should make one think of pneumonia, while jaundice would make one think of hepatitis.

DIAGNOSTIC WORKUP

Routine studies include a CBC, sedimentation rate, chemistry panel, VDRL test, and tuberculin skin test. Serial blood cultures should be done on all patients. Febrile agglutinins usually should be done. An antistreptolysin-O titer or streptozyme test should be done to exclude rheumatic fever. RNA, antinuclear antibody, and DNA tests should be done to look for lupus and other connective tissue disease. An HIV antibody titer may need to be ordered.

The next step is to culture any discharge or various body fluids that might be suspect. Thus, a urinalysis and urine culture should be done. A nose and throat culture should be done. A sputum smear and culture may need to be done. The next consideration is to do various serologic tests. A heterophile antibody titer should be done in teenagers. Febrile agglutinin tests may need to be done. Acute and convalescent phase sera for viral studies may need to be done.

Next one should do skin testing. Thus, histoplasmin, coccidioidin, and blastomycin skin testing should be done on patients with a cough. *Trichinella* skin testing may need to be done, as well as brucellin skin testing. A Kveim test might need to be done for suspected sarcoidosis.

The next step is to do plain x-rays of suspected areas. For instance, x-rays of the teeth may disclose an abscessed tooth. X-rays of the long bones may disclose a metastatic carcinoma.

The next step is contrast x-ray studies of various organ systems. An intravenous pyelogram may show a hypernephroma. A cholecystogram may show gallstones. An upper GI series and barium enema may show chronic pancreatitis or diverticulitis. Angiography may disclose periarteritis nodosa, aortitis or giant cell arteritis.

Next, consider biopsying various organ systems. For instances, a lymph node biopsy may disclose a lymphoma or sarcoidosis. A muscle biopsy may disclose periarteritis nodosa, polymyositis, or trichinella.

The next step is to do a CT scan of the abdomen and pelvis. If this is negative, consider a CT scan of the chest and mediastinum. Echocardiography may disclose valvular vegetations or an atrial myxoma.

Next one should do bone scans and gallium scans for possible metastasis, osteomyelitis, or localized abscesses.

If all these procedures fail to turn up a lesion, then an exploratory laparotomy may need to be done. A fibrin test may indicate Mediterranean fever, or urine for etiocholanolone may also indicate a relapsing type of fever. A urine test for porphobilinogen may diagnose porphyria.

The wisest move is to conduct this investigation with the help of an infectious disease specialist or a specialist in the body organ system most likely suspected of harboring the infection.

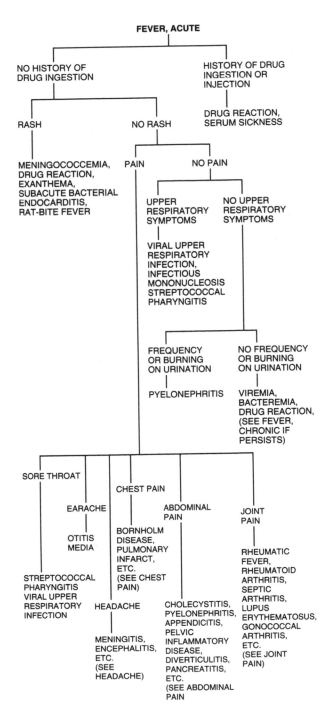

FEVER, ACUTE

NO HISTORY OF DRUG INGESTION

HISTORY OF DRUG INGESTION OR INJECTION

DRUG REACTION, SERUM SICKNESS

RASH

NO RASH

MENINGOCOCCEMIA, DRUG REACTION, EXANTHEMA, SUBACUTE BACTERIAL ENDOCARDITIS, RAT-BITE FEVER

PAIN

NO PAIN

UPPER RESPIRATORY SYMPTOMS

NO UPPER RESPIRATORY SYMPTOMS

VIRAL UPPER RESPIRATORY INFECTION, INFECTIOUS MONONUCLEOSIS STREPTOCOCCAL PHARYNGITIS

FREQUENCY OR BURNING ON URINATION

NO FREQUENCY OR BURNING ON URINATION

PYELONEPHRITIS

VIREMIA, BACTEREMIA, DRUG REACTION, (SEE FEVER, CHRONIC IF PERSISTS)

SORE THROAT

CHEST PAIN

EARACHE

ABDOMINAL PAIN

JOINT PAIN

OTITIS MEDIA

BORNHOLM DISEASE, PULMONARY INFARCT, ETC. (SEE CHEST PAIN)

RHEUMATIC FEVER, RHEUMATOID ARTHRITIS, SEPTIC ARTHRITIS, LUPUS ERYTHEMATOSUS, GONOCOCCAL ARTHRITIS, ETC. (SEE JOINT PAIN)

STREPTOCOCCAL PHARYNGITIS VIRAL UPPER RESPIRATORY INFECTION

HEADACHE

CHOLECYSTITIS, PYELONEPHRITIS, APPENDICITIS, PELVIC INFLAMMATORY DISEASE, DIVERTICULITIS, PANCREATITIS, ETC. (SEE ABDOMINAL PAIN

MENINGITIS, ENCEPHALITIS, ETC. (SEE HEADACHE)

FEVER, CHRONIC

Ask the following questions:

1. Is there a history of drug ingestion or injection? Of course, the history should reveal that the patient has been on a certain drug or has received certain antitoxins, serums, or vaccines.
2. Is there a rash? If there is a rash, one should suspect subacute bacterial endocarditis, Rocky Mountain spotted fever, secondary syphilis, rat-bite fever, pemphigus, a drug reaction, lupus erythematosus, dermatomyositis, or typhoid fever. There are other conditions associated with a rash also.
3. Is there a characteristic pattern to the fever? The various forms of malaria give a characteristic pattern of the fever, as well as undulant fever in Hodgkin's disease.
4. Is there localized pain? Abdominal pain should suggest a cholecystitis, hepatic abscess, diverticulitis, etc. A sore throat should suggest infectious mononucleosis, leukemia, and subacute thyroiditis. Joint pain should suggest rheumatoid arthritis, rheumatic fever, or gonococcal arthritis. Earache should suggest otitis media or mastoiditis. Chest pain should suggest tuberculosis, pleurisy, or empyema.
5. Is there a localized discharge? Purulent sputum should suggest pneumonia, tuberculosis, or chronic fungal disease in the lung. A urethral discharge would suggest gonorrhea or Reiter's disease.
6. Is there a localized mass or swelling? An abdominal mass would suggest hepatic abscess, pancreatic cyst, or diverticular abscess. A flank mass might suggest hypernephroma or perinephric abscess.

DIAGNOSTIC WORKUP

The diagnostic workup is similar to that for acute fever on page 218.

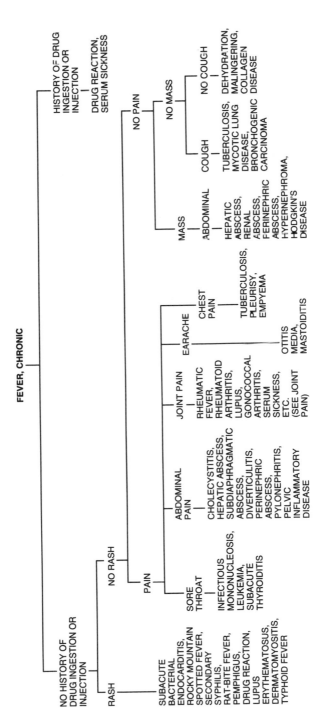

FEVER, CHRONIC

FEVER, CHRONIC
├── NO HISTORY OF DRUG INGESTION OR INJECTION
│   ├── RASH
│   │   └── SUBACUTE BACTERIAL ENDOCARDITIS, ROCKY MOUNTAIN SPOTTED FEVER, SECONDARY SYPHILIS, RAT-BITE FEVER, PEMPHIGUS, DRUG REACTION, LUPUS ERYTHEMATOSUS, DERMATOMYOSITIS, TYPHOID FEVER
│   └── NO RASH
│   ├── PAIN
│   │   ├── SORE THROAT
│   │   │   └── INFECTIOUS MONONUCLEOSIS, LEUKEMIA, SUBACUTE THYROIDITIS
│   │   ├── ABDOMINAL PAIN
│   │   │   └── CHOLECYSTITIS, HEPATIC ABSCESS, SUBDIAPHRAGMATIC ABSCESS, DIVERTICULITIS, PERINEPHRIC ABSCESS, PYLONEPHRITIS, PELVIC INFLAMMATORY DISEASE
│   │   ├── JOINT PAIN
│   │   │   └── RHEUMATIC FEVER, RHEUMATOID ARTHRITIS, LUPUS, GONOCOCCAL ARTHRITIS, SERUM SICKNESS, ETC. (SEE JOINT PAIN)
│   │   └── EARACHE
│   │   ├── CHEST PAIN
│   │   │   └── TUBERCULOSIS, PLEURISY, EMPYEMA
│   │   └── OTITIS MEDIA, MASTOIDITIS
│   └── NO PAIN
│   ├── MASS
│   │   └── ABDOMINAL
│   │   └── HEPATIC ABSCESS, RENAL ABSCESS, PERINEPHRIC ABSCESS, HYPERNEPHROMA, HODGKIN'S DISEASE
│   └── NO MASS
│   ├── COUGH
│   │   └── TUBERCULOSIS, MYCOTIC LUNG DISEASE, BRONCHOGENIC CARCINOMA
│   └── NO COUGH
│   └── DEHYDRATION, MALINGERING, COLLAGEN DISEASE
└── HISTORY OF DRUG INGESTION OR INJECTION
    └── DRUG REACTION, SERUM SICKNESS

Fever, Chronic   223

FLANK MASS

Ask the following questions:

1. Are there bilateral flank masses? If the masses are bilateral, one should consider polycystic kidney or early bilateral hydronephrosis.
2. Is there associated hypertension? If there is hypertension, one should consider polycystic kidneys, hypernephroma, pheochromocytoma, or adrenocortical carcinoma.
3. Is the mass painful? A painful flank mass should make one think of perinephric abscess, hydronephrosis with partial obstruction, or tuberculosis.
4. Is there blood in the urine? Hematuria should make one think of hypernephroma, a Wilms' tumor, tuberculosis, renal calculus, or polycystic kidneys.

DIAGNOSTIC WORKUP

If the mass is unilateral, the most cost-effective approach would be to refer the patient to a urologist at the outset. If a urologist is not available or if the mass is bilateral, one might proceed with a workup. This should include a CBC, chemistry panel, VDRL test, urinalysis or urine culture, and a flat plate of the abdomen. Catheterization for residual urine may be done to determine if there is bladder neck obstruction with associated hydronephrosis. An intravenous pyelogram would be the next step.

If these tests fail to make a definitive diagnosis, perhaps abdominal ultrasound may help with the diagnosis of a renal cyst. A CT scan of the abdomen would be the next logical step in confusing cases. Renal angiography and cystoscopy with retrograde pyelography are not usually necessary.

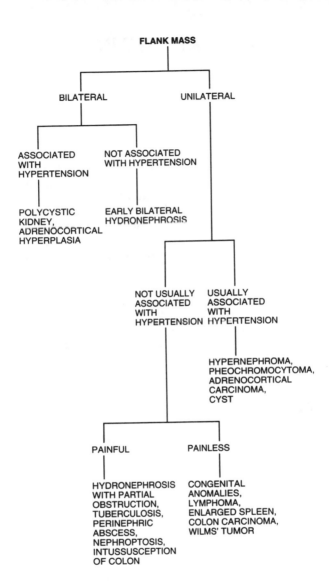

FLANK MASS

BILATERAL

UNILATERAL

ASSOCIATED WITH HYPERTENSION

NOT ASSOCIATED WITH HYPERTENSION

POLYCYSTIC KIDNEY, ADRENOCORTICAL HYPERPLASIA

EARLY BILATERAL HYDRONEPHROSIS

NOT USUALLY ASSOCIATED WITH HYPERTENSION

USUALLY ASSOCIATED WITH HYPERTENSION

HYPERNEPHROMA, PHEOCHROMOCYTOMA, ADRENOCORTICAL CARCINOMA, CYST

PAINFUL

PAINLESS

HYDRONEPHROSIS WITH PARTIAL OBSTRUCTION, TUBERCULOSIS, PERINEPHRIC ABSCESS, NEPHROPTOSIS, INTUSSUSCEPTION OF COLON

CONGENITAL ANOMALIES, LYMPHOMA, ENLARGED SPLEEN, COLON CARCINOMA, WILMS' TUMOR

FLANK PAIN

Ask the following questions:

1. Is there associated fever? The presence of fever along with chest pain should make one think of a perinephric abscess or pyelonephritis. Occasionally, however, hypernephroma can cause fever and flank pain, as can bilateral hydronephrosis.
2. Is there a flank mass? The presence of flank pain along with a flank mass should make one think of a hypernephroma, hydronephrosis, polycystic kidneys, or perinephric abscess.
3. Is there hematuria? The presence of pain and hematuria should make one think of renal calculus first, but the possibility of a renal infarction, polycystic kidneys, and tuberculosis of the kidneys must be considered also. Hematuria is also found in a hypernephroma.

DIAGNOSTIC WORKUP

Routine tests include a CBC, sedimentation rate, chemistry panel, urinalysis, and urine culture. An intravenous pyelogram is the next logical step. If these fail to make a definitive diagnosis, one should consider ordering an abdominal ultrasound or a CT scan of the abdomen. If a renal infarction is suspected, aortography and renal angiography may be ordered. When the above tests are all negative, one should consider x-rays of the lumbosacral spine and MRI of the thoracic and lumbar spine. Consulting a urologist is prudent before ordering expensive diagnostic tests.

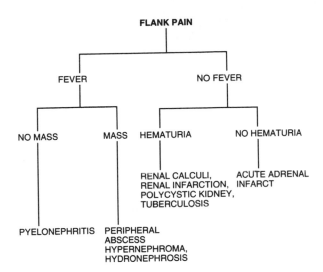

FLATULENCE

Ask the following questions:

1. Is the excessive gas eructated or passed rectally? If the gas is eructated, then the flatulence is gastric in origin and may be due to reflux esophagitis, gastritis, duodenal ulcer, gastric dilatation, or aerophagia. If the gas is passed rectally, an intestinal disorder such as intestinal obstruction, steatorrhea, or diverticulitis should be considered.
2. Is the flatulence associated with heartburn or regurgitation? The presence of flatulence with heartburn or regurgitation should suggest reflux esophagitis, gastric or duodenal ulcer, or chronic cholecystitis.
3. Is there a history of a gastrectomy? History of a gastrectomy may indicate that there is gastric dilatation due to the fact that the stomach fails to drain adequately.
4. Is there abdominal pain or distention? The presence of abdominal pain or distention would indicate the possibility of partial intestinal obstruction, steatorrhea, or diverticulitis.
5. Are there other signs of a nervous disorder? If there is a history of emotional trauma or there is hyperkinesis, increased sweating, insomnia, loss of appetite, or other signs of a nervous disorder, then aerophagia should be considered.

DIAGNOSTIC WORKUP

If the gas is eructated, stools for occult blood and an upper GI series and esophagram should be ordered. These may disclose a hiatal hernia and esophagitis, a gastric or duodenal ulcer, and other upper intestinal disorders. A gallbladder series may be done if the upper GI series is unremarkable. Gastroscopy and esophagoscopy may be necessary, as well as a gastric analysis.

If the excessive gas is passed rectally, stools for occult blood, stools for ovum and parasite, and stool cultures should be done. A flat plate of the abdomen may disclose evidence of intestinal obstruction. If these are negative, a barium enema may be done and that may be followed with a small bowel series. A quantitative stool fat analysis should be done to determine if there is steatorrhea and if so, the workup would proceed for steatorrhea (page 539). A lactose tolerance test can be done in cases suspected of lactase deficiency. When extensive testing is negative, a psychiatrist may need to be consulted.

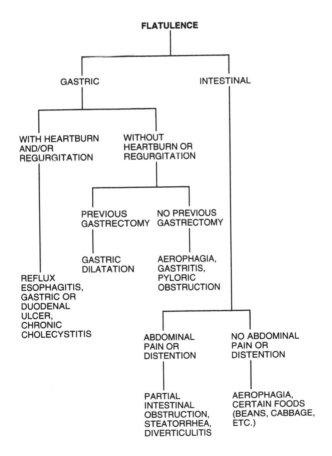

FOOT DEFORMITIES

Ask the following question:

Are there signs of a neurologic disease? Many foot deformities are associated with neurologic disease. For example, a pes cavus may be associated with a peroneal muscular atrophy, poliomyelitis, and Friedreich's ataxia. Muscular dystrophy produces an equinovarus deformity. Friedreich's ataxia may produce a talipes equinovarus. Amyotrophic lateral sclerosis and progressive muscular atrophy may also cause foot deformities.

DIAGNOSTIC WORKUP

Rather than undertaking an extensive diagnostic workup, it is wise to refer the patient to the appropriate specialist. If there are neurologic signs, the patient should be referred to a neurologist. Otherwise, the patient should be referred to an orthopedic surgeon or podiatrist.

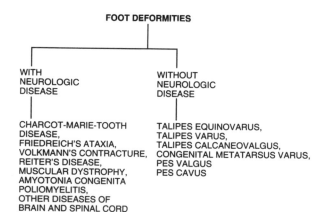

FOOT DEFORMITIES

WITH NEUROLOGIC DISEASE

CHARCOT-MARIE-TOOTH DISEASE,
FRIEDREICH'S ATAXIA,
VOLKMANN'S CONTRACTURE,
REITER'S DISEASE,
MUSCULAR DYSTROPHY,
AMYOTONIA CONGENITA
POLIOMYELITIS,
OTHER DISEASES OF
BRAIN AND SPINAL CORD

WITHOUT NEUROLOGIC DISEASE

TALIPES EQUINOVARUS,
TALIPES VARUS,
TALIPES CALCANEOVALGUS,
CONGENITAL METATARSUS VARUS,
PES VALGUS
PES CAVUS

FOOT AND TOE PAIN

Ask the following questions:

1. Is there fever or localized erythema? Localized erythema would suggest phlebitis, gout, osteomyelitis, cellulitis, ingrown toenail, and paronychia. The presence of fever would make one suspect osteomyelitis and cellulitis.
2. Is there associated deformity of the foot? Hallux valgus, hammertoe, hallux rigidus, arthritis, and displaced fracture are the main causes of a deformity of the foot.
3. Are the peripheral pulses palpable? Diminished arterial pulses would make one think of arterial embolism, peripheral arteriosclerosis, and diabetes.
4. Are there associated neurologic findings? The presence of loss of sensation to touch and pain should make one think of peripheral neuropathy and tarsal tunnel syndrome.

DIAGNOSTIC WORKUP

Routine diagnostic tests include a CBC, sedimentation rate, chemistry panel, VDRL test, and an x-ray of the foot. If the peripheral pulses are diminished, Doppler studies and angiography should be considered. If there is diffuse swelling and erythema, venography may need to be done. If there are neurologic findings, nerve conduction velocity studies and electromyograms (EMGs) may be helpful. Consider bone scans, CT scans and arthroscopy if the above tests are negative. It is wise to refer the patient to an orthopedic surgeon or podiatrist before ordering expensive diagnostic tests.

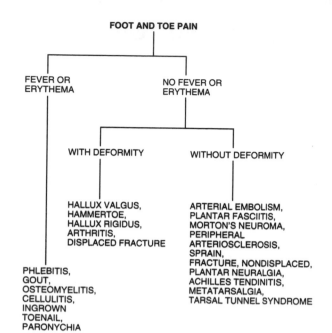

FOOT AND TOE PAIN

FEVER OR ERYTHEMA

NO FEVER OR ERYTHEMA

WITH DEFORMITY

WITHOUT DEFORMITY

HALLUX VALGUS,
HAMMERTOE,
HALLUX RIGIDUS,
ARTHRITIS,
DISPLACED FRACTURE

ARTERIAL EMBOLISM,
PLANTAR FASCIITIS,
MORTON'S NEUROMA,
PERIPHERAL
ARTERIOSCLEROSIS,
SPRAIN,
FRACTURE, NONDISPLACED,
PLANTAR NEURALGIA,
ACHILLES TENDINITIS,
METATARSALGIA,
TARSAL TUNNEL SYNDROME

PHLEBITIS,
GOUT,
OSTEOMYELITIS,
CELLULITIS,
INGROWN
TOENAIL,
PARONYCHIA

FOOT ULCERATION

Ask the following questions:

1. Are there diminished or absent peripheral pulses? The finding of poor peripheral pulses would suggest that the lesion is secondary to ischemia from arteriosclerosis, Buerger's disease, diabetic arteriolar sclerosis, familial hyperlipidemia, and cryoproteinemia.
2. Are there abnormalities on neurologic examination? The presence of good peripheral pulses should make one look for a neurologic explanation for the ulcer and if there is diminished sensation to touch and pain in the periphery, then peripheral neuropathy is very likely. Ulcers may also form in paraplegia of any cause, leprosy, and tabes dorsalis.
3. Is there a history of diabetes? A history of diabetes makes the diagnosis of diabetic arteriolar sclerosis very likely. Remember, the pulses may be normal in this condition.
4. Is there a positive smear or culture? The presence of good peripheral pulses should prompt one to do a smear and culture of material from the lesion and if this is positive, then the diagnosis is made. We would consider, in addition to the normal bacteria, blastomycosis, sporotrichosis, maduromycosis, and syphilis.

DIAGNOSTIC WORKUP

This includes a CBC, sedimentation rate, urinalysis, chemistry panel, VDRL test, and glucose tolerance test. An x-ray of the involved foot should be done to rule out osteomyelitis. A bone scan is even more sensitive to osteomyelitis and other disorders of the bone that may be causing the ulcer. A smear should be made of the ulcer material and a culture done also, not just for the common pathogens, but for acid-fast bacilli and fungi. A dark field preparation may be necessary. Skin testing for blastomycosis and other fungi should be done. A nerve conduction velocity study of the lower extremities will be helpful in differentiating neurologic causes. Femoral angiography may be valuable in determining the exact level of the lesion and whether it can be approached surgically.

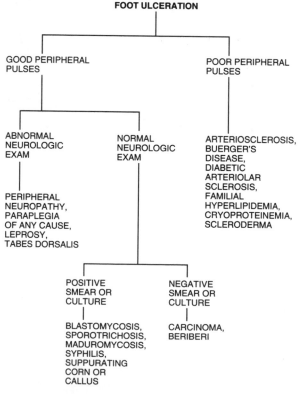

FOOT ULCERATION

GOOD PERIPHERAL PULSES

POOR PERIPHERAL PULSES

ABNORMAL NEUROLOGIC EXAM

NORMAL NEUROLOGIC EXAM

ARTERIOSCLEROSIS, BUERGER'S DISEASE, DIABETIC ARTERIOLAR SCLEROSIS, FAMILIAL HYPERLIPIDEMIA, CRYOPROTEINEMIA, SCLERODERMA

PERIPHERAL NEUROPATHY, PARAPLEGIA OF ANY CAUSE, LEPROSY, TABES DORSALIS

POSITIVE SMEAR OR CULTURE

NEGATIVE SMEAR OR CULTURE

BLASTOMYCOSIS, SPOROTRICHOSIS, MADUROMYCOSIS, SYPHILIS, SUPPURATING CORN OR CALLUS

CARCINOMA, BERIBERI

FOREHEAD ENLARGEMENT

In adults, forehead enlargement is seen in Paget's disease, fibrous dysplasia, leontiasis ossea, and acromegaly. It may also be a normal process as the frontal air sinuses develop over the years. In children, forehead enlargement may be due to hydrocephalus, rickets, congenital syphilis, and a large hematoma.

DIAGNOSTIC WORKUP

X-ray of the skull, tests for calcium, phosphorus and acid alkaline phosphatase, and a VDRL test should be performed in all cases. When other signs of acromegaly are present, serum growth hormone level should be measured. Children may need a referral to a pediatrician.

FREQUENCY OF URINATION

Ask the following questions:

1. Is the 24-hr urine volume increased? If the 24-hr urine volume is increased, then one has identified polyuria. The differential diagnosis of this condition is found on page 449.
2. Is there dysuria? If there is dysuria, one should consider cystitis, urethritis, prostatitis, bladder calculi, and tuberculosis of the bladder. If there is no dysuria, then a bladder neck obstruction, from conditions such as prostatic hypertrophy or urethral stricture might be considered.
3. Is there fever? If there is fever along with frequency of urination, this could be due to a systemic condition, but it is more important to look for pyelonephritis.

DIAGNOSTIC WORKUP

The first thing to do is a urinalysis and examine the urinary sediment. This will help determine if there is a urinary tract infection and if there is diabetes or one of the other causes of polyuria. A sterile sample of the urine should be sent to the lab for culture regardless of whether the urinalysis is normal or not.

If these studies are unremarkable, a 24-hr urine volume is determined. If the urine volume is substantially increased, the workup may proceed for polyuria (see page 449). If the 24-hr urine volume is normal, a pelvic and rectal examination must be done for a mass that might be pressing on the bladder. Even if the pelvic and rectal exam is negative, pelvic ultrasound may disclose a pelvic mass.

The next step would be to catheterize for residual urine. If the residual urine is large, bladder neck obstruction is probably the problem and prostatic hypertrophy, median bar hypertrophy, and urethral stricture must be considered.

Further studies include an intravenous pyelogram, cystogram, cystoscopy, and retrograde pyelography, but these should be done in consultation with a urologist.

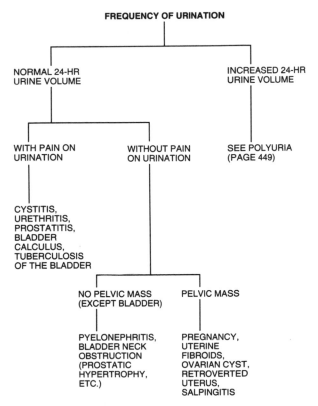

FREQUENCY OF URINATION

NORMAL 24-HR URINE VOLUME

INCREASED 24-HR URINE VOLUME

WITH PAIN ON URINATION

WITHOUT PAIN ON URINATION

SEE POLYURIA (PAGE 449)

CYSTITIS, URETHRITIS, PROSTATITIS, BLADDER CALCULUS, TUBERCULOSIS OF THE BLADDER

NO PELVIC MASS (EXCEPT BLADDER)

PELVIC MASS

PYELONEPHRITIS, BLADDER NECK OBSTRUCTION (PROSTATIC HYPERTROPHY, ETC.)

PREGNANCY, UTERINE FIBROIDS, OVARIAN CYST, RETROVERTED UTERUS, SALPINGITIS

FRIGIDITY

Ask the following questions:

1. Are there abnormalities on the vaginal examination? Imperforated hymen, a mass in the cul-de-sac, a retroverted uterus, pregnancy, pelvic inflammatory disease, and cystitis are just a few of the conditions that might be found.
2. Are there abnormalities on the rectal examination? The rectal examination may disclose anal fissures, hemorrhoids, or perirectal abscess.
3. Are there abnormalities of the secondary sexual characteristics? Turner's syndrome and testicular feminization are two of the conditions that may be associated with these abnormalities.
4. Is there a history of emotional trauma? Childhood sexual molestations and marital difficulties are among the conditions that may be found on a careful history.

DIAGNOSTIC WORKUP

First, one should do is a good pelvic and rectal examination. If abnormalities are found on these examinations, referral to a gynecologist or proctologist can be made. If the pelvic and rectal examinations are normal, the patient should probably be referred to a psychiatrist or psychologist for treatment. If there are abnormalities of the secondary sexual characteristics, the clinician may undertake studies of these disorders, but referral to an endocrinologist is probably more cost-effective.

FRIGIDITY

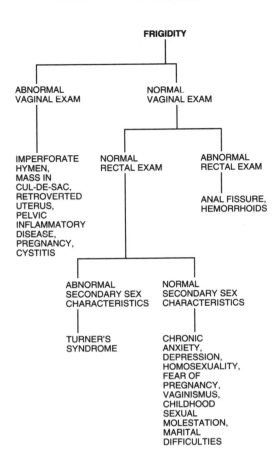

GAIT DISTURBANCES

Ask the following questions:

1. Are there abnormalities on neurologic examination? An abnormal neurologic examination should make one think of multiple sclerosis, peripheral neuropathy, muscular dystrophy, Parkinson's disease, Huntington's chorea, and a host of degenerative neurologic conditions.
2. Is there a painful limp? The findings of a painful limp should make one suspect hip, knee, or ankle joint pathology. A herniated lumbar disk may also cause a characteristic antalgic gait.
3. Is the gait characteristic of a particular type? Characteristic gaits include the short-stepped shuffling gait of Parkinson's disease, the ataxic gait of multiple sclerosis and cerebellar disorders, the reeling, clownish gait of Huntington's chorea, the pelvic tilt of muscular dystrophy, and the steppage gait of peripheral neuropathy.
4. Could the gait disturbance be due to malingering or hysteria? The gait of conversion hysteria is quite remarkable. The patient has a normal neurologic examination and has no difficulty maintaining balance while sitting down, but there is total inability to walk or stand without reeling about.

DIAGNOSTIC WORKUP

Routine orders would include a CBC, sedimentation rate, chemistry panel, VDRL test, and urinalysis. If there is a painful limp, then x-rays of the hip, knee, or ankle on the affected side should be performed. An x-ray of the lumbar spine will not usually be of great assistance, however. If plain x-rays are negative, a CT scan or MRI of the lumbar spine, the hip, knee, or ankle may be of assistance in the diagnosis. A bone scan may pick up obscure fractures and other pathology.

If there are abnormalities on the neurologic examination, MRI or CT scan of the appropriate level of suspected pathology will be done. A spastic gait with abnormal cranial nerve findings would suggest a cerebral tumor or other brain disease and a CT scan or MRI of the brain should be done. Keep in mind that the MRI is almost double the cost of a CT scan and the diagnostic yield is not that much greater in many cases.

A spastic gait without cranial nerve signs or papilledema would suggest a spinal cord disorder and an MRI or CT scan of the appropriate level of the spinal cord should be done. A CT scan of the cervical spine, however, is not very useful and MRI is preferred.

If multiple sclerosis is suspected, a spinal tap for myelin basic protein or gamma globulin levels should be done. A visual evoked potential study, a brain stem evoked potential study, or a somatosensory evoked potential study will also be useful in diagnosing multiple sclerosis.

If there is an ataxic gait, cerebellar disorder should be suspected and a CT scan of the brain may be done. However, an ataxic gait may also suggest multiple sclerosis, pernicious anemia, and tabes dorsalis. If the VDRL test is negative, a fluorescent treponemal antibody-absorption (FTA-ABS) test should be done. Blood levels for vitamin B_{12} and folic acid will help diagnose pernicious anemia. A Schilling test, however, is sometimes necessary to facilitate this diagnosis. If muscular dystrophy is suspected, electromyographic examination and muscle biopsy will help confirm the diagnosis. If the patient has a steppage gait, the workup of peripheral neuropathy should be done, as noted on page 425.

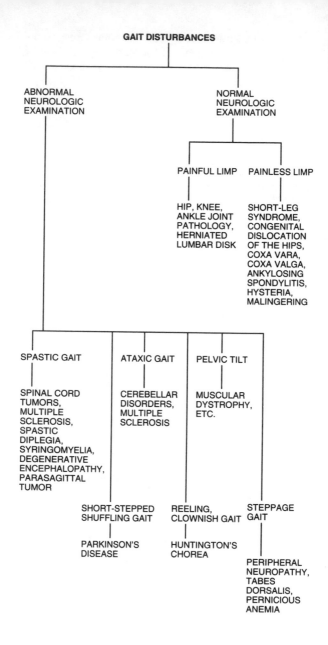

GAIT DISTURBANCES

ABNORMAL NEUROLOGIC EXAMINATION

NORMAL NEUROLOGIC EXAMINATION

PAINFUL LIMP

PAINLESS LIMP

HIP, KNEE, ANKLE JOINT PATHOLOGY, HERNIATED LUMBAR DISK

SHORT-LEG SYNDROME, CONGENITAL DISLOCATION OF THE HIPS, COXA VARA, COXA VALGA, ANKYLOSING SPONDYLITIS, HYSTERIA, MALINGERING

SPASTIC GAIT

ATAXIC GAIT

PELVIC TILT

SPINAL CORD TUMORS, MULTIPLE SCLEROSIS, SPASTIC DIPLEGIA, SYRINGOMYELIA, DEGENERATIVE ENCEPHALOPATHY, PARASAGITTAL TUMOR

CEREBELLAR DISORDERS, MULTIPLE SCLEROSIS

MUSCULAR DYSTROPHY, ETC.

SHORT-STEPPED SHUFFLING GAIT

REELING, CLOWNISH GAIT

STEPPAGE GAIT

PARKINSON'S DISEASE

HUNTINGTON'S CHOREA

PERIPHERAL NEUROPATHY, TABES DORSALIS, PERNICIOUS ANEMIA

GANGRENE

Ask the following questions:

1. Does it involve the upper or lower extremity? Involvement of the upper extremities should suggest Raynaud's disease, scleroderma, and other collagen diseases.
2. Are there good peripheral pulses? The complete absence of a peripheral pulse, particularly if it is sudden onset should suggest an arterial embolism. If it is gradual onset, suspect arteriosclerosis or diabetic ulcer.
3. Are there signs of systemic disease? If there are other signs of systemic disease, then collagen disease, macroglobulinemia, and cryoglobulinemia should be suspected.
4. Is the gangrene sudden in onset? A sudden onset of the gangrene should make one suspect clostridia infections or arterial embolism.
5. Is there a positive culture? The culture will be positive in clostridia infections, anthrax, and cancrum oris.

DIAGNOSTIC WORKUP

Routine orders include a CBC, sedimentation rate, chemistry panel, VDRL test, serum protein electrophoresis, antinuclear antibody titer, and glucose tolerance test. The gangrenous area should be cultured. Plain x-rays of the area sometimes are helpful. If there are diminished pulses, especially if the onset is acute, angiography will be useful. A muscle biopsy or skin biopsy will be useful in diagnosing collagen diseases. The Sia water test and serum immunoelectrophoresis will be useful in diagnosing macroglobulinemia and cryoglobulinemia.

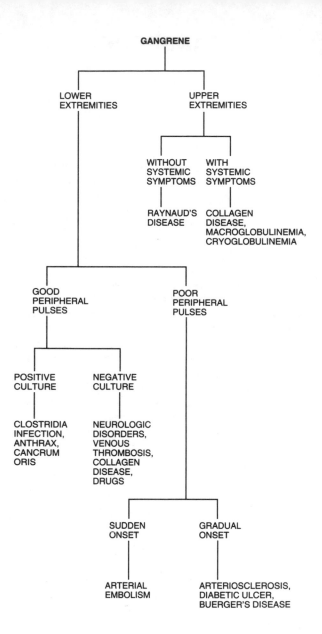

GANGRENE

LOWER EXTREMITIES

UPPER EXTREMITIES

WITHOUT SYSTEMIC SYMPTOMS

WITH SYSTEMIC SYMPTOMS

RAYNAUD'S DISEASE

COLLAGEN DISEASE, MACROGLOBULINEMIA, CRYOGLOBULINEMIA

GOOD PERIPHERAL PULSES

POOR PERIPHERAL PULSES

POSITIVE CULTURE

NEGATIVE CULTURE

CLOSTRIDIA INFECTION, ANTHRAX, CANCRUM ORIS

NEUROLOGIC DISORDERS, VENOUS THROMBOSIS, COLLAGEN DISEASE, DRUGS

SUDDEN ONSET

GRADUAL ONSET

ARTERIAL EMBOLISM

ARTERIOSCLEROSIS, DIABETIC ULCER, BUERGER'S DISEASE

GIGANTISM

Ask the following questions:

1. Are there abnormal secondary sex characteristics? Patients with Klinefelter's syndrome, supermale, superfemale, sexual precocity, and virilism have abnormal secondary sex characteristics and a tall stature.
2. Is there arachnodactyly? Arachnodactyly is associated with Marfan's syndrome and homocystinuria.
3. Is there a family history? Patients with a family history of tall stature often have constitutional tall stature and not pituitary gigantism.

DIAGNOSTIC WORKUP

X-rays of the skull and a CT scan will help identify a pituitary eosinophilic adenoma, but serum growth hormone will also be elevated early and FSH and LH may be depressed later. Serum FSH and LH will be elevated in Klinefelter's syndrome. A chromosome study should be done to identify Klinefelter's syndrome, supermale, and superfemale. A serum testosterone, dihydrotestosterone and dehydroepiandrosterone sulfate will be helpful in diagnosing sexual precocity and virilism caused by tumors and hyperplasia of the adrenal gland. Echocardiography and urinary hydroxyproline will help identify Marfan's syndrome, while a urine for homocystine will help diagnose homocystinuria. A thyroid profile should be done to rule out thyrotoxicosis.

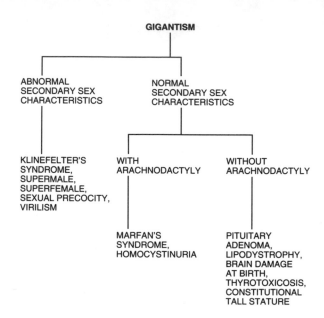

GIRDLE PAIN

Ask the following questions:

1. Is there an associated rash? Presence of a rash, whether it is macular or vesicular, especially if it is in a dermatomal distribution, would suggest herpes zoster. Occasionally, herpes zoster occurs without a rash and should still be considered in the differential diagnosis.
2. Are there pyramidal tract or other long tract signs? The findings of long tract signs would indicate compression, degeneration, or inflammation of the spinal cord, and conditions such as multiple sclerosis, acute transverse myelitis, spinal cord tumor, herniated disk, and pernicious anemia should be considered. If there are no long tract signs and no rash, then one should consider early spinal cord tumor or herniated disk, intercostal neuralgia, fractured ribs, and sometimes a compression fracture of the vertebra.

DIAGNOSTIC WORKUP

Patients with a rash, particularly if it is vesicular and in a dermatomal distribution, may be treated for herpes zoster before doing an extensive diagnostic workup. However, one should remember that herpes zoster may be associated with an underlying neoplasm, particularly Hodgkin's disease.

If a patient does not have a rash, then routine laboratory tests include a CBC, chemistry panel, sedimentation rate, VDRL test, serum B_{12}, and folic acid. In addition, x-rays of the chest, ribs, and thoracic spine should be done. If these are normal and the diagnosis remains in doubt, one should consult a neurologist. If none is available, MRI of the thoracic spine may be ordered. A spinal tap may be done to help rule out multiple sclerosis and tabes dorsalis. Somatosensory evoked potential studies can be done to diagnose multiple sclerosis. A thoracic myelogram is occasionally necessary in confusing cases.

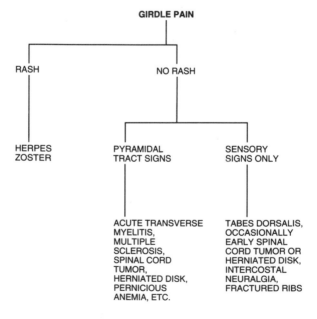

GIRDLE PAIN

RASH

NO RASH

HERPES ZOSTER

PYRAMIDAL TRACT SIGNS

SENSORY SIGNS ONLY

ACUTE TRANSVERSE MYELITIS, MULTIPLE SCLEROSIS, SPINAL CORD TUMOR, HERNIATED DISK, PERNICIOUS ANEMIA, ETC.

TABES DORSALIS, OCCASIONALLY EARLY SPINAL CORD TUMOR OR HERNIATED DISK, INTERCOSTAL NEURALGIA, FRACTURED RIBS

GYNECOMASTIA

Ask the following questions:

1. Is there a history of drug ingestion? Digitalis, phenothiazine, amphetamine, marijuana, and many other drugs may cause gynecomastia.
2. Is there a testicular mass? Leydig's cell and Sertoli's cell tumors of the testicle may cause gynecomastia.
3. Are there abnormal secondary sex characteristics? Klinefelter's syndrome, male pseudohermaphroditism, and testicular feminization syndrome may cause gynecomastia.
4. Is there a bronze skin? If there is a bronze skin, one should consider hemochromatosis, as this may be associated with gynecomastia.
5. Are there other endocrine abnormalities? Cushing's syndrome, Addison's syndrome, and hyperthyroidism may cause gynecomastia.
6. Are there abnormalities on neurologic examination? Myotonic dystrophy, paraplegias of various types, and Friedreich's ataxia are among the many neurologic disorders that may be associated with gynecomastia.

DIAGNOSTIC WORKUP

A urine drug screen and thyroid profile should be done at the outset. Liver function studies, liver biopsy, and serum iron and iron binding capacity will help rule out hemochromatosis and cirrhosis of the liver. A serum FSH, LH, human chorionic gonadotrophin, and estradiol will help diagnose testicular tumors, Klinefelter's syndrome, and testicular feminization syndrome. A serum cortisol, cortisol suppression test, and rapid ACTH test will help diagnose Cushing's syndrome and Addison's disease. There is a specific beta–human chorionic gonadotropin assay that can be done to rule out an HCG-secreting tumor such as carcinoma of the lung.

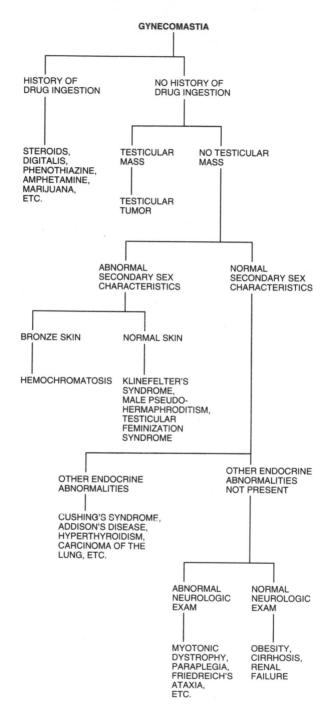

GYNECOMASTIA

HISTORY OF DRUG INGESTION

STEROIDS, DIGITALIS, PHENOTHIAZINE, AMPHETAMINE, MARIJUANA, ETC.

NO HISTORY OF DRUG INGESTION

TESTICULAR MASS

TESTICULAR TUMOR

NO TESTICULAR MASS

ABNORMAL SECONDARY SEX CHARACTERISTICS

NORMAL SECONDARY SEX CHARACTERISTICS

BRONZE SKIN

HEMOCHROMATOSIS

NORMAL SKIN

KLINEFELTER'S SYNDROME, MALE PSEUDO-HERMAPHRODITISM, TESTICULAR FEMINIZATION SYNDROME

OTHER ENDOCRINE ABNORMALITIES

CUSHING'S SYNDROME, ADDISON'S DISEASE, HYPERTHYROIDISM, CARCINOMA OF THE LUNG, ETC.

OTHER ENDOCRINE ABNORMALITIES NOT PRESENT

ABNORMAL NEUROLOGIC EXAM

MYOTONIC DYSTROPHY, PARAPLEGIA, FRIEDREICH'S ATAXIA, ETC.

NORMAL NEUROLOGIC EXAM

OBESITY, CIRRHOSIS, RENAL FAILURE

HALITOSIS

Ask the following questions:

1. Is there a history of ingestion or use of a foul substance? Such a history may suggest that the cause is onions, garlic, alcohol, tobacco, paraldehyde, mercury, or other substances.
2. Are there abnormalities of examination of the mouth, nose, and throat? Abnormalities that may be found on examination of the mouth, nose, and throat include gingivitis, carious teeth, pyorrhea, stomatitis, sinusitis, pharyngitis, and tonsillitis.
3. Is there a chronic productive cough? The presence of a chronic productive cough should suggest bronchiectasis, lung abscess, gangrene of the lungs, tuberculosis, and other lung infections.
4. Is there esophageal regurgitation? The history of esophageal regurgitation should suggest reflux esophagitis, peptic ulcer, partial intestinal obstruction, and esophageal diverticula. If there are none of these findings, one should look for uremia or cirrhosis.

DIAGNOSTIC WORKUP

Routine tests include a CBC and sedimentation rate to rule out chronic inflammation; a chemistry panel to rule out uremia and cirrhosis; and sputum, nose, and throat cultures to rule out chronic infections of the sinuses, nose, throat, and lungs. Cultures of any suspicious area of inflammation in the mouth, nose, and throat should be done. X-rays of the teeth, sinuses, and chest should also be done. An upper GI series and esophagram will help diagnose reflux esophagitis, peptic ulcer, partial intestinal obstruction, and esophageal diverticula.

A 24-hr sputum collection may help differentiate bronchiectasis and lung abscesses. A tuberculin test and sputum for acid-fast bacilli (AFB) smear, culture, and possible guinea pig inoculation may identify tuberculosis.

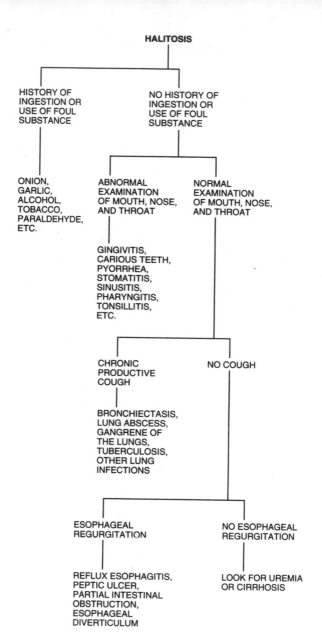

HALLUCINATIONS

Ask the following questions:

1. Is there a history of drug or alcohol ingestion? Hallucinations are common during alcohol withdrawal, but also may be noted in cocaine addiction, marijuana addiction, LSD intoxication, and PCP intoxication.
2. Are the hallucinations primarily visual in nature? This would suggest an organic cause such as organic brain syndrome, epilepsy, brain tumor, etc.
3. Are the hallucinations episodic? If the hallucinations occur in episodes with normal behavior in between, one should consider epilepsy or narcolepsy.
4. Are the hallucinations associated with early stages of falling asleep or awakening? These types of hallucinations are called hypnagogic and are common in narcolepsy, but may also be seen in normal people.
5. Are the hallucinations primarily auditory in nature? This is the type of hallucination most commonly associated with schizophrenia.

DIAGNOSTIC WORKUP

A blood alcohol level and urine drug screen are essential at the outset. Most physicians will want to refer the patient to a psychiatrist if these studies are negative. However, the interested physician may proceed further with a wake and sleep EEG to identify psychomotor epilepsy or a CT scan and MRI to identify brain tumors and other causes of organic brain syndrome. Remember, the MRI costs twice as much as a CT scan. A spinal tap will be helpful in diagnosing central nervous system lues. A sleep study will help diagnose narcolepsy. Psychometric testing will help identify schizophrenia and other psychiatric disorders.

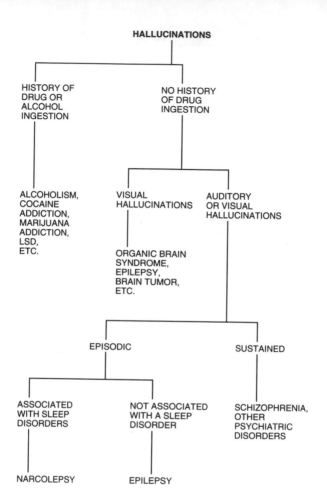

HALLUCINATIONS

HISTORY OF
DRUG OR
ALCOHOL
INGESTION

NO HISTORY
OF DRUG
INGESTION

ALCOHOLISM,
COCAINE
ADDICTION,
MARIJUANA
ADDICTION,
LSD,
ETC.

VISUAL
HALLUCINATIONS

AUDITORY
OR VISUAL
HALLUCINATIONS

ORGANIC BRAIN
SYNDROME,
EPILEPSY,
BRAIN TUMOR,
ETC.

EPISODIC

SUSTAINED

ASSOCIATED
WITH SLEEP
DISORDERS

NOT ASSOCIATED
WITH A SLEEP
DISORDER

SCHIZOPHRENIA,
OTHER
PSYCHIATRIC
DISORDERS

NARCOLEPSY

EPILEPSY

HEADACHE

Ask the following questions:

1. Is there a history of drug, caffeine, or alcohol ingestion? The hangover headache is well known and should not present a problem in diagnosis. Caffeine withdrawal headaches are also common because of the large amount of caffeine consumed in coffee, various soft drinks, and chocolate. Drugs that may induce headache include the nonsteroidal anti-inflammatory drugs such as indomethacin (Indocin®) and the antihypertensives such as clonidine, aspirin, quinidine, and bromides.

2. Is there a history of trauma? Trauma may cause concussion and postconcussion headaches, intracranial neoplasms such as subdural hematoma, and cervical sprain, all of which can induce headaches.

3. Is the headache acute or chronic? An acute onset of a headache can be a serious problem. It should be taken seriously because it may mean a subarachnoid hemorrhage or meningitis. This can be easily confirmed by checking for nuchal rigidity. Whenever there is an acute onset of a headache this must be done. Chronic headaches, on the other hand, are most likely due either to migraine if they occur in exacerbations or remissions, or to tension headaches if they are fairly constant, mild, and chronic. The headache of a brain tumor is rarely severe and is rarely the presenting symptom of a brain tumor. Headaches that occur in clusters almost daily for 6 to 8 weeks with interruptions of several months must make one consider cluster headaches. Unilateral headaches in the elderly with acute onset should make one think of temporal arteritis.

4. Is there nuchal rigidity? The presence of nuchal rigidity should make one think of a subarachnoid hemorrhage or meningitis, but it may also be due to cerebral hemorrhage or cerebral abscess.

5. Is there fever? If the headache is associated with

fever, the possibility of acute sinusitis should be considered and the sinuses should be transilluminated. Other sources for the fever should be looked for and meningitis or encephalitis should be considered.

6. Is there papilledema or focal neurologic signs? With acute headache and focal neurologic signs and/or papilledema, one should consider cerebral abscess or cerebral hemorrhage. With a chronic headache and papilledema or focal neurologic signs, one should consider a space-occupying lesion such as a primary brain tumor or metastatic neoplasm.

7. Do the sinuses transilluminate well? A sinus transilluminator should be in the armamentarium of every physician who expects to diagnose headache. If the sinuses fail to transilluminate, one should consider acute sinusitis as the diagnosis.

8. Is there tenderness of the superficial temporal artery? The presence of a tender superficial temporal artery should make one think of temporal arteritis, particularly in the elderly, but it may also be related to a longstanding migraine attack.

9. Is the headache relieved by superficial temporal artery compression? Relief of the headache on superficial temporal artery compression should suggest classical or common migraine. If one can relieve the headache by compression of the occipital artery, then occipital migraine should be considered. When there is no relief on compression of the superficial temporal artery, one should consider tension headaches, occipital neuralgia, cervical spondylosis, and cluster headaches as the cause.

DIAGNOSTIC WORKUP

Routine diagnostic tests include a CBC to rule out severe anemia, a sedimentation rate to rule out temporal arteritis, a chemistry panel to rule out liver and kidney disease, a VDRL test to rule out central nervous system syphilis, an x-ray of the sinuses to rule out sinusitis, and an x-ray of the cervical spine to exclude cervical spondylosis. A chest x-ray should also be done to rule out the possibility of metastatic neoplasm. A tonometry study may be done if glaucoma is suspected.

If there are focal neurologic signs, referral should be made to a neurologist or neurosurgeon as soon as possible. If one is not readily available, a CT scan or MRI may be done, the CT scan being the preferred procedure if the expense is a consideration.

If there is nuchal rigidity, a CT scan should be done to rule out a space-occupying lesion before proceeding with a spinal tap. If the CT scan is negative, a spinal tap can be done and this will ascertain whether there is intracranial bleeding or meningitis. It is usually best to refer the patient to a neurologist or neurosurgeon if there is nuchal rigidity.

If the headaches are chronic and episodic and there are no focal neurologic signs, papilledema, or nuchal rigidity, an imaging study can be postponed for a while until the response to treatment is evaluated. However, if the response to treatment is poor, one should not hesitate to order a CT scan or MRI.

Difficult cases of headache should also be studied with 24-hr blood pressure monitoring, a 24-hr urine for catecholamines, and lumbar puncture to diagnose central nervous system lues. Histamine phosphate 0.5 cc subcutaneously may help diagnose cluster headaches. Response to beta-blockers may help diagnose migraine. Cerebral angiography may be necessary to diagnose aneurysms and arteriovenous malformations. Patients with chronic headache unresponsive to therapy should be referred to a psychiatrist.

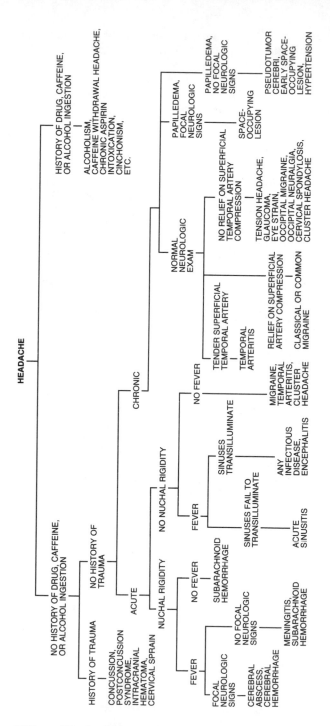

HEADACHE

- **NO HISTORY OF DRUG, CAFFEINE, OR ALCOHOL INGESTION**
  - **HISTORY OF TRAUMA**
    - CONCUSSION, POSTCONCUSSION SYNDROME, INTRACRANIAL HEMATOMA, CERVICAL SPRAIN
  - **NO HISTORY OF TRAUMA**
    - **ACUTE**
      - **NUCHAL RIGIDITY**
        - **FEVER**
          - **FOCAL NEUROLOGIC SIGNS**
            - CEREBRAL ABSCESS, CEREBRAL HEMORRHAGE
          - **NO FOCAL NEUROLOGIC SIGNS**
            - MENINGITIS, SUBARACHNOID HEMORRHAGE
        - **NO FEVER**
          - SUBARACHNOID HEMORRHAGE
      - **NO NUCHAL RIGIDITY**
        - **FEVER**
          - **SINUSES FAIL TO TRANSILLUMINATE**
            - ACUTE SINUSITIS
          - **SINUSES TRANSILLUMINATE**
            - ANY INFECTIOUS DISEASE, ENCEPHALITIS
        - **NO FEVER**
          - MIGRAINE, TEMPORAL ARTERITIS, CLUSTER HEADACHE
    - **CHRONIC**
      - **NORMAL NEUROLOGIC EXAM**
        - **TENDER SUPERFICIAL TEMPORAL ARTERY**
          - TEMPORAL ARTERITIS
        - **NO RELIEF ON SUPERFICIAL TEMPORAL ARTERY COMPRESSION**
          - TENSION HEADACHE, GLAUCOMA, EYE STRAIN, OCCIPITAL NEURALGIA, CERVICAL SPONDYLOSIS, CLUSTER HEADACHE
        - **RELIEF ON SUPERFICIAL ARTERY COMPRESSION**
          - CLASSICAL OR COMMON MIGRAINE
      - **PAPILLEDEMA, FOCAL NEUROLOGIC SIGNS**
        - SPACE-OCCUPYING LESION
      - **PAPILLEDEMA, NO FOCAL NEUROLOGIC SIGNS**
        - PSEUDOTUMOR CEREBRI, EARLY SPACE-OCCUPYING LESION, HYPERTENSION
- **HISTORY OF DRUG, CAFFEINE, OR ALCOHOL INGESTION**
  - ALCOHOLISM, CAFFEINE WITHDRAWAL HEADACHE, CHRONIC ASPIRIN INTOXICATION, CINCHONISM, ETC.

258   Headache

HEAD MASS OR SWELLING

Smaller localized, freely movable masses are the sebaceous cysts, hematomas, lipomas, and lymph nodes. Masses that seem to be attached to the skull are osteomas, dermoid cysts, and sarcomas. Brain tumor tissue may occasionally protrude out beneath the scalp through a craniotomy defect. Mastoiditis may spread to the subcutaneous tissues also. In the newborn there may be edema of the scalp (called caput succedaneum) following a vertex delivery due to molding or a large hematoma over one or both parietal bones (called cephalhematoma) due to the trauma of delivery. There may be meningoceles or encephalomeningoceles due to imperfect closure of the skull (cranium bifidum). Vascular abnormalities of the skin may be found and include angiomas, arteriovenous fistulas, and telangiectasis.

DIAGNOSTIC WORKUP

A skull x-ray will help distinguish the bone lesions, while aspiration or biopsy will help distinguish the others. Referral to the appropriate specialist would be the most cost-effective approach.

HEARTBURN

Ask the following questions:

1. Is there frequent regurgitation? If there is frequent regurgitation, the most likely diagnosis is reflux esophagitis and hiatal hernia. Gastritis and a previous gastrectomy will also cause frequent regurgitation.
2. Is there recurrent nausea or vomiting? If there is recurrent nausea or vomiting, the most likely diagnosis is cholecystitis and cholelithiasis. Chronic pancreatitis can cause the same symptoms, however.
3. Is the heartburn precipitated by exercise and/or relieved by nitroglycerin? These findings suggest coronary insufficiency.
4. Is there associated hematemesis or recurrent black stool? The presence of hematemesis or recurrent black stools should suggest a peptic ulcer.
5. Is there relief with lidocaine hydrochloride (Xylocaine® Viscous Solution)? The relief of the pain on Viscous lidocaine suggests reflux esophagitis, hiatal hernia, and previous gastrectomy with bile esophagitis. Gastritis is not usually relieved by Viscous Xylocaine.

DIAGNOSTIC WORKUP

The workup begins with an upper GI series and esophagram and stools for occult blood. If there is recurrent vomiting and right upper quadrant pain, then a gallbladder ultrasound or cholecystogram should be done. If these are negative, it is best to refer the patient to a gastroenterologist for esophagoscopy and gastroscopy. He may do a Bernstein test, which will reproduce symptoms by an infusion of dilute hydrochloric acid into the distal esophagus. He may also perform esophageal manometry or pH monitoring of the distal esophagus. An exercise tolerance test and coronary angiography also have their place in the diagnostic armamentarium.

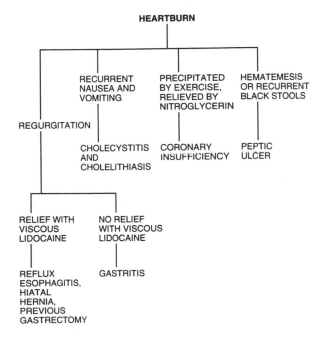

HEARTBURN

REGURGITATION

RECURRENT NAUSEA AND VOMITING

PRECIPITATED BY EXERCISE, RELIEVED BY NITROGLYCERIN

HEMATEMESIS OR RECURRENT BLACK STOOLS

CHOLECYSTITIS AND CHOLELITHIASIS

CORONARY INSUFFICIENCY

PEPTIC ULCER

RELIEF WITH VISCOUS LIDOCAINE

NO RELIEF WITH VISCOUS LIDOCAINE

REFLUX ESOPHAGITIS, HIATAL HERNIA, PREVIOUS GASTRECTOMY

GASTRITIS

HEEL PAIN

Ask the following questions:

1. Are there abnormalities on inspection of the heel? Inspection of the heel may disclose an ulcer, foreign body, cellulitis, plantar wart, and other disorders.
2. Is the patient a child? Children often have Sever's disease (osteochondritis of the heel).
3. Is there tenderness or deformity of the Achilles tendon? Tenderness or deformity of the Achilles tendon should suggest Achilles tendinitis, rupture, or bursitis.
4. Are there abnormalities on x-ray examination? An x-ray may disclose a calcaneal fracture, osteomyelitis, a tumor, or calcaneal spur. If the x-ray is negative, plantar fasciitis is the most likely diagnosis, but one should also consider gout.

DIAGNOSTIC WORKUP

In addition to a plain x-ray of the foot, a CBC, sedimentation rate, chemistry panel, and arthritis panel should be done. A bone scan may disclose an occult fracture. Response to a trigger point injection should be evaluated. If the diagnosis is still in doubt, referral to an orthopedic surgeon or podiatrist should be made before ordering expensive diagnostic tests such as a CT scan or MRI.

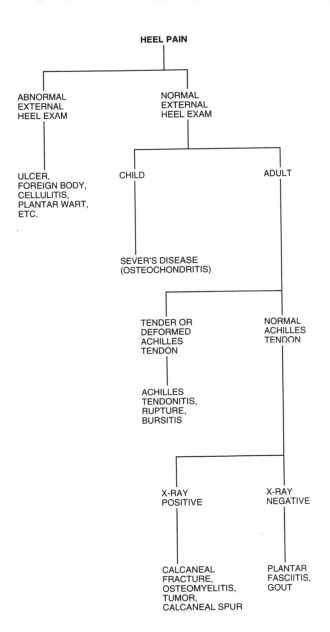

HEEL PAIN

ABNORMAL EXTERNAL HEEL EXAM

NORMAL EXTERNAL HEEL EXAM

ULCER, FOREIGN BODY, CELLULITIS, PLANTAR WART, ETC.

CHILD

ADULT

SEVER'S DISEASE (OSTEOCHONDRITIS)

TENDER OR DEFORMED ACHILLES TENDON

NORMAL ACHILLES TENDON

ACHILLES TENDONITIS, RUPTURE, BURSITIS

X-RAY POSITIVE

X-RAY NEGATIVE

CALCANEAL FRACTURE, OSTEOMYELITIS, TUMOR, CALCANEAL SPUR

PLANTAR FASCIITIS, GOUT

Heel Pain   263

HEMATEMESIS

Ask the following questions:

1. Is there fever? The presence of fever should suggest scarlet fever, measles, malaria, leptospirosis, yellow fever, and other acute and chronic infectious diseases.
2. Is there a history of ingestion of poison, drugs, or alcohol? Poison, many drugs, and alcohol may cause acute gastritis, gastric ulcer, and corrosive esophagitis.
3. Is there associated abdominal pain? Abdominal pain associated with the hematemesis suggests the possibility of gastric or duodenal ulcer, a hiatal hernia, and esophagitis or carcinoma of the stomach. Of course, any of these conditions may occur without abdominal pain.
4. Was the hematemesis preceded by blood-free vomitus? If in the initial stages of vomiting the vomitus was blood-free, one should consider Mallory-Weiss syndrome, which is a tear of the distal esophagus due to severe vomiting.
5. Is there hepatomegaly or splenomegaly? Hepatomegaly would suggest cirrhosis of the liver, while a portal vein thrombosis may occur without hepatomegaly, but almost certainly is associated with splenomegaly. Splenomegaly should suggest Banti's syndrome with depression of platelets, leukocytes, and anemia. Splenomegaly also suggests other blood dyscrasias.
6. Is there a positive tourniquet test or IVY skin bleeding time? These tests may indicate thrombocytopenia and other blood dyscrasias. If these tests are negative and there is no hepatomegaly, splenomegaly or abdominal pain, one should consider hereditary hemorrhagic telangiectasia, an aortic aneurysm, and pseudoxanthoma elasticum.

DIAGNOSTIC WORKUP

Hematemesis, no matter how small, is a clear indication for immediate consultation with a gastroenterologist and esophagoscopy, gastroscopy, and duo-denoscopy. To delay this while ordering an upper GI series and other diagnostic tests may place the patient in serious jeopardy. The clinician would be prudent to order a CBC and coagulation profile, type, and cross-match of several units of blood while waiting for the gastroenterologist to see the patient.

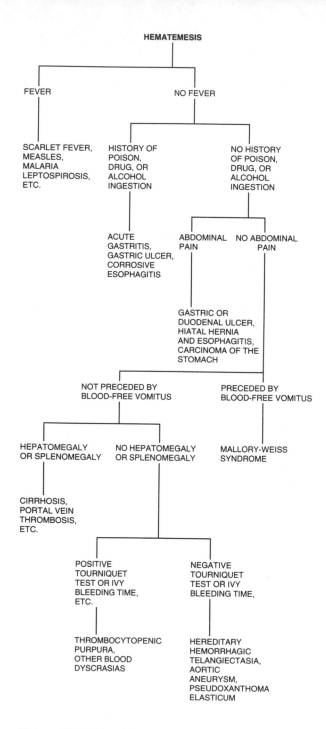

HEMATEMESIS

- **FEVER**
  - SCARLET FEVER, MEASLES, MALARIA LEPTOSPIROSIS, ETC.
- **NO FEVER**
  - **HISTORY OF POISON, DRUG, OR ALCOHOL INGESTION**
    - ACUTE GASTRITIS, GASTRIC ULCER, CORROSIVE ESOPHAGITIS
  - **NO HISTORY OF POISON, DRUG, OR ALCOHOL INGESTION**
    - **ABDOMINAL PAIN**
      - GASTRIC OR DUODENAL ULCER, HIATAL HERNIA AND ESOPHAGITIS, CARCINOMA OF THE STOMACH
    - **NO ABDOMINAL PAIN**
      - **NOT PRECEDED BY BLOOD-FREE VOMITUS**
        - **HEPATOMEGALY OR SPLENOMEGALY**
          - CIRRHOSIS, PORTAL VEIN THROMBOSIS, ETC.
        - **NO HEPATOMEGALY OR SPLENOMEGALY**
          - **POSITIVE TOURNIQUET TEST OR IVY BLEEDING TIME, ETC.**
            - THROMBOCYTOPENIC PURPURA, OTHER BLOOD DYSCRASIAS
          - **NEGATIVE TOURNIQUET TEST OR IVY BLEEDING TIME,**
            - HEREDITARY HEMORRHAGIC TELANGIECTASIA, AORTIC ANEURYSM, PSEUDOXANTHOMA ELASTICUM
      - **PRECEDED BY BLOOD-FREE VOMITUS**
        - MALLORY-WEISS SYNDROME

HEMATURIA

Ask the following questions:

1. Is there abdominal pain? The presence of abdominal pain with hematuria should first suggest renal calculus, but other causes such as renal embolism, renal contusion, or laceration must be considered.
2. Is there dysuria or frequency of micturition associated with the hematuria? The presence of dysuria and frequency with the hematuria should suggest a bladder stone, prostatic disease, or a urinary tract infection.
3. Is there fever? The presence of fever with the hematuria would suggest pyelonephritis.
4. Is there a flank mass? The presence of bilateral flank masses with hematuria should suggest polycystic kidneys and hydronephrosis, while a unilateral flank mass would suggest a hypernephroma or unilateral hydronephrosis. A solitary cyst or renal vein thrombosis may also present with a flank mass and hematuria.
5. Is there hypertension? The presence of hypertension with the hematuria suggests glomerulonephritis, polycystic kidneys, and collagen diseases.
6. Are there other systemic signs and symptoms? If there are other systemic signs and symptoms, one should be looking for collagen disease, coagulation disorders, leukemia, and sickle cell anemia. When there is no hypertension or other signs and symptoms of systemic diseases, one should be looking for a benign or malignant tumor of the bladder, tuberculosis, or parasitic infection.

DIAGNOSTIC WORKUP

The workup begins with a urinalysis and microscopic examination of the urinary sediment. The physician can easily do this in his office. If there is proteinuria, granular cast, and red cell cast, then glomerulonephritis or collagen disease should be suspected. A culture and sensitivity and colony count should be done if a urinary tract infection is suspected. If this is negative, an anaerobic culture should be done also and then an acid-fast bacilli (AFB) smear and culture and guinea pig inoculation to rule out tuberculosis. An intravenous pyelogram will also usually have to be done. A CBC, sedimentation rate, chemistry panel, coagulation profile, and antinuclear antibody test will help rule out blood dyscrasias, collagen diseases, and other systemic diseases.

If the above are not revealing, referral to a urologist is indicated. He will probably do a cystoscopy and retrograde pyelography. He may also want to order a CT scan of the abdomen and pelvis and a renal biopsy. Renal angiography and aortography may be necessary to evaluate renovascular hypertension and renal embolism.

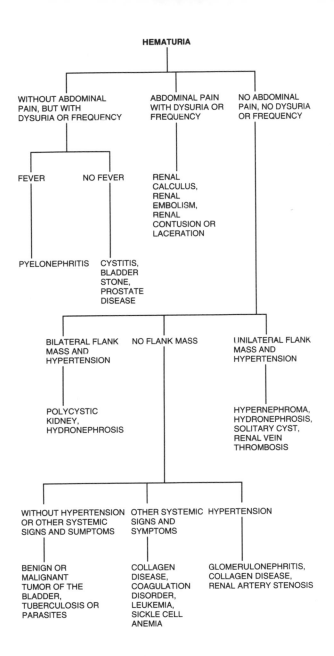

HEMIANOPSIA

Ask the following questions:

1. Is it intermittent? Intermittent hemianopsia, whether it is bitemporal or homonymous in type, would suggest migraine, carotid artery insufficiency, or vertebral basilar artery insufficiency.
2. Is the hemianopsia of sudden or gradual onset? Sudden onset of hemianopsia would suggest a vascular disorder such as cerebral thrombosis, embolism, or hemorrhage, but it may also suggest multiple sclerosis or a ruptured aneurysm. Gradual onset of hemianopsia would suggest a space-occupying lesion.
3. What type of hemianopsia is it? A bitemporal hemianopsia often suggests a pituitary tumor, especially if there are endocrine changes, but it may also be due to an aneurysm compressing the optic chiasm. Homonymous hemianopsia suggests involvement of the optic tract or occipital cortex. This may be by a space-occupying lesion, an aneurysm, arterial thrombosis, an embolism, or a hemorrhage.
4. Are there long tract signs? Neurologic signs of pyramidal tract involvement or posterior column involvement would suggest anterior or middle cerebral artery occlusion, epidural hematoma, or multiple sclerosis if it is acute and compression of the cortex by a subdural hematoma or brain tumor if it is chronic.
5. Are there endocrine changes? The presence of weight loss, hair loss, or diabetes insipidus would suggest a chromophobe adenoma of the pituitary. On the other hand, a protruding jaw, enlargement of the hands and fingers, and hypertrophy of the other tissues suggest acromegaly.
6. Is there macular sparing? The presence of macular sparing suggests that the lesion is in the optic cortex. This is most often a space-occupying lesion.

DIAGNOSTIC WORKUP

Referral to an ophthalmologist for a thorough visual field examination is suggested at the outset. A neurology consultation also needs to be obtained. The neurologist will probably order a CT scan of the brain to rule out a space-occupying lesion unless multiple sclerosis is suspected.

If multiple sclerosis is suspected, MRI would be the study of choice, even though it is more expensive. In addition, visual evoked potential studies and spinal fluid analysis may be ordered to rule out multiple sclerosis.

A carotid duplex scan will help diagnose carotid vascular insufficiency, but four-vessel cerebral angiography will most likely be done so that both carotid and vertebral basilar artery disease can be evaluated. If there are endocrine changes, an endocrinologist should be consulted.

If a cerebral embolism is suspected, a source for the embolism should be looked for. A cardiologist can best determine what tests to order to search for an embolic source.

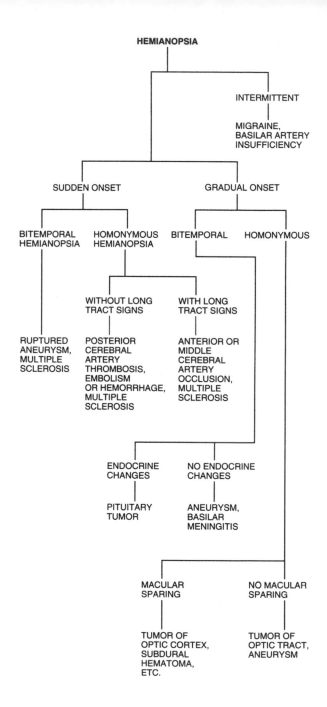

HEMIPARESIS/HEMIPLEGIA

Ask the following questions:

1. Is it intermittent? Intermittent hemiparesis or hemiplegia would suggest migraine or transient ischemic attacks from basilar artery or carotid artery disease.

2. Is it sudden or gradual in onset? Sudden onset of hemiparesis would suggest a cerebral thrombosis, hemorrhage, or embolism. However, contusion or concussion of the spinal cord can occasionally produce a sudden onset of hemiparesis or hemiplegia. If there is a history of trauma, a subdural or epidural hematoma must be suspected. Gradual onset of hemiparesis or hemiplegia would suggest a space-occupying lesion.

3. Is there facial paralysis or other cranial nerve signs? If there is a central facial palsy or other cranial nerve signs, one would look for a lesion above the foramen magnum (i.e., in the brain). If there are no cranial nerve signs, a spinal cord lesion should be suspected.

4. Is there a fever? The presence of fever should suggest a cerebral abscess, venous sinus thrombosis, or encephalitis.

5. Is there a history of trauma? The history of trauma with hemiparesis or hemiplegia would suggest a subdural, epidural hematoma or a hemorrhage in the brain itself.

6. Is there a history of hypertension? The history of hypertension along with hemiparesis or hemiplegia suggests a cerebral hemorrhage. However, a cerebral thrombosis or cerebral aneurysm may also occur with a history of hypertension.

7. Is there auricular fibrillation or another embolic source? The presence of auricular fibrillation, cardiac murmur, or other signs of an embolic source would suggest a cerebral embolism.

DIAGNOSTIC WORKUP

A neurologist should be consulted at the outset because he can best determine what type of imaging study should be done. A spinal tap is no longer done without first doing an imaging study. Carotid scans can be done to rule out carotid artery insufficiency. Four vessel cerebral angiography may be indicated, especially in transient ischemic attacks. Electrocardiography, echocardiography, and blood cultures will help identify an embolic source, but a cardiologist should be consulted to investigate this further. Somatosensory evoked potentials, brain stem evoked potentials, and visual evoked potential studies along with a spinal tap will help diagnose multiple sclerosis.

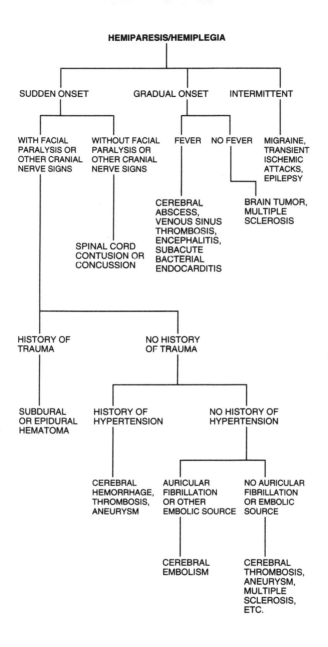

HEMIPARESIS/HEMIPLEGIA

SUDDEN ONSET

GRADUAL ONSET

INTERMITTENT

WITH FACIAL PARALYSIS OR OTHER CRANIAL NERVE SIGNS

WITHOUT FACIAL PARALYSIS OR OTHER CRANIAL NERVE SIGNS

FEVER

NO FEVER

MIGRAINE, TRANSIENT ISCHEMIC ATTACKS, EPILEPSY

CEREBRAL ABSCESS, VENOUS SINUS THROMBOSIS, ENCEPHALITIS, SUBACUTE BACTERIAL ENDOCARDITIS

BRAIN TUMOR, MULTIPLE SCLEROSIS

SPINAL CORD CONTUSION OR CONCUSSION

HISTORY OF TRAUMA

NO HISTORY OF TRAUMA

SUBDURAL OR EPIDURAL HEMATOMA

HISTORY OF HYPERTENSION

NO HISTORY OF HYPERTENSION

CEREBRAL HEMORRHAGE, THROMBOSIS, ANEURYSM

AURICULAR FIBRILLATION OR OTHER EMBOLIC SOURCE

NO AURICULAR FIBRILLATION OR EMBOLIC SOURCE

CEREBRAL EMBOLISM

CEREBRAL THROMBOSIS, ANEURYSM, MULTIPLE SCLEROSIS, ETC.

Hemiparesis/Hemiplegia   275

HEMOPTYSIS

Ask the following questions:

1. Is there chest pain? If there is chest pain along with the hemoptysis, one should suspect a pulmonary embolism.
2. Is there fever and/or purulent sputum? The presence of fever and purulent sputum suggests pneumonia, lung abscess, tuberculosis, and bronchiectasis. However, bronchiectasis does not usually occur with fever.
3. Is there dyspnea, cardiomegaly, or a heart murmur? These findings suggest congestive heart failure or mitral stenosis.
4. Is there copious sputum? The presence of copious sputum should suggest bronchiectasis or lung abscess. If there is fever along with it, lung abscess is more likely. Copious foamy sputum suggests congestive heart failure.

DIAGNOSTIC WORKUP

Routine diagnostic tests include a CBC, sedimentation rate, chemistry panel, coagulation profile, sputum smear, culture and sensitivity, a chest x-ray, and an EKG.

If a pulmonary embolism or infarction is suspected, arterial blood gases and a ventilation-perfusion scan should be ordered. In some cases a pulmonary angiogram may be necessary.

If tuberculosis is suspected, one should order a sputum or gastric washings for acid-fast bacilli (AFB) smear, culture, and guinea pig inoculation. A tuberculin test should also be done. Apical lordotic views of the lung as well as lateral and oblique views may help identify a tuberculous cavity. There are serologic tests for antibodies against specific mycobacterial antigens.

Sputum cultures for fungi and skin tests for the various fungi may need to be done. If congestive heart failure is suspected, venous pressure and circulation time should be measured and a pulmonary function test should be done. Echocardiography will help diagnose mitral stenosis.

A consultation with a pulmonologist and bronchoscopy need to be done if bronchogenic carcinoma or bronchiectasis is suspected. Other studies that are helpful in diagnosing bronchogenic carcinoma are sputa for Papanicolaou smear, transbronchial needle biopsy, and tomography. A bronchogram will be helpful in diagnosing bronchiectasis and foreign bodies.

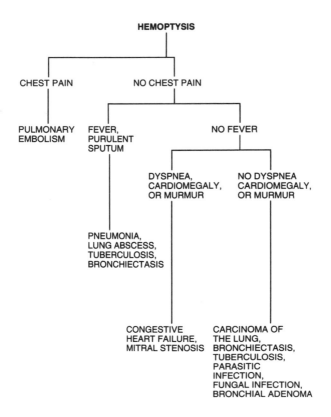

HEMORRHOIDS

Hemorrhoids are dilated perianal veins which become thrombosed or can rupture producing subcutaneous or submucosal hematomas. They are usually due to chronic constipation, but may be the cause of constipation also. While they are usually considered to be a disease, it is important to remember that they may be a sign of cirrhosis of the liver and other conditions associated with portal hypertension. As such, they may point to the diagnosis of esophageal varices in cases of hematemesis and their absence would make this diagnosis unlikely.

HEPATOMEGALY

Ask the following questions:

1. Is there jaundice? Hepatomegaly with jaundice may make one think of hemolytic anemias; toxic or infectious hepatitis; bile duct obstruction due to stones, carcinoma of the pancreas, or ampulla of Vater; and biliary cirrhosis.
2. Is there fever? Hepatomegaly with fever should make one think of viral hepatitis, infectious mononucleosis, ascending cholangitis, and other infectious diseases.
3. Is there splenomegaly? Hepatomegaly and splenomegaly should make one think of alcoholic cirrhosis, amyloidosis, reticuloendotheliosis, various hemolytic anemias, biliary cirrhosis, and myeloid metaplasia. It should also make one think of various parasitic diseases.
4. Is there an enlarged gallbladder? The presence of hepatomegaly with jaundice and enlarged gallbladder is characteristic of bile duct obstruction due to carcinoma of the pancreas, bile ducts, or ampulla of Vater. The clinician should remember that hydrops of the gallbladder with a common duct stone can mimic the same clinical presentation.
5. Is the splenomegaly massive? Massive splenomegaly is characteristic of Gaucher's disease, kala azar, and myeloid metaplasia. Occasionally, other forms of reticuloendotheliosis may also be associated with massive splenomegaly.
6. Is there another abdominal mass? The presence of another abdominal mass suggests metastatic carcinoma.
7. Is the liver tender? Tenderness of the liver is seen with viral or toxic hepatitis, congestive heart failure, and ascending cholangitis.

DIAGNOSTIC WORKUP

Routine diagnostic studies include a CBC, sedimentation rate, antinuclear antibody test, Monospot test, chemistry panel, chest x-ray, EKG, and flat plate of the abdomen.

If viral hepatitis is suspected, a hepatitis profile should be ordered. If congestive heart failure is suspected, a venous pressure and circulation time and pulmonary function tests should be done. A CT scan of the abdomen will assist in the diagnosis of metastatic carcinoma and often find a primary source for the metastasis. Metastatic neoplasms and the various forms of cirrhosis may be diagnosed by liver biopsy, but one should keep in mind that it is dangerous to do a liver biopsy if biliary cirrhosis is suspected. Gallbladder ultrasound or cholecystography should be done if cholecystitis and cholelithiasis are suspected. Transhepatic cholangiography or endoscopic retrograde cholangiopancreatography (ERCP) may need to be done.

The various infectious diseases will need antibody titers and skin tests to pin down the diagnosis. For example, a brucellin antibody titer or a Monospot test can be done. Skin tests for the various fungi and tuberculosis can be done.

The various hemolytic anemias may be diagnosed by blood smears, a sickle cell preparation, serum haptoglobin, and hemoglobin electrophoresis. The reticuloendothelioses require liver biopsy. Hemochromatosis is also diagnosed by liver biopsy, but a test for serum iron and iron binding capacity should also be done. Wilson's disease is diagnosed by serum copper and ceruloplasmin tests. Venography will diagnose hepatic vein thrombosis.

Most physicians prefer to refer the patient with hepatomegaly to a gastroenterologist once the preliminary studies have been done. This would be the most cost-effective approach.

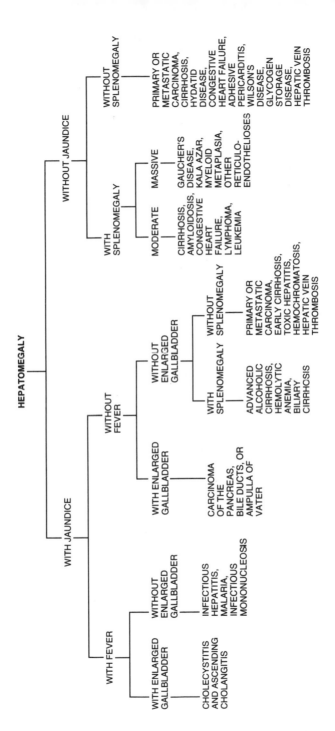

HEPATOMEGALY

- WITH JAUNDICE
  - WITH FEVER
    - WITH ENLARGED GALLBLADDER
      - CHOLECYSTITIS AND ASCENDING CHOLANGITIS
    - WITHOUT ENLARGED GALLBLADDER
      - INFECTIOUS HEPATITIS, MALARIA, INFECTIOUS MONONUCLEOSIS
  - WITHOUT FEVER
    - WITH ENLARGED GALLBLADDER
      - CARCINOMA OF THE PANCREAS, BILE DUCTS, OR AMPULLA OF VATER
    - WITHOUT ENLARGED GALLBLADDER
      - WITH SPLENOMEGALY
        - ADVANCED ALCOHOLIC CIRRHOSIS, HEMOLYTIC ANEMIA, BILIARY CIRRHOSIS
      - WITHOUT SPLENOMEGALY
        - PRIMARY OR METASTATIC CARCINOMA, EARLY CIRRHOSIS, TOXIC HEPATITIS, HEMOCHROMATOSIS, HEPATIC VEIN THROMBOSIS
- WITHOUT JAUNDICE
  - WITH SPLENOMEGALY
    - MODERATE
      - CIRRHOSIS, AMYLOIDOSIS, CONGESTIVE HEART FAILURE, LYMPHOMA, LEUKEMIA
    - MASSIVE
      - GAUCHER'S DISEASE, KALA AZAR, MYELOID METAPLASIA, OTHER RETICULO-ENDOTHELIOSES
  - WITHOUT SPLENOMEGALY
    - PRIMARY OR METASTATIC CARCINOMA, CIRRHOSIS, HYDATID DISEASE, CONGESTIVE HEART FAILURE, ADHESIVE PERICARDITIS, WILSON'S DISEASE, GLYCOGEN STORAGE DISEASE, HEPATIC VEIN THROMBOSIS

Hepatomegaly   281

HICCUPS

Ask the following questions:

1. Is there a history of alcoholism? Alcoholic gastritis is a frequent cause of hiccups.
2. Is there a fever? The presence of fever should make one think of pneumonia with pleurisy, pericarditis, subdiaphragmatic abscess, and peritonitis. It should also make one think of epidemic hiccups.
3. Is there heartburn or regurgitation? The presence of heartburn and regurgitation should make one think of a hiatal hernia and esophagitis.
4. Is there a mediastinal mass? Because they irritate the phrenic nerve, mediastinal masses such as Hodgkin's disease, bronchogenic carcinoma, and esophageal carcinoma may cause hiccups.
5. Are there abnormalities on neurologic examination? Hiccups may occur in tabes dorsalis, syringomyelia, encephalitis, chorea, and cerebral hemorrhage.

DIAGNOSTIC WORKUP

The basic workup includes a CBC, sedimentation rate, chemistry panel, a VDRL test, tuberculin test, EKG, chest x-ray, and a flat plate of the abdomen. If these are negative, an upper GI series and esophagram should be done.

If there is still confusion at this point, a gastroenterologist should be consulted before ordering other expensive diagnostic tests. He will probably do an esophagoscopy, gastroscopy, and duodenoscopy and may order a CT scan of the abdomen and mediastinum. A Bernstein test may help diagnose reflux esophagitis. Esophageal manometry and pH monitoring of the distal esophagus may also help in this regard.

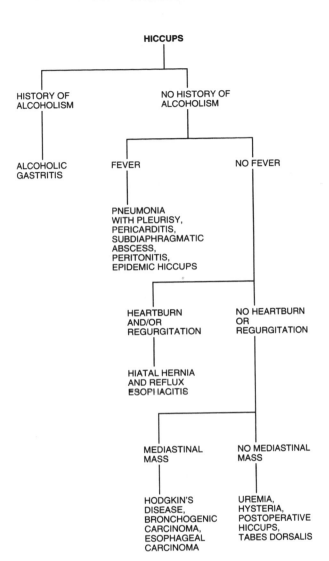

HICCUPS

- **HISTORY OF ALCOHOLISM**
  - **ALCOHOLIC GASTRITIS**
- **NO HISTORY OF ALCOHOLISM**
  - **FEVER**
    - **PNEUMONIA WITH PLEURISY, PERICARDITIS, SUBDIAPHRAGMATIC ABSCESS, PERITONITIS, EPIDEMIC HICCUPS**
  - **NO FEVER**
    - **HEARTBURN AND/OR REGURGITATION**
      - **HIATAL HERNIA AND REFLUX ESOPHAGITIS**
    - **NO HEARTBURN OR REGURGITATION**
      - **MEDIASTINAL MASS**
        - **HODGKIN'S DISEASE, BRONCHOGENIC CARCINOMA, ESOPHAGEAL CARCINOMA**
      - **NO MEDIASTINAL MASS**
        - **UREMIA, HYSTERIA, POSTOPERATIVE HICCUPS, TABES DORSALIS**

HIP PAIN

Ask the following questions:

1. Is there a positive straight leg raising test or other neurologic signs? The presence of positive straight leg raising tests or other neurologic signs would suggest a herniated disk, a cauda equina tumor, or other neurologic disorders of the lumbar spine. Meralgia paresthetica will cause characteristic loss of sensation in the distribution of the lateral femoral cutaneous nerve.
2. Is there a positive Patrick's test or limitation of the range of motion of the hip? These findings suggest a greater trochanter bursitis or hip joint pathology such as fracture, osteoarthritis, rheumatoid arthritis, metastasis, slipped femoral epiphysis, Legg-Perthes disease, rheumatic fever, or transient synovitis.
3. Is there tenderness of the greater trochanter bursa? Tenderness of the greater trochanter bursa will help differentiate greater trochanter bursitis. It is also seen in hysteria.
4. Is the patient a child or an adult? If the patient is a child, transient synovitis, slipped femoral epiphysis, Legg-Perthes disease, and rheumatic fever should be considered. If the patient is an adult, it is more likely that the problem is osteoarthritis, a fracture, rheumatoid arthritis, metastasis, or avascular necrosis.
5. Is there a history of trauma? A history of trauma would suggest that there is a fracture or a sprain of the hip joint, but the clinician should remember that a fracture in the elderly often occurs with no history of trauma.

DIAGNOSTIC WORKUP

A CBC, sedimentation rate, chemistry panel, arthritis panel, tuberculin test, and x-rays of the lumbosacral spine and hip will diagnose 90% of the cases. These are relatively expensive in comparison to MRI. A serum protein electrophoresis will help diagnose multiple myeloma. A trigger point injection of the greater trochanter bursa or ischiogluteal bursa will assist in the diagnosis of these conditions. An orthopedic surgeon should be consulted before ordering MRI of the lumbar spine or hip. However, MRI is especially important if the diagnosis of avascular necrosis is suspected.

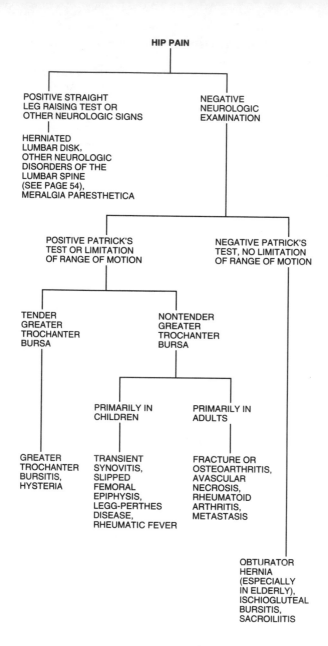

HIP PAIN

POSITIVE STRAIGHT LEG RAISING TEST OR OTHER NEUROLOGIC SIGNS

HERNIATED LUMBAR DISK, OTHER NEUROLOGIC DISORDERS OF THE LUMBAR SPINE (SEE PAGE 54), MERALGIA PARESTHETICA

NEGATIVE NEUROLOGIC EXAMINATION

POSITIVE PATRICK'S TEST OR LIMITATION OF RANGE OF MOTION

NEGATIVE PATRICK'S TEST, NO LIMITATION OF RANGE OF MOTION

TENDER GREATER TROCHANTER BURSA

NONTENDER GREATER TROCHANTER BURSA

PRIMARILY IN CHILDREN

PRIMARILY IN ADULTS

GREATER TROCHANTER BURSITIS, HYSTERIA

TRANSIENT SYNOVITIS, SLIPPED FEMORAL EPIPHYSIS, LEGG-PERTHES DISEASE, RHEUMATIC FEVER

FRACTURE OR OSTEOARTHRITIS, AVASCULAR NECROSIS, RHEUMATOID ARTHRITIS, METASTASIS

OBTURATOR HERNIA (ESPECIALLY IN ELDERLY), ISCHIOGLUTEAL BURSITIS, SACROILIITIS

HIRSUTISM

Ask the following questions:

1. Is there clitoral enlargement or other signs of virilism? These findings would suggest an ovarian tumor, an adrenal tumor or hyperplasia, chromosome mosaicism, and true hermaphroditism, which is rare.
2. Is there obesity? The presence of obesity and hirsutism should bring to mind Cushing's syndrome. However, it is also a sign of polycystic ovaries.
3. Is there a history of the use of the steroids or other drugs? Adrenocortical steroids, testosterone, phenytoin, minoxidil, and diazoxide are just a few of the drugs that may cause hirsutism.
4. Is there an ovarian mass? The presence of an ovarian mass should make one think of polycystic ovaries, an arrhenoblastoma, or granulosis cell tumor.

DIAGNOSTIC WORKUP

The routine diagnostic workup includes a serum free testosterone, free cortisol, prolactin, a skull x-ray (much more economical than a CT scan or MRI of the brain), and a urinary gonadotrophin assay. Pelvic ultrasound and CT scan of the abdomen would complete the workup, but why order these expensive diagnostic tests before consulting a gynecologist or endocrinologist?

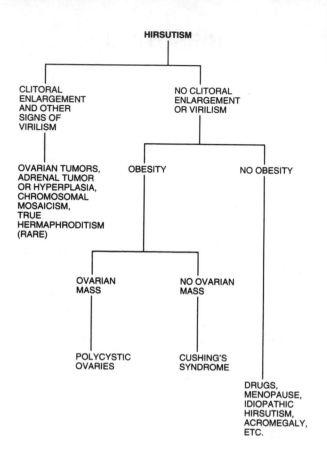

HIRSUTISM

- CLITORAL ENLARGEMENT AND OTHER SIGNS OF VIRILISM
  - OVARIAN TUMORS, ADRENAL TUMOR OR HYPERPLASIA, CHROMOSOMAL MOSAICISM, TRUE HERMAPHRODITISM (RARE)
- NO CLITORAL ENLARGEMENT OR VIRILISM
  - OBESITY
    - OVARIAN MASS
      - POLYCYSTIC OVARIES
    - NO OVARIAN MASS
      - CUSHING'S SYNDROME
  - NO OBESITY
    - DRUGS, MENOPAUSE, IDIOPATHIC HIRSUTISM, ACROMEGALY, ETC.

HOARSENESS

Ask the following questions:

1. Is it acute? Acute hoarseness is usually due to a viral upper respiratory infection, but acute simple laryngitis and acute subglottic laryngitis or rarely laryngeal diphtheria may be responsible. Simple strain may be responsible due to the patient's occupation.
2. Is it intermittent? Intermittent hoarseness would suggest myasthenia gravis, urticaria, occupational causes, reflux esophagitis, tobacco, and alcoholism.
3. Are there abnormalities on the neurologic examination? If there are other abnormalities on the neurologic examination, one should consider peripheral neuropathy, poliomyelitis, Guillain-Barré syndrome, brain stem tumors, and cerebrovascular disease.
4. Are there abnormalities on the laryngoscopic examination? Laryngoscopy will identify many intrinsic lesions of the vocal cords such as carcinoma, singer's nodes, polyps, tuberculosis, or syphilis. It will also identify vocal cord paralysis due to carcinoma of the lung, aortic aneurysm, cardiac enlargement, or other mediastinal tumors.

   A normal laryngoscopic examination would suggest hysteria, myxedema, or acromegaly.

DIAGNOSTIC WORKUP

Acute hoarseness will require only a CBC, sedimentation rate, nose and throat culture, and sputum culture if sputum is available. A chest x-ray may also be ordered. Laryngoscopic examination is rarely necessary unless the acute hoarseness becomes chronic.

The laryngoscopic examination is the single most important test for chronic hoarseness. It will identify most intrinsic lesions. If vocal cord paralysis is found, a chest x-ray and possibly a CT scan of the mediastinum may be ordered. However, an ear, nose and throat specialist should be consulted before ordering these expensive tests. If there are other neurologic abnormalities, a referral to a neurologist should be made before ordering a CT scan or MRI of the brain. In cases of intermittent hoarseness, a Tensilon test or acetylcholine receptor antibody titer should be done.

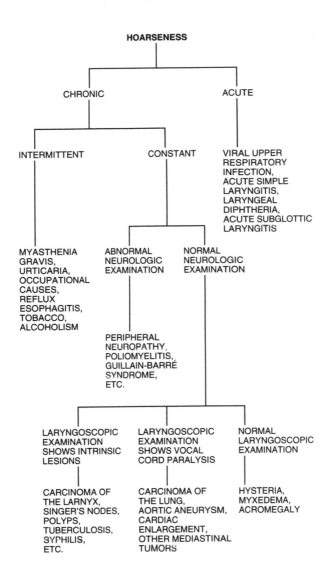

HORNER'S SYNDROME

Ask the following questions:

1. Is there pain in the ipsilateral upper extremity? If there is pain in the ipsilateral upper extremity, one should consider brachial plexus neuritis, thoracic outlet syndrome, Pancoast's tumor, and spinal cord tumor.
2. Is there hemiplegia or other long tract neurologic signs? If there is hemiplegia or other long tract signs, one should consider carotid artery thrombosis, Wallenberg's syndrome, or syringomyelia.
3. Is there a mediastinal mass? A chest x-ray or an imaging study may be necessary to disclose a mediastinal mass, but this will establish the diagnosis of Horner's syndrome and carcinoma of the lung, lymphoma, aortic aneurysms, and mediastinitis. If there is no pain in the extremities and the neurologic examination is normal and there is no mediastinal mass, one should consider the possibility of migraine and histamine headaches.

DIAGNOSTIC WORKUP

A neurologist should probably be consulted at the outset. If there is pain in the upper extremities along with the Horner's syndrome, x-rays of the chest should be done to rule out a Pancoast's tumor and x-rays of the cervical spine should be done to rule out a cervical rib. Nerve conduction velocity studies, somatosensory evoked potential studies, and electromyograms of the upper extremities may help diagnosis a brachial plexus neuralgia. MRI will be necessary to diagnose a tumor of the cervical spinal cord.

If there is hemiplegia or other long tract neurologic signs, then a CT scan or MRI of the brain or cervical spinal cord needs to be done. If these tests are negative and there is an isolated Horner's syndrome, a CT scan of the mediastinum should be ordered. Esophagrams, aortography, and mediastinoscopy may all be necessary to establish the diagnosis in difficult cases.

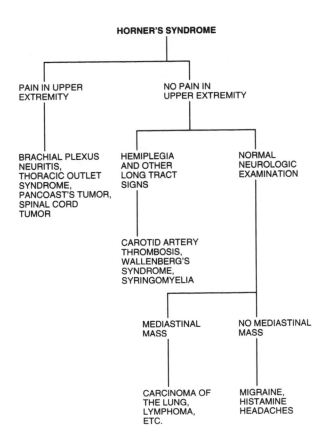

HORNER'S SYNDROME

PAIN IN UPPER EXTREMITY

NO PAIN IN UPPER EXTREMITY

BRACHIAL PLEXUS NEURITIS, THORACIC OUTLET SYNDROME, PANCOAST'S TUMOR, SPINAL CORD TUMOR

HEMIPLEGIA AND OTHER LONG TRACT SIGNS

NORMAL NEUROLOGIC EXAMINATION

CAROTID ARTERY THROMBOSIS, WALLENBERG'S SYNDROME, SYRINGOMYELIA

MEDIASTINAL MASS

NO MEDIASTINAL MASS

CARCINOMA OF THE LUNG, LYMPHOMA, ETC.

MIGRAINE, HISTAMINE HEADACHES

HYPERACTIVE REFLEXES

Ask the following questions:

1. Are they intermittent or persistent? If the hyperactive reflexes are intermittent, one should consider multiple sclerosis and cerebral vascular insufficiency.
2. Are they focal? If the hyperactive reflexes are focal, and especially if they are unilateral, one should consider vascular diseases, space-occupying lesions, or multiple sclerosis. Certain degenerative diseases such as amyotrophic lateral sclerosis may also present with focal hyperactive reflexes.
3. If the hyperactive reflexes are focal, are they unilateral? Unilateral hyperactive reflexes are characteristic of hemiplegia. Hemiplegia is usually associated with a cerebral vascular disease or space-occupying lesion of the brain, especially if there are cranial nerve signs. However, early spinal cord tumors may present with unilateral hyperactive reflexes.
4. Are there cranial nerve signs? The presence of cranial nerve signs suggests that the lesion is above the foramen magnum and a cerebral or brain stem tumor is the first thing to be considered. A cerebral vascular lesion or multiple sclerosis must also be considered.
5. Is there dementia? The presence of dementia along with the hyperactive reflexes, especially if they are diffuse, suggests Alzheimer's disease, Pick's disease, general paresis, and Korsakoff's syndrome. There are many other causes of dementia to consider.
6. Are there other long tract signs? The presence of hyperactive reflexes with sensory changes should suggest pernicious anemia, syringomyelia, and Friedreich's ataxia. It may also indicate multiple sclerosis, a spinal cord tumor, a brain stem tumor, or basilar artery insufficiency.

DIAGNOSTIC WORKUP

Hyperactive reflexes, especially if they are unilateral, are a clear indication for an imaging study. It is wise to consult a neurologist or neurosurgeon before determining which imaging study to order. If there are cranial nerve findings and dementia, a CT scan or MRI of the brain should be ordered.

If there are hyperactive reflexes of all four extremities without dementia or cranial nerve signs, MRI of the cervical spine would probably be the most appropriate procedure. It may, however, be necessary to get a CT scan or MRI of the brain anyway.

If only the lower extremities are involved, MRI of the thoracic cord would probably be most appropriate, but then MRI of the cervical spine should be done if the thoracic MRI is negative. Spinal fluid analysis will help diagnose multiple sclerosis, central nervous system syphilis, cerebral hemorrhages, or abscess. A CBC, serum B_{12} and folic acid, and Schilling test will help diagnose pernicious anemia. Plain films of the appropriate level of the spine are necessary in trauma cases. An electroencephalogram and psychometric testing should be done in cases of dementia. Somatosensory evoked potential studies, visual evoked potentials, and brain stem evoked potentials are helpful in diagnosing multiple sclerosis. Carotid duplex scans and four-vessel angiography may be necessary for diagnosing cerebral vascular disease.

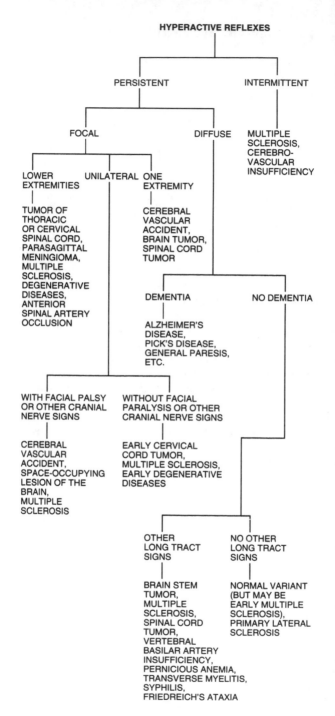

HYPERACTIVE REFLEXES

PERSISTENT

INTERMITTENT

FOCAL

DIFFUSE

MULTIPLE SCLEROSIS, CEREBRO-VASCULAR INSUFFICIENCY

LOWER EXTREMITIES

TUMOR OF THORACIC OR CERVICAL SPINAL CORD, PARASAGITTAL MENINGIOMA, MULTIPLE SCLEROSIS, DEGENERATIVE DISEASES, ANTERIOR SPINAL ARTERY OCCLUSION

UNILATERAL ONE EXTREMITY

CEREBRAL VASCULAR ACCIDENT, BRAIN TUMOR, SPINAL CORD TUMOR

DEMENTIA

ALZHEIMER'S DISEASE, PICK'S DISEASE, GENERAL PARESIS, ETC.

NO DEMENTIA

WITH FACIAL PALSY OR OTHER CRANIAL NERVE SIGNS

CEREBRAL VASCULAR ACCIDENT, SPACE-OCCUPYING LESION OF THE BRAIN, MULTIPLE SCLEROSIS

WITHOUT FACIAL PARALYSIS OR OTHER CRANIAL NERVE SIGNS

EARLY CERVICAL CORD TUMOR, MULTIPLE SCLEROSIS, EARLY DEGENERATIVE DISEASES

OTHER LONG TRACT SIGNS

BRAIN STEM TUMOR, MULTIPLE SCLEROSIS, SPINAL CORD TUMOR, VERTEBRAL BASILAR ARTERY INSUFFICIENCY, PERNICIOUS ANEMIA, TRANSVERSE MYELITIS, SYPHILIS, FRIEDREICH'S ATAXIA

NO OTHER LONG TRACT SIGNS

NORMAL VARIANT (BUT MAY BE EARLY MULTIPLE SCLEROSIS), PRIMARY LATERAL SCLEROSIS

HYPERKINESIS

Ask the following questions:

1. Is there a positive drug history? Phenothiazines, amphetamines, tricyclic drugs, lithium, and other substances may cause hyperkinesis.
2. Is there a tremor, a goiter, or tachycardia? The findings would suggest hyperthyroidism.
3. Are there other neurologic signs and symptoms? The presence of other neurologic signs and symptoms would suggest Wilson's disease, Huntington's chorea, Sydenham's chorea, and Parkinson's disease. If there are no other neurologic signs and symptoms, one should look for an attention deficit disorder or Gilles de la Tourette's syndrome.

DIAGNOSTIC WORKUP

Routine studies include a CBC, sedimentation rate, antistreptolysin-O (ASO) titer, chemistry panel, urine drug screen, and a thyroid panel. A serum copper and ceruloplasmin will usually diagnose Wilson's disease. If all of the above studies are negative, MRI of the brain may be done to rule out tumors or degenerative disease of the nervous system, but why not consult a neurologist first? An EEG may identify epilepsy and brain damage. Referral to a psychiatrist or psychologist is made if all of the above studies are normal.

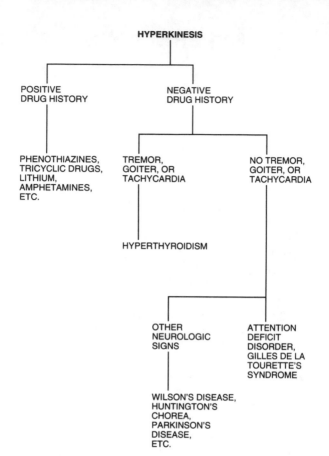

HYPERKINESIS

POSITIVE DRUG HISTORY

NEGATIVE DRUG HISTORY

PHENOTHIAZINES, TRICYCLIC DRUGS, LITHIUM, AMPHETAMINES, ETC.

TREMOR, GOITER, OR TACHYCARDIA

NO TREMOR, GOITER, OR TACHYCARDIA

HYPERTHYROIDISM

OTHER NEUROLOGIC SIGNS

ATTENTION DEFICIT DISORDER, GILLES DE LA TOURETTE'S SYNDROME

WILSON'S DISEASE, HUNTINGTON'S CHOREA, PARKINSON'S DISEASE, ETC.

HYPERPIGMENTATION

Ask the following questions:

1. Is there a history of drug ingestion? Argyria, arsenic poisoning, and methemoglobinemia are among the considerations in taking a drug history.
2. Is there hepatomegaly? The presence of hepatomegaly would make one think of hemochromatosis.
3. Is there significant weight loss? The presence of significant weight loss would suggest Addison's disease, pellagra, hyperthyroidism, or an ectopic hormone-secreting tumor.
4. Is there a history of seizures or neuropathy? The history of seizures or neuropathy should make one consider porphyria.

DIAGNOSTIC WORKUP

The serum iron and iron binding capacity should be measured to rule out hemochromatosis. A thyroid profile will exclude hyperthyroidism. A serum cortisol and cortisol stimulation test will identify Addison's disease. A urine for porphyrins and porphobilinogen will diagnose porphyria. A urine N-methyl niacinamide will help diagnose pellagra.

If there is still doubt after these studies are done, a liver biopsy may be done to rule out hemochromatosis and a CT scan of the abdomen will help identify Addison's disease.

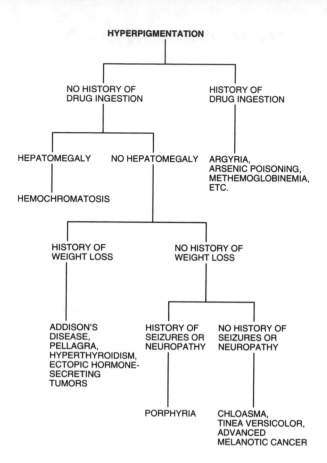

HYPERSOMNIA

Ask the following questions:

1. Is there a history of drug or alcohol use? Alcoholism and barbiturate intoxication are just two of the causes of hypersomnia.
2. Are there hallucinations, sleep paralysis, and cataplexy? These findings suggest narcolepsy.
3. Is there associated loss of appetite and/or libido? These findings suggest endogenous depression.
4. Are there abnormalities on the neurologic examination? Abnormal neurologic findings suggest multiple sclerosis, encephalitis, neurosyphilis, and other disorders.

DIAGNOSTIC WORKUP

The routine workup includes a CBC, sedimentation rate, chemistry panel, VDRL test, and urine drug screen. If there are abnormal neurologic signs, then MRI of the brain and spinal tap can be done, but it is advisable to consult a neurologist first. An EEG and sleep study complete the workup.

If all of the above studies are normal, referral to a psychiatrist would be in order.

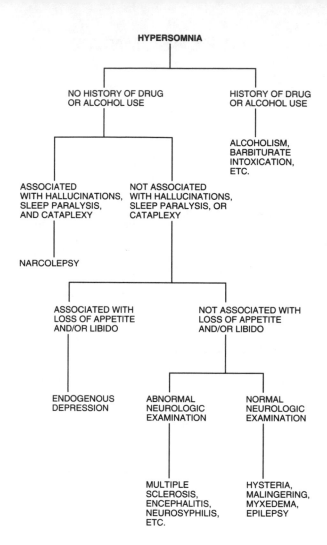

HYPERSOMNIA

NO HISTORY OF DRUG
OR ALCOHOL USE

HISTORY OF DRUG
OR ALCOHOL USE

ALCOHOLISM,
BARBITURATE
INTOXICATION,
ETC.

ASSOCIATED
WITH HALLUCINATIONS,
SLEEP PARALYSIS,
AND CATAPLEXY

NOT ASSOCIATED
WITH HALLUCINATIONS,
SLEEP PARALYSIS, OR
CATAPLEXY

NARCOLEPSY

ASSOCIATED WITH
LOSS OF APPETITE
AND/OR LIBIDO

NOT ASSOCIATED WITH
LOSS OF APPETITE
AND/OR LIBIDO

ENDOGENOUS
DEPRESSION

ABNORMAL
NEUROLOGIC
EXAMINATION

NORMAL
NEUROLOGIC
EXAMINATION

MULTIPLE
SCLEROSIS,
ENCEPHALITIS,
NEUROSYPHILIS,
ETC.

HYSTERIA,
MALINGERING,
MYXEDEMA,
EPILEPSY

HYPERTENSION

Ask the following questions:

1. Is there systolic hypertension only? The presence of an elevated systolic pressure only would suggest hyperthyroidism, aortic insufficiency, and atherosclerotic aortitis.
2. Is the hypertension paroxysmal? The presence of paroxysmal hypertension should suggest a pheochromocytoma.
3. Is there a blood pressure in the lower extremities? These findings would suggest a coarctation of the aorta.
4. Is there a flank mass? The presence of a flank mass should suggest hypernephroma, hydronephrosis, and polycystic kidneys.
5. Are there abnormalities of the urinary sediment? These findings suggest glomerulonephritis, collagen disease, Henoch-Schönlein purpura, and chronic nephritis. All primary care physicians should have this capability in their office.

DIAGNOSTIC WORKUP

Routine diagnostic tests include a CBC, sedimentation rate, chemistry panel, a VDRL test, urinalysis including microscopic, a urine culture with colony count and sensitivity, and an EKG, chest x-ray, and flat plate of the abdomen for kidney size.

If these are normal, a nephrologist should be consulted before undertaking expensive diagnostic tests. It may be wise to observe the results of treatment before further testing also.

Additional tests that may be ordered are an intravenous pyelogram, a 24-hr urine catecholamine, a serum cortisol, a plasma renin level, a 24-hr urine aldosterone determination, a cystoscopy, and retrograde pyelography. Renal angiography used to be done more frequently, but should be considered in sudden onset of hypertension in the elderly and in hypertension which is resistant to treatment.

Twenty-four hour blood pressure monitoring can be useful both in diagnosis and in evaluating the results of therapy.

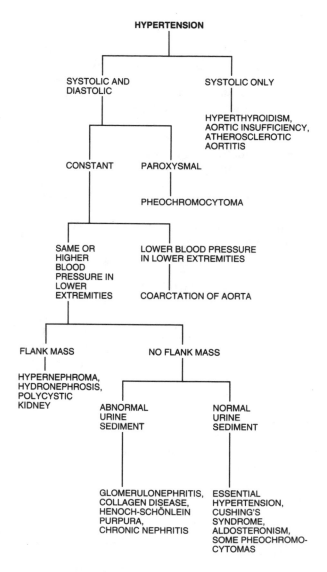

HYPOACTIVE REFLEXES

Ask the following questions:

1. Is it focal? Hypoactive reflexes limited to one extremity suggest a herniated disk, plexopathy, or early cauda equina or spinal cord tumor.
2. If focal, are the hypoactive reflexes involving both the upper and lower extremity? If the hypoactive reflexes are in both the upper and lower extremity on one side, this may be a normal phenomenon suggesting that the opposite side is pathologic. It may also be a finding in early cerebral vascular accident.
3. If the hypoactive reflexes are diffuse, was there a sudden onset? Sudden onset of hypoactive reflexes would suggest acute spinal cord conditions such as spinal fractures, transverse myelitis, Guillain-Barré syndrome, poliomyelitis, or acute central nervous system disorders such as toxic metabolic disease of the central nervous system, concussion, subdural hematoma, or acute increased intercranial pressure. Early basilar artery thrombosis may be associated with hypoactive reflexes also.
4. Are there other neurologic signs? The presence of other neurologic signs, particularly cranial nerve involvement, would suggest an early basilar artery thrombosis, cerebral vascular accident, or subdural hematoma. If there are no other neurologic findings or there is simply a disordered state of consciousness, then a head injury or toxic metabolic disease of the central nervous system, increased intercranial pressure, or poliomyelitis might be suspected.

DIAGNOSTIC WORKUP

Focal hypoactive reflexes of the lower extremity require plane x-rays of the lumbosacral spine, a CT scan or MRI of the lumbosacral spine, nerve conduction velocity and EMG studies. Dermatomal somatosensory evoked potential studies will occasionally show radiculopathy when EMGs are negative.

Hypoactive reflexes of one upper extremity can be worked up with x-rays of the cervical spine, MRI of the cervical spine, nerve conduction velocity studies, EMGs, and dermatomal somatosensory evoked potential studies. X-rays of the chest may be useful to rule out a Pancoast's tumor.

Diffuse hypoactive reflexes require a neuropathy workup (see page 425). A serum B_{12} and folic acid and possibly a Schilling test may need to be done to rule out pernicious anemia. An EMG and muscle biopsy may be done to rule out muscular dystrophy. A spinal tap will be helpful in cases of poliomyelitis and Guillain-Barré syndrome. If the hypoactive reflexes are part of a toxic metabolic or inflammatory disease of the nervous system, the workup will be similar to that of coma (page 100).

HYPOACTIVE REFLEXES

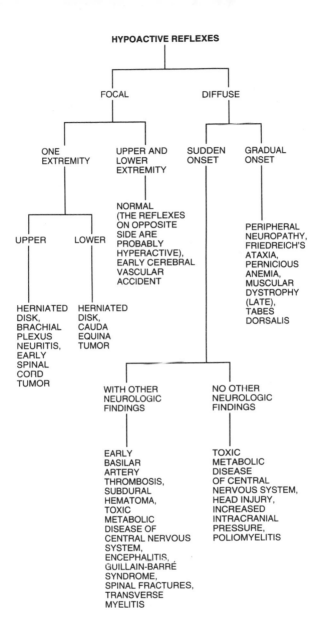

HYPOCHONDRIASIS

Ask the following questions:

1. Is there loss of libido and/or appetite? The findings of loss of libido and appetite would suggest endogenous depression. There may also be insomnia.
2. Is there loss of memory or concentration? These findings suggest the possibility of an organic brain syndrome or cerebral arteriosclerosis. Epilepsy may also be involved.
3. Does extensive testing fail to convince the patient he or she is well? If extensive testing fails to convince the patient he/she is well, then the diagnoses of delusional hypochondriasis and schizophrenia must be considered.

DIAGNOSTIC WORKUP

The diagnostic workup need not be extensive, but certain routine tests should be done. These include a CBC, sedimentation rate, chemistry panel, thyroid profile, EKG, chest x-ray, and flat plate of the abdomen. If there are complaints of memory loss and/or poor concentration, an EEG and CT scan of the brain may be done. A neurologist should be consulted. If the above tests fail to disclose an organic cause for the complaints and the patient is still not convinced he/she is well, referral to a psychiatrist is indicated.

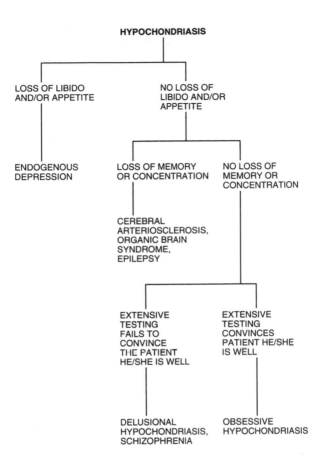

HYPOCHONDRIASIS

LOSS OF LIBIDO
AND/OR APPETITE

NO LOSS OF
LIBIDO AND/OR
APPETITE

ENDOGENOUS
DEPRESSION

LOSS OF MEMORY
OR CONCENTRATION

NO LOSS OF
MEMORY OR
CONCENTRATION

CEREBRAL
ARTERIOSCLEROSIS,
ORGANIC BRAIN
SYNDROME,
EPILEPSY

EXTENSIVE
TESTING
FAILS TO
CONVINCE
THE PATIENT
HE/SHE IS WELL

EXTENSIVE
TESTING
CONVINCES
PATIENT HE/SHE
IS WELL

DELUSIONAL
HYPOCHONDRIASIS,
SCHIZOPHRENIA

OBSESSIVE
HYPOCHONDRIASIS

Hypochondriasis   309

HYPOTENSION, CHRONIC

Ask the following questions:

1. Is the hypotension found only on standing? The finding of hypotension on standing suggests orthostatic hypotension, which may be due to several causes, including hypopituitarism, diabetic neuropathy, anemia, and various cardiovascular disorders.
2. Is there a history of drug ingestion? Many drugs induce hypotension, including nitroglycerin and its analogues, vasodilators, quinidine, and tricyclic drugs.
3. Is there cardiomegaly or a heart murmur? These findings suggest mitral valvular disease, aortic stenosis, and congestive heart failure.
4. Is there pallor? The findings of pallor suggest anemia.
5. Is there hyperpigmentation? The presence of hyperpigmentation suggests Addison's disease.

DIAGNOSTIC WORKUP

Routine studies include a CBC, sedimentation rate, chemistry panel, urinalysis, thyroid panel, EKG, and chest x-ray. Blood volume and arterial blood gas studies may be useful. If there is cardiomegaly or a murmur, echocardiography and venous pressure and circulation time should be done. A cardiologist should also be consulted.

If there is hyperpigmentation, a serum cortisol and cortisol stimulation test should be done. A skull x-ray can be done to rule out pituitary tumors. A visual field examination by a qualified ophthalmologist may be helpful in this regard also. Twenty-four hour blood pressure monitoring may be useful in the workup also.

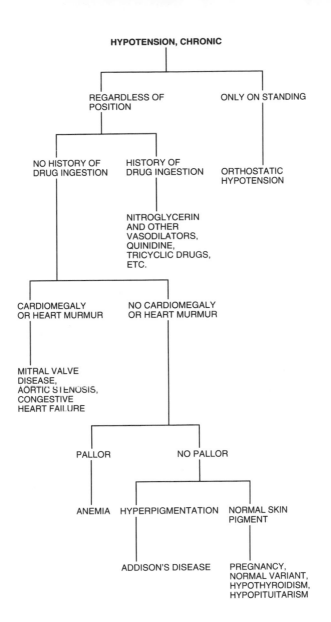

HYPOTENSION, CHRONIC

REGARDLESS OF POSITION

ONLY ON STANDING

NO HISTORY OF DRUG INGESTION

HISTORY OF DRUG INGESTION

ORTHOSTATIC HYPOTENSION

NITROGLYCERIN AND OTHER VASODILATORS, QUINIDINE, TRICYCLIC DRUGS, ETC.

CARDIOMEGALY OR HEART MURMUR

NO CARDIOMEGALY OR HEART MURMUR

MITRAL VALVE DISEASE, AORTIC STENOSIS, CONGESTIVE HEART FAILURE

PALLOR

NO PALLOR

ANEMIA

HYPERPIGMENTATION

NORMAL SKIN PIGMENT

ADDISON'S DISEASE

PREGNANCY, NORMAL VARIANT, HYPOTHYROIDISM, HYPOPITUITARISM

HYPOTHERMIA

Ask the following questions:

1. Is there a history of drug or alcohol ingestion? Alcoholic intoxication, opium poisoning, the tricyclic antidepressants, and phenothiazine may cause hypothermia.
2. Is there a history of severe vomiting or diarrhea? Severe vomiting or diarrhea may induce dehydration and electrolyte disturbances, which will induce hypothermia. Intestinal obstruction, cholera, and peritonitis are among the many disorders that may lead to severe vomiting or diarrhea.
3. Are there endocrine abnormalities? Signs of hypothyroidism and Addison's disease may be obvious, but hypopituitarism, hypoglycemia, and diabetes mellitus may also be the cause of hypothermia.
4. Are there abnormalities on the neurologic examination? Focal neurologic findings may be seen in a cerebral vascular accident, epidural or subdural hematoma. However, thiamine deficiency may also result in hypothermia.

DIAGNOSTIC WORKUP

Routine laboratory tests include a CBC and differential count, a sedimentation rate and chemistry panel, electrolytes, thyroid profile, blood cultures, urinalysis, and a urine drug screen. An EKG and chest x-ray should also be done. A CT scan of the brain is done if there are focal neurologic abnormalities or disorders of consciousness.

An infusion of dextrose intravenously and thiamine are given as soon as blood studies are drawn in case there is hypoglycemia or thiamine deficiency.

If the above studies are normal, a thorough endocrine workup is indicated, including tests for serum cortisol, follicle-stimulating hormone (FSH), lutein-stimulating hormone (LSH), and growth hormone. A cardiologist, neurologist, or endocrinologist may need to be consulted to help solve the diagnostic dilemma.

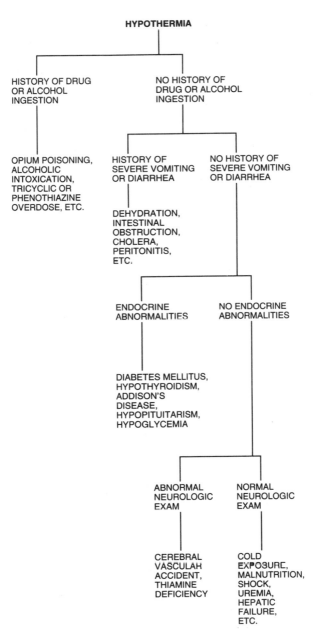

HYPOTHERMIA

HISTORY OF DRUG OR ALCOHOL INGESTION → OPIUM POISONING, ALCOHOLIC INTOXICATION, TRICYCLIC OR PHENOTHIAZINE OVERDOSE, ETC.

NO HISTORY OF DRUG OR ALCOHOL INGESTION

HISTORY OF SEVERE VOMITING OR DIARRHEA → DEHYDRATION, INTESTINAL OBSTRUCTION, CHOLERA, PERITONITIS, ETC.

NO HISTORY OF SEVERE VOMITING OR DIARRHEA

ENDOCRINE ABNORMALITIES → DIABETES MELLITUS, HYPOTHYROIDISM, ADDISON'S DISEASE, HYPOPITUITARISM, HYPOGLYCEMIA

NO ENDOCRINE ABNORMALITIES

ABNORMAL NEUROLOGIC EXAM → CEREBRAL VASCULAR ACCIDENT, THIAMINE DEFICIENCY

NORMAL NEUROLOGIC EXAM → COLD EXPOSURE, MALNUTRITION, SHOCK, UREMIA, HEPATIC FAILURE, ETC.

Hypothermia   313

IMPOTENCE

Ask the following questions:

1. Is there a history of alcohol or drug ingestion? A host of antihypertensive drugs including the beta-blockers may cause impotence. In addition, tricyclic drugs, nicotine, and alcohol intoxication may cause impotence.
2. Is there loss of secondary sex characteristics? These findings suggest Fröhlich's syndrome, Klinefelter's syndrome, and other congenital disorders.
3. Are there abnormalities on urologic examination? Various conditions such as Peyronie's disease, atrophied testes, prostatitis, and Leriche's syndrome may be found on urologic examination.
4. Are there abnormalities on the neurologic examination? Neurologic examination may reveal diabetic neuropathy, spinal cord tumor, multiple sclerosis, and other neurologic disorders.

DIAGNOSTIC WORKUP

Routine tests include a CBC and differential count, a urinalysis, a urine culture and colony count, a chemistry panel, VDRL test, thyroid profile, serum testosterone, and gonadotrophin assay. A referral to a urologist is probably wise at this point. He will work up the patient further with a nocturnal tumescent study and penile blood pressure studies. In addition, he may want to do a cystoscopy.

Nerve conduction velocity studies and EMGs may be needed to rule out diabetic neuropathy. Magnetic resonance imaging of the spine, cystometric studies, and somatosensory evoked potential studies will help to rule out multiple sclerosis and other spinal cord lesions. A spinal tap may help rule out central nervous system lues. Angiography may be needed to exclude a Leriche's syndrome.

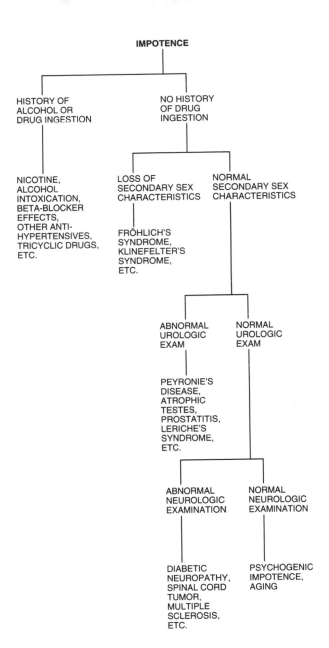

IMPOTENCE

- **HISTORY OF ALCOHOL OR DRUG INGESTION**
  - NICOTINE, ALCOHOL INTOXICATION, BETA-BLOCKER EFFECTS, OTHER ANTI-HYPERTENSIVES, TRICYCLIC DRUGS, ETC.

- **NO HISTORY OF DRUG INGESTION**
  - **LOSS OF SECONDARY SEX CHARACTERISTICS**
    - FRÖHLICH'S SYNDROME, KLINEFELTER'S SYNDROME, ETC.
  - **NORMAL SECONDARY SEX CHARACTERISTICS**
    - **ABNORMAL UROLOGIC EXAM**
      - PEYRONIE'S DISEASE, ATROPHIC TESTES, PROSTATITIS, LERICHE'S SYNDROME, ETC.
    - **NORMAL UROLOGIC EXAM**
      - **ABNORMAL NEUROLOGIC EXAMINATION**
        - DIABETIC NEUROPATHY, SPINAL CORD TUMOR, MULTIPLE SCLEROSIS, ETC.
      - **NORMAL NEUROLOGIC EXAMINATION**
        - PSYCHOGENIC IMPOTENCE, AGING

INCONTINENCE OF FECES

Ask the following questions:

1. Is the stool volume small or large? A small volume of stool should suggest anal fissure; hemorrhoids, diarrhea, or postoperative incontinence from a fistulectomy; or other types of surgery in the perirectal area.
2. Is the incontinence intermittent? Intermittent incontinence suggests epilepsy or organic brain syndrome.
3. Are there hyperactive reflexes in the lower extremities? Presence of hyperactive reflexes in the lower extremities should suggest a spinal cord tumor or trauma to the spinal cord, multiple sclerosis, a parasagittal meningioma, transverse myelitis, and syringomyelia.
4. Are there hypoactive reflexes in the lower extremities? The presence of hypoactive reflexes in the lower extremities should suggest tabes dorsalis, a cauda equina tumor, spinal stenosis, and other conditions of the lumbar spine and lumbosacral area.

DIAGNOSTIC WORKUP

Routine studies include a CBC, sedimentation rate, chemistry panel, and VDRL test. The anorectal area should be carefully inspected for lesions and the sphincter competence determined by a digital exam. If these findings are normal, it would be wise to consult a neurologist. If one is not available, further workup may be done.

If there are hyperactive reflexes with cranial nerve signs, then a CT scan or MRI of the brain should be done. If there are hyperactive reflexes of all four extremities with no cranial nerve signs, MRI of the cervical spine should be done. With hyperactive reflexes of the lower extremities only, MRI of the thoracic cord should be done. If there are hypoactive reflexes in the lower extremities, MRI or CT scan of the lumbar spine should be done. If increased intracranial pressure has been excluded, a spinal tap may be done to help diagnose multiple sclerosis or tabes dorsalis.

If the general physical examination and neurologic examination are negative, psychogenic causes should be considered and cystometric studies might be helpful. The patient should be referred to a psychiatrist.

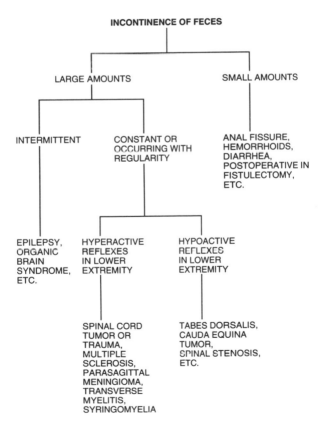

INCONTINENCE OF FECES

LARGE AMOUNTS — SMALL AMOUNTS

INTERMITTENT — CONSTANT OR OCCURRING WITH REGULARITY

ANAL FISSURE, HEMORRHOIDS, DIARRHEA, POSTOPERATIVE IN FISTULECTOMY, ETC.

EPILEPSY, ORGANIC BRAIN SYNDROME, ETC.

HYPERACTIVE REFLEXES IN LOWER EXTREMITY

HYPOACTIVE REFLEXES IN LOWER EXTREMITY

SPINAL CORD TUMOR OR TRAUMA, MULTIPLE SCLEROSIS, PARASAGITTAL MENINGIOMA, TRANSVERSE MYELITIS, SYRINGOMYELIA

TABES DORSALIS, CAUDA EQUINA TUMOR, SPINAL STENOSIS, ETC.

INCONTINENCE OF URINE

Ask the following questions:

1. Is the volume of urine large or small? If the volume of urine released is small, stress incontinence and vesicovaginal fistula should be considered. If the amounts released are large, one should consider a neurologic condition or an enlarged prostate with bladder neck obstruction as the cause.
2. Are there abnormalities on the neurologic examination? Neurologic disorders to be considered are spastic neurogenic bladder due to multiple sclerosis, spinal cord tumor, and spinal cord trauma, as well as incompetent sphincter due to cauda equina syndrome, spinal stenosis, poliomyelitis, diabetic neuropathy, and tabes dorsalis.
3. Are there hyperactive reflexes? This helps distinguish the disorders of the spinal cord and parasagittal area, such as spastic neurogenic bladder from multiple sclerosis, spinal cord tumor, spinal cord trauma, and parasagittal meningioma.
4. Are the reflexes hypoactive? Hypoactive reflexes suggest poliomyelitis, cauda equina syndrome, spinal stenosis, diabetic neuropathy, and tabes dorsalis.
5. Is there an enlarged bladder or prostate? If an enlarged bladder or prostate is palpated, one should consider overflow incontinence from bladder neck obstruction, prostatic hypertrophy, and tuberculosis of the bladder.

DIAGNOSTIC WORKUP

Routine laboratory tests include a CBC, a urinalysis, a urine culture and sensitivity, a chemistry panel, and a VDRL test. An intravenous pyelogram and a voiding cystogram may be helpful. A Q-tip test or stress test may be helpful in diagnosing stress incontinence. The bladder may be catheterized for residual urine or abdominal ultrasonography may be employed to evaluate residual urine. Cystoscopy may also be necessary to determine if there is chronic bladder inflammation or bladder neck obstruction. Office cystometrography can be considered, but it is usually best to refer the patient to a urologist for cystometric studies. Prostatic size can be determined by transrectal prostatic ultrasonography.

The simplest and most cost-effective approach is to refer the patient to a neurologist if there are abnormalities on the neurologic examination and refer the patient to a urologist if there are not. If there is stress incontinence and a cystocele is found on vaginal examination, the patient should be referred to a gynecologist. It is not cost-effective to begin ordering MRIs or CT scans of the brain and spinal cord without the assistance of these specialists.

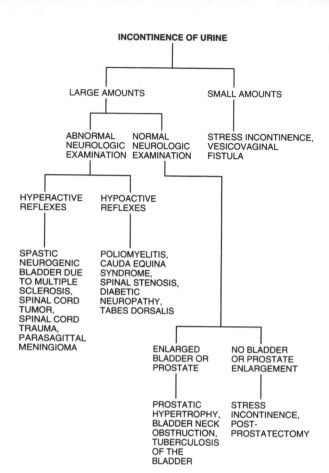

INCONTINENCE OF URINE

LARGE AMOUNTS

SMALL AMOUNTS

ABNORMAL
NEUROLOGIC
EXAMINATION

NORMAL
NEUROLOGIC
EXAMINATION

STRESS INCONTINENCE,
VESICOVAGINAL
FISTULA

HYPERACTIVE
REFLEXES

HYPOACTIVE
REFLEXES

SPASTIC
NEUROGENIC
BLADDER DUE
TO MULTIPLE
SCLEROSIS,
SPINAL CORD
TUMOR,
SPINAL CORD
TRAUMA,
PARASAGITTAL
MENINGIOMA

POLIOMYELITIS,
CAUDA EQUINA
SYNDROME,
SPINAL STENOSIS,
DIABETIC
NEUROPATHY,
TABES DORSALIS

ENLARGED
BLADDER OR
PROSTATE

NO BLADDER
OR PROSTATE
ENLARGEMENT

PROSTATIC
HYPERTROPHY,
BLADDER NECK
OBSTRUCTION,
TUBERCULOSIS
OF THE
BLADDER

STRESS
INCONTINENCE,
POST-
PROSTATECTOMY

INDIGESTION

Ask the following questions:

1. Is there a history of drug or alcohol ingestion? Alcohol, tobacco, aspirin, other nonsteroidal anti-inflammatory drugs, steroids, caffeine, and antibiotics are just a few of the drugs that may irritate the stomach.
2. Is the indigestion brought on by exertion? A history of indigestion brought on by exertion should suggest angina pectoris.
3. Is there a loss of appetite and weight? These findings would suggest not only a gastrointestinal neoplasm, but also pernicious anemia, chronic pancreatitis and pyloric obstruction, and chronic gastritis. Chronic organ failure should also be entertained, such as uremia, cirrhosis, or congestive heart failure.
4. Is the indigestion or pain relieved by food or antacids? These findings would suggest a duodenal ulcer, hiatal hernia, and esophagitis.
5. Is the indigestion or pain brought on by food? These findings would suggest cholecystitis, gastric ulcer, or toxins in food such as monosodium glutamate or sulfites.
6. Is the indigestion or pain unrelated to meals? These findings would suggest a chronic appendicitis, chronic intestinal obstruction, or tabes dorsalis.
7. Is there no pain associated with the indigestion? This finding would suggest functional dyspepsia.

DIAGNOSTIC WORKUP

Routine tests include a CBC, urinalysis, chemistry panel, VDRL, thyroid profile, serum B_{12} and folic acid, an upper GI series, esophagram, and stools for occult blood and ovum and parasites. The next step is a cholecystogram or gallbladder ultrasound.

If these studies are negative, a gastroenterologist

should be consulted. He will do esophagoscopy, gastroscopy, and duodenoscopy. He may also perform esophageal motility studies or esophageal pH monitoring. A Bernstein test may be of value in solving the diagnostic dilemma. He may also want to order a CT scan of the abdomen or a small bowel series.

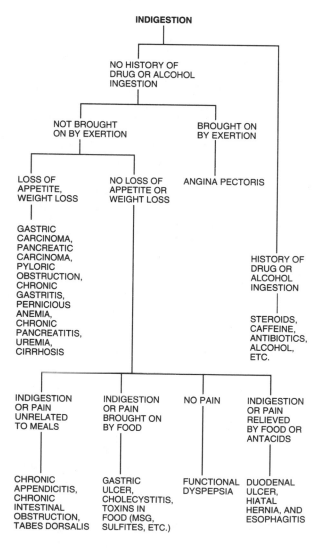

INFERTILITY, FEMALE

Ask the following questions:

1. Are there abnormalities on pelvic examination? Abnormalities found on the pelvic examination are cervicitis, stenosis of the cervix, fibroids, retroverted uterus, tubo-ovarian abscesses, and polycystic ovaries.
2. Are there abnormal secondary sex characteristics? Patients with Turner's syndrome, Simmonds' disease, Fröhlich's syndrome, and virilism may exhibit abnormal secondary sex characteristics.
3. Are there other abnormalities in endocrine examination? The physical examination may disclose hypothyroidism, hyperthyroidism, Simmonds' disease, or acromegaly.

DIAGNOSTIC WORKUP

Routine studies include a CBC, urinalysis, urine culture and colony count, a chemistry panel, a thyroid profile, VDRL test, and a vaginal smear and culture. The next logical step is to obtain a specimen of semen from the husband for sperm count.

If the above tests are negative, referral to a gynecologist is in order. If one is not available, further workup can be done, including a serum FSH and LH, a serum estradiol, and a serum progesterone to determine the presence of pituitary or ovarian causes of ovulatory dysfunction. A hysterosalpingogram can be done. The patient can keep a temperature chart to determine if ovulation occurs. Cervical mucus studies can be done for spinnbarkheit testing and the presence of significant white blood cell counts should be noted. Pelvic ultrasound may be done and laparoscopy may be necessary to rule out other conditions that may affect fertility. A trial of clomiphene citrate may be given. Endometrial biopsy may also contribute to solving the diagnostic dilemma.

INFERTILITY, FEMALE

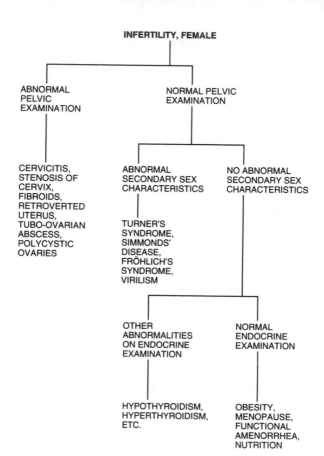

ABNORMAL PELVIC EXAMINATION

CERVICITIS, STENOSIS OF CERVIX, FIBROIDS, RETROVERTED UTERUS, TUBO-OVARIAN ABSCESS, POLYCYSTIC OVARIES

NORMAL PELVIC EXAMINATION

ABNORMAL SECONDARY SEX CHARACTERISTICS

TURNER'S SYNDROME, SIMMONDS' DISEASE, FRÖHLICH'S SYNDROME, VIRILISM

NO ABNORMAL SECONDARY SEX CHARACTERISTICS

OTHER ABNORMALITIES ON ENDOCRINE EXAMINATION

HYPOTHYROIDISM, HYPERTHYROIDISM, ETC.

NORMAL ENDOCRINE EXAMINATION

OBESITY, MENOPAUSE, FUNCTIONAL AMENORRHEA, NUTRITION

INFERTILITY, MALE

Ask the following questions:

1. Are there abnormalities on examination of the external genitalia and prostate? Abnormalities that need to be looked for are Klinefelter's syndrome, epididymitis, testicular atrophy, urethritis, and prostatitis.
2. Are there abnormalities on the endocrine examination? The general endocrine examination may turn up hypothyroidism, hyperthyroidism, or hypopituitarism.
3. Are there stress factors that need to be considered such as marital difficulties or overwork? Overwork and marital difficulties may lead to drug addiction and alcoholism, among other problems. All these affect fertility.

DIAGNOSTIC WORKUP

Routine laboratory tests include a CBC, urinalysis, chemistry panel, thyroid profile, VDRL test, and sperm count. If there is a urethral discharge, a smear and culture should be done. If the sperm count reveals oligospermia on two separate specimens, referral should be made to a urologist for further evaluation.

Additional tests that can be ordered include blood tests for LH, FSH, and testosterone. If these are normal, a testicular biopsy may need to be done. Ultrasonography of the testicles may be helpful.

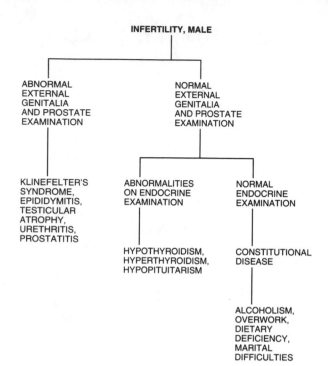

INFERTILITY, MALE

ABNORMAL EXTERNAL GENITALIA AND PROSTATE EXAMINATION

NORMAL EXTERNAL GENITALIA AND PROSTATE EXAMINATION

KLINEFELTER'S SYNDROME, EPIDIDYMITIS, TESTICULAR ATROPHY, URETHRITIS, PROSTATITIS

ABNORMALITIES ON ENDOCRINE EXAMINATION

NORMAL ENDOCRINE EXAMINATION

HYPOTHYROIDISM, HYPERTHYROIDISM, HYPOPITUITARISM

CONSTITUTIONAL DISEASE

ALCOHOLISM, OVERWORK, DIETARY DEFICIENCY, MARITAL DIFFICULTIES

INGUINAL SWELLING

Ask the following questions:

1. Is it reducible? If the inguinal swelling is reducible, a femoral hernia or inguinal hernia should be suspected.
2. Does it transilluminate? If the mass transilluminates, it is probably a hydrocele and may be a hydrocele of the cord or a hydrocele of Nuck's canal.
3. Is it tender? Tenderness in the groin may signify an abscess, hematoma, lymphadenitis, a strangulated hernia, or an obturated hernia.

DIAGNOSTIC WORKUP

The routine workup includes a CBC, sedimentation rate, chemistry panel, VDRL test, and an x-ray of the hips and pelvis. A bone scan may be helpful in ruling out a psoas abscess. Arteriography may be helpful for diagnosing aneurysm. Venography will help diagnose saphenous varix. Needle aspiration may be necessary to diagnose an abscess. Exploratory surgery will be necessary in most cases for both diagnosis and treatment.

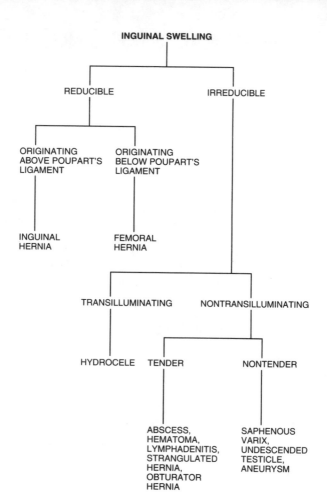

INSOMNIA

Ask the following questions:

1. Is there dyspnea? If there is a history of dyspnea, then heart disease or lung disease should be suspected.
2. Is there a history of drug or alcohol ingestion? There are many drugs that may cause insomnia, including the amphetamines, theophylline, caffeine, anticonvulsants, nicotine, thyroid hormones, and the sympathomimetics. Alcohol may induce sleep, but the patients complain of early morning wakening.
3. Is there a history of a painful condition? Abscessed teeth, arthritis, sciatica, bone metastasis, hiatal hernia, and esophagitis are just a few of the conditions that may keep a patient awake because of pain.
4. Are there other psychiatric symptoms? Anxiety, loss of libido, loss of appetite, and depression may be associated with hyperthyroidism, general paresis, organic brain syndrome, chronic anxiety, and endogenous depression.

DIAGNOSTIC WORKUP

Routine studies include a CBC, a sedimentation rate, a urinalysis and drug screen, a chemistry panel, a thyroid profile, VDRL test, EKG, and chest x-ray. Arterial blood gases and pulmonary function testing should be done to rule out pulmonary disease. A venous pressure and circulation time will help rule out early congestive heart failure. Blood pressure monitoring can be used to rule out paroxysmal hypertension. If an organic brain syndrome is suspected, a CT scan or MRI of the brain should be done. When all of the above diagnostic tests are negative, a sleep study must be done.

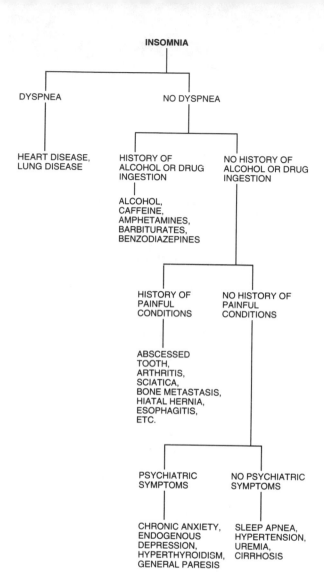

INTRACRANIAL OR
CERVICAL BRUIT

Intracranial bruit may be due to a carotid-cavernous sinus fistula or a cerebral angioma. It may also be due to a congenital arteriovenous anomaly. A cerebral aneurysm is rarely big enough to cause a bruit. Severe anemia may cause intracranial bruits without localized pathology being responsible. All intracranial bruits should be investigated with MRI and angiography unless some systemic disease is found (e.g., anemia) that would explain the sign.

Cervical bruits may be due to carotid stenosis, hyperthyroidism, a venous hum, or aortic stenosis with transmission of the bruit to the vessels in the neck. If hyperthyroidism and aortic stenosis can be excluded, a carotid duplex scan and possibly carotid angiography should be done to look for significant carotid stenosis. There is considerable controversy over whether asymptomatic carotid stenosis should be operated on. Nevertheless, a thorough workup should be done so the clinician knows what he is dealing with.

JAUNDICE

Ask the following questions:

1. Is the jaundice associated with hepatomegaly? There is little or no hepatomegaly associated with hemolytic anemias, pernicious anemia, Gilbert's disease, and Dubin-Johnson syndrome.
2. Is the hepatomegaly massive? Massive hepatomegaly is associated with Gaucher's disease.
3. Is there associated fever, right upper quadrant pain, or a tender liver? These findings would suggest viral hepatitis, cholecystitis, infectious mononucleosis, leptospirosis, ascending cholangitis, hepatic vein thrombosis, and toxic hepatitis.
4. Is the gallbladder enlarged? The finding of an enlarged gallbladder with the jaundice suggests obstructive jaundice, carcinoma of the pancreas, carcinoma of the bowel ducts or ampulla of Vater.
5. Is there skin pigmentation? The presence of skin pigmentation that is not bilirubin suggests hemochromatosis.
6. Is there splenomegaly? The presence of significant splenomegaly suggests infectious mononucleosis, cirrhosis of the liver, hemolytic anemia, Gaucher's disease, kala azar, or agnogenic myeloid metaplasia.
7. Is there edema and ascites? The presence of edema and ascites suggests alcoholic cirrhosis.

DIAGNOSTIC WORKUP

The basic workup includes a CBC, sedimentation rate, reticulocyte count, red cell fragility test, urinalysis, chemistry panel, VDRL test, EKG, a chest x-ray, and flat plate of the abdomen.

If infectious hepatitis is suspected, a hepatitis profile, febrile agglutinins, monospot test, cytomegalic virus antibody titer, and leptospirosis antibody titer should be done. If lupoid hepatitis is suspected, a test for antinuclear antibodies and a smooth muscle antibody should be done.

If hemochromatosis is suspected, a serum iron, iron binding capacity, and ferritin should be done.

If hemolytic anemia is suspected, serum haptoglobins, hemoglobin electrophoresis, and sickle cell preparations may be done.

If obstructive jaundice is suspected, then gallbladder ultrasound should be done to rule out gallstones and a CT scan of the abdomen may be done to look for gastrointestinal neoplasm. An upper GI series may assist in finding a primary neoplasm in the GI tract.

Endoscopic retrograde cholangiopancreatography (ERCP) or percutaneous transhepatic cholangiography will assist in determining whether there is definitely obstructive jaundice and whether it is due to a surgically resectable lesion. Peritoneoscopy can also be helpful. An exploratory laparotomy will probably be necessary regardless of whether one performs the above tests.

Hepatocellular jaundice will often require a needle biopsy of the liver to pin down the diagnosis. Antimitochondrial antibodies will need to be ordered to screen for biliary cirrhosis. By the time you have reached this point, you have gone to considerable expense in the diagnostic workup. It would be much more prudent to ask for a gastroenterology consultation before ordering all these expensive diagnostic tests.

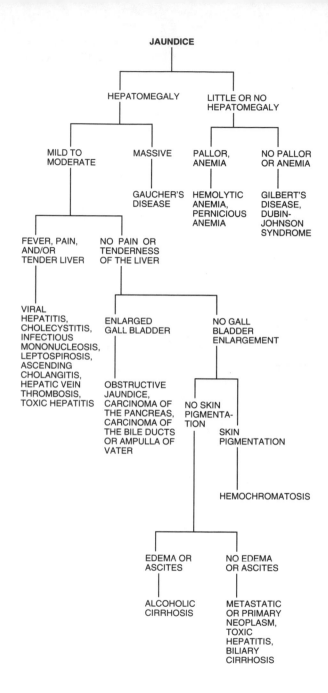

JAW PAIN

Ask the following questions:

1. Are there abnormalities on examination of the teeth or gums? A thorough examination of the teeth and gums may disclose dental caries, gingivitis, oral tumors, or alveolar abscess.
2. Is the pain intermittent? Intermittent pain should suggest a trigeminal neuralgia or glossopharyngeal neuralgia.
3. Is there a rash? The presence of a rash would suggest herpes zoster. Be sure to examine the ear drum for Ramsay Hunt's syndrome.

DIAGNOSTIC WORKUP

Routine diagnostic studies include a CBC, sedimentation rate, chemistry panel, arthritis panel, and an x-ray of the teeth and jaw. X-ray of the sinuses may be helpful. At this point referral to a dentist or oral surgeon should be made if there is still diagnostic difficulty.

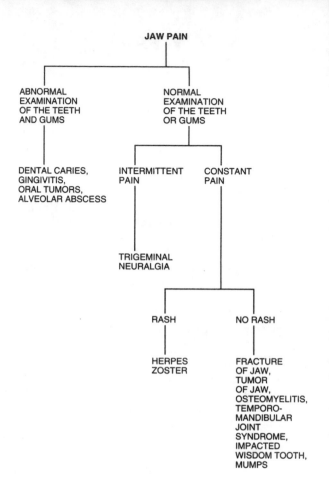

JAW PAIN

ABNORMAL
EXAMINATION
OF THE TEETH
AND GUMS

NORMAL
EXAMINATION
OF THE TEETH
OR GUMS

DENTAL CARIES,
GINGIVITIS,
ORAL TUMORS,
ALVEOLAR ABSCESS

INTERMITTENT
PAIN

CONSTANT
PAIN

TRIGEMINAL
NEURALGIA

RASH

NO RASH

HERPES
ZOSTER

FRACTURE
OF JAW,
TUMOR
OF JAW,
OSTEOMYELITIS,
TEMPORO-
MANDIBULAR
JOINT
SYNDROME,
IMPACTED
WISDOM TOOTH,
MUMPS

JAW SWELLING

Ask the following questions:

1. Is the swelling focal or diffuse? Focal jaw swelling should suggest alveolar abscess, gingivitis, adamantinoma, actinomycosis, epithelioma, a cyst, osteoma, odontoma, or epulis.
2. Is it painful? Painful jaw swelling should suggest alveolar abscess, gingivitis, actinomycosis, adamantinoma, cellulitis, fracture, hematoma, necrosis of the jaw, or osteomyelitis.
3. Is there enlargement of the hands and feet? Enlargement of the hands and feet should suggest acromegaly.

DIAGNOSTIC WORKUP

Routine tests include a CBC, urinalysis, sedimentation rate, chemistry panel, and x-ray of the jaw and teeth. X-rays of the skull and long bones and a serum growth hormone should be done if acromegaly is suspected. Parathyroid hormone assay and x-ray of the skull and long bones should be done if osteitis fibrosa cystica is suspected. Referral to a dentist or oral surgeon should be made if there is still diagnostic confusion at this point.

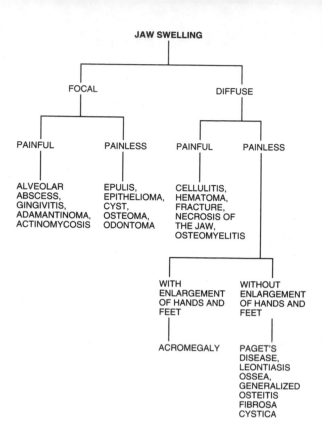

JOINT PAIN

Ask the following questions:

1. Is the joint pain localized to a single joint? Localization to a single joint should suggest a septic arthritis, gout, tuberculosis, hemophilia, sickle cell disease, trauma, avascular necrosis, and pseudogout.
2. Is there fever? The presence of fever should make one think of septic arthritis, rheumatic fever, gonococcal arthritis, Reiter's syndrome, lupus erythematosus, Lyme arthritis, polymyalgia rheumatica, Still's disease, and rheumatoid arthritis.
3. Is there a urethral discharge? The presence of a urethral discharge should make one think of Reiter's syndrome or gonococcal arthritis.
4. Is there low back pain? The presence of low back pain should suggest rheumatoid spondylitis, ochronosis, and gout.
5. Is the arthritis migratory? The presence of migratory arthritis should make one think of rheumatic fever and rat-bite fever.
6. What is the age of the patient? Younger patients may have sickle cell disease, hemophilia, trauma, rheumatic fever, Still's disease, and gonococcal arthritis. Older patients are more likely to have osteoarthritis, polymyalgia rheumatica, and gout. It should be noted that there is considerable overlap here.

DIAGNOSTIC WORKUP

Routine studies include a CBC, sedimentation rate, antistreptolysin-O titer, cross-reacting protein (CRP), urinalysis, chemistry panel, arthritis panel, and x-rays of the involved joints. It is also wise at times to order a bone survey. Synovial fluid analysis and culture should be done if there is sufficient joint effusion. A trial of therapy may be initiated at this point and will assist in the diagnosis. For example, a course of colchicine may be given to rule out gout.

339

If there is still doubt, a rheumatology consultation should be made. Other tests that may be made include a gonococcal antibody titer and a coagulation profile. If there is a urethral discharge, a smear and culture of the material should be made. If there is fever, febrile agglutinins, serologic tests for Lyme disease, brucellin antibody titer, blood cultures, and a Monospot test may be done. If collagen disease is suspected, antinuclear antibodies and anti-DNA antibodies may be looked for. If sickle cell anemia is suspected, a sickle cell preparation should be done. A bone scan will help diagnose rheumatoid spondylitis and ochronosis. A urine for homogentisic acid will diagnose ochronosis also.

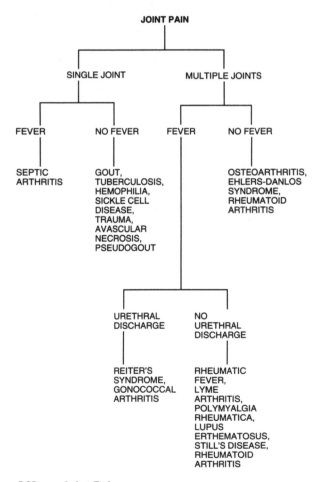

JOINT SWELLING

Ask the following questions:

1. Is it painless? The presence of joint swelling without pain, especially on motion, would suggest Charcot's disease.
2. Is the involvement primarily in small or large joints? Involvement of the small joints is characteristic of rheumatoid arthritis, gonococcal arthritis, and Reiter's syndrome. Involvement of the larger joints is more characteristic of gout and osteoarthritis. However, osteoarthritis and rheumatoid arthritis may involve both.
3. Is the involvement symmetrical or asymmetrical? Asymmetrical involvement is more typical of gout, rheumatic fever, hemophilia, neoplasm, septic arthritis, and trauma. Symmetrical involvement is more characteristic of rheumatoid arthritis and osteoarthritis.
4. Is there fever? The presence of fever should make one think of rheumatic fever, gonococcal arthritis or other types of septic arthritis, Reiter's syndrome, rheumatoid arthritis, and lupus erythematosus.
5. What is the age of the patient? The younger patients with joint swelling most likely have gonococcal arthritis, lupus erythematosus, rheumatoid arthritis, and hemophilia. Gout, osteoarthritis, and neoplasm are more common in older patients. However, there is considerable overlap here.

DIAGNOSTIC WORKUP

Routine tests include a CBC, sedimentation rate, antistreptolysin-O titer, CRP, urinalysis, chemistry panel, arthritis panel, and x-rays of the involved joints. It is also wise to do a bone survey when there is multiple joint involvement. A synovial fluid analysis and culture may be done if there is sufficient joint fluid. A trial of therapy can be initiated and may be diagnostic. At this point it is wise to refer the patient to a rheumatologist for further evaluation. Additional tests that may be ordered are found on page 340.

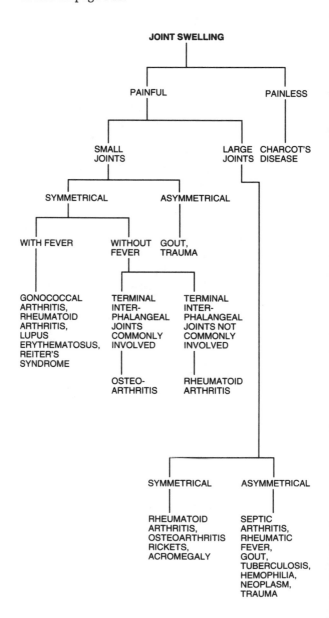

KNEE PAIN

Ask the following questions:

1. Is it transient? Transient knee pain may be due to rheumatic fever, sarcoidosis, palindromic rheumatism, or trauma.
2. Is it unilateral or bilateral? Unilateral knee pain would suggest gout, septic arthritis, bursitis, hemophilia, pseudogout, osteogenic sarcoma, and traumatic conditions such as torn meniscus, hemarthrosis, sprain of collateral ligaments, and fracture.
3. Is there a history of trauma? History of trauma would suggest a sprain, torn meniscus, bruise, or fracture.
4. Are there prominent systemic symptoms? If there are prominent systemic symptoms, one should consider lupus erythematosus, Reiter's disease, rheumatoid arthritis, other collagen disease, scurvy, and rheumatic fever.
5. What is the age of the patient? Younger patients are more likely to have traumatic conditions such as fracture, sprains, bruises, or a torn meniscus. Osgood-Schlatter disease would be more typical of patients in their early teens. Patients in their twenties are more likely to have rheumatoid arthritis, Reiter's disease, and lupus erythematosus, while patients in the fourth or fifth decade and higher would be more likely to have osteoarthritis, gout, and pseudogout.

DIAGNOSTIC WORKUP

Routine studies include a CBC, sedimentation rate, antistreptolysin-O titer, CRP, urinalysis, chemistry panel, arthritis panel, and x-rays of the involved joint. It is also wise to do a bone survey. Synovial fluid analysis and culture may be done if there is sufficient joint fluid. A trial of therapy can be initiated and may be diagnostic.

If further diagnostic workup need be done at this point, it is most cost-effective to refer the patient to a rheumatologist or orthopedic surgeon before ordering MRI or other studies. He may want to do an arthroscopic examination before proceeding with other tests for arthritic conditions. For further workup of knee pain, see page 340.

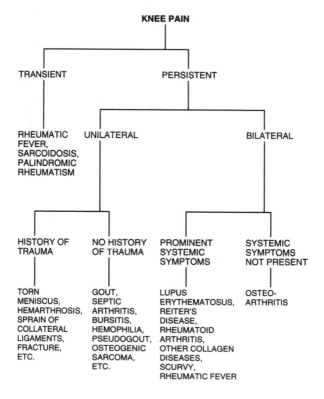

KNEE PAIN

TRANSIENT

PERSISTENT

RHEUMATIC FEVER, SARCOIDOSIS, PALINDROMIC RHEUMATISM

UNILATERAL

BILATERAL

HISTORY OF TRAUMA

NO HISTORY OF TRAUMA

PROMINENT SYSTEMIC SYMPTOMS

SYSTEMIC SYMPTOMS NOT PRESENT

TORN MENISCUS, HEMARTHROSIS, SPRAIN OF COLLATERAL LIGAMENTS, FRACTURE, ETC.

GOUT, SEPTIC ARTHRITIS, BURSITIS, HEMOPHILIA, PSEUDOGOUT, OSTEOGENIC SARCOMA, ETC.

LUPUS ERYTHEMATOSUS, REITER'S DISEASE, RHEUMATOID ARTHRITIS, OTHER COLLAGEN DISEASES, SCURVY, RHEUMATIC FEVER

OSTEO-ARTHRITIS

KNEE SWELLING

Ask the following questions:

1. Is it painless? Painless swelling of the knee is probably a Charcot's joint.
2. Is it unilateral or bilateral? Unilateral knee swelling is most likely due to trauma, gout, pseudogout, hemophilia, septic arthritis, tuberculosis, osteogenic sarcoma, torn meniscus, or osteomyelitis. Bilateral swelling of the knee is more commonly seen in osteoarthritis, lupus erythematosus, Reiter's disease, and rheumatoid arthritis.
3. Is there fever? The presence of fever suggests septic arthritis, rheumatic fever, rheumatoid arthritis, osteomyelitis, lupus erythematosus, and Reiter's disease.
4. Are there systemic symptoms? Systemic symptoms suggest lupus erythematosus, rheumatoid arthritis, and Reiter's disease, as well as rheumatic fever.
5. What is the age of the patient? Knee swelling in younger patients is more likely to be due to rheumatic fever, septic arthritis, lupus erythematosus, Reiter's disease, and rheumatoid arthritis. Older patients are more likely to be affected with gout, pseudogout, and osteoarthritis. Osteogenic sarcoma seems to occur between the ages of 5 and 25 years in most cases.

DIAGNOSTIC WORKUP

Routine diagnostic tests include CBC, sedimentation rate, urinalysis, chemistry panel, arthritis panel, VDRL test, and x-rays of the involved joint or joints. A bone survey should probably also be done. If there is significant swelling, an arthrocentesis for synovial fluid should be done and the fluid analyzed and cultured. A therapeutic trial may be initiated at this point and can assist in the diagnosis.

If there is still doubt about the diagnosis, referral to a rheumatologist or orthopedic surgeon should be made before ordering MRI or expensive diagnostic tests. Additional diagnostic tests to order in cases of knee swelling may be found on page 340.

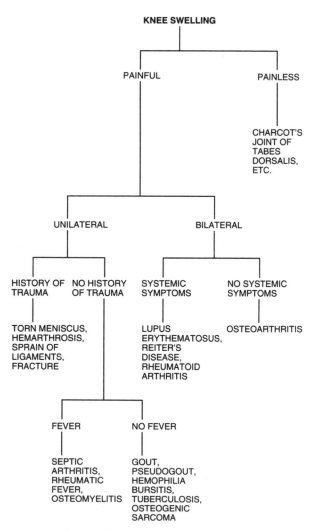

KYPHOSIS

Ask the following questions:

1. Is there a history of chronic cough? A history of cough would suggest tuberculosis of the spine, emphysema, and metastatic carcinoma.
2. What is the sex of the patient? If the patient is a woman in her forties, then menopausal osteoporosis should be suspected.
3. What is the age of the patient? Children more likely have kyphosis due to rickets, leukopolysaccharidosis, Hurler's disease, Scheuermann's disease, Pott's disease, or Morquio's disease. Adults are more likely to suffer from osteoarthritis, Paget's disease, Parkinson's disease, osteomalacia, osteoporosis, and ankylosing spondylitis.

DIAGNOSTIC WORKUP

Routine diagnostic studies include a CBC, sedimentation rate, urinalysis, chemistry panel, arthritis panel, tuberculin test, chest x-ray, x-rays of the thoracic spine, the lumbar spine, and the hips. If there is a productive cough, a sputum for acid-fast bacilli smear and culture should be made.

If muscular disease is suspected, a muscle biopsy may be done. If menopause is suspected, a serum follicle-stimulating hormone (FSH) and luteinizing hormone (LH) and serum estradiol can be done. A bone scan may identify pathologic fractures and ankylosing spondylitis. An HLA-B27 antigen test should be ordered if ankylosing spondylitis is suspected. A bone biopsy may clear up the diagnostic dilemma.

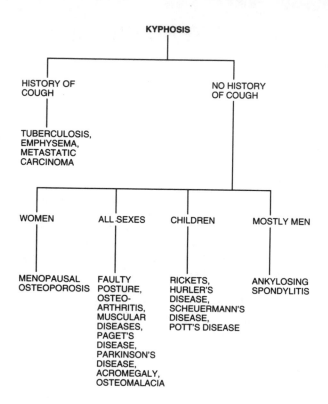

KYPHOSIS

HISTORY OF COUGH

TUBERCULOSIS, EMPHYSEMA, METASTATIC CARCINOMA

NO HISTORY OF COUGH

WOMEN

MENOPAUSAL OSTEOPOROSIS

ALL SEXES

FAULTY POSTURE, OSTEO-ARTHRITIS, MUSCULAR DISEASES, PAGET'S DISEASE, PARKINSON'S DISEASE, ACROMEGALY, OSTEOMALACIA

CHILDREN

RICKETS, HURLER'S DISEASE, SCHEUERMANN'S DISEASE, POTT'S DISEASE

MOSTLY MEN

ANKYLOSING SPONDYLITIS

LEG ULCERATION

Ask the following questions:

1. Are the peripheral pulses diminished or absent? Presence of poor peripheral pulses suggests arteriosclerosis, diabetes mellitus, Buerger's disease, and femoral artery thrombosis.
2. Are there abnormalities on the neurologic examination? Neurologic disorders associated with leg ulceration include tabes dorsalis, diabetic neuropathy, hemiplegia, and many other disorders.
3. Is there a positive smear or culture of the material from the ulcer? A positive smear or culture of material from the ulcer may be found in osteomyelitis, tuberculosis, syphilis, anthrax, and other fungal diseases.

DIAGNOSTIC WORKUP

Routine studies include a CBC, sedimentation rate, sickle cell preparation, urinalysis, chemistry panel, VDRL test, smear and culture of the material from the ulcer, and x-rays of the involved area. A biopsy may be necessary to establish the diagnosis. Rarely a dark field examination will be necessary. Arteriography or venography may establish the level of arterial or venous obstruction. A bone scan will help pin down the diagnosis of osteomyelitis.

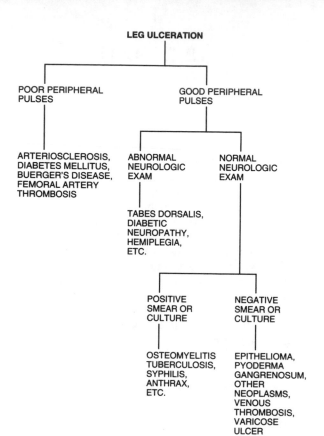

LEG ULCERATION

POOR PERIPHERAL
PULSES

GOOD PERIPHERAL
PULSES

ARTERIOSCLEROSIS,
DIABETES MELLITUS,
BUERGER'S DISEASE,
FEMORAL ARTERY
THROMBOSIS

ABNORMAL
NEUROLOGIC
EXAM

NORMAL
NEUROLOGIC
EXAM

TABES DORSALIS,
DIABETIC
NEUROPATHY,
HEMIPLEGIA,
ETC.

POSITIVE
SMEAR OR
CULTURE

NEGATIVE
SMEAR OR
CULTURE

OSTEOMYELITIS
TUBERCULOSIS,
SYPHILIS,
ANTHRAX,
ETC.

EPITHELIOMA,
PYODERMA
GANGRENOSUM,
OTHER
NEOPLASMS,
VENOUS
THROMBOSIS,
VARICOSE
ULCER

LIP PAIN

Ask the following questions:

1. Is there ulceration or swelling? Presence of an ulceration would suggest herpes simplex, syphilis, and carcinoma. A swelling would suggest there was trauma, a carbuncle, insect bites or stings, and angioneurotic edema.
2. Is there a rash? The presence of a rash would suggest herpes zoster, particularly if it is unilateral.
3. Is there a history of trauma, insect bite or sting? These historical findings are important in determining if the swelling is due to trauma, insect bites or stings.

DIAGNOSTIC WORKUP

Routine studies include a CBC, sedimentation rate, urinalysis, chemistry panel, VDRL test, and culture of any material that can be obtained from an ulceration if present. A therapeutic trial of antibiotics or antiviral medication can be done at this point. If this is unsuccessful, the patient should be referred to an oral surgeon or dermatologist.

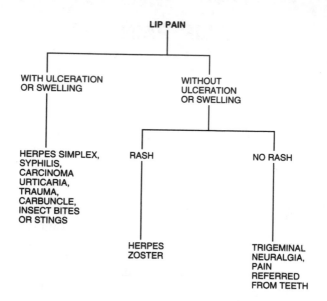

LIP PAIN

WITH ULCERATION OR SWELLING

WITHOUT ULCERATION OR SWELLING

HERPES SIMPLEX, SYPHILIS, CARCINOMA URTICARIA, TRAUMA, CARBUNCLE, INSECT BITES OR STINGS

RASH

NO RASH

HERPES ZOSTER

TRIGEMINAL NEURALGIA, PAIN REFERRED FROM TEETH

LIP SWELLING

Ask the following question:
Is it painful or nonpainful? Painful swelling of the lip is more likely to be herpes zoster, herpes simplex, pyoderma granulosa, insect bites or stings, alveolar abscess, and trauma. Painless swellings of the lip are more likely to be due to syphilis, allergic urticaria, angioneurotic edema, contact dermatitis, carcinoma, myxedema, and cretinism.

DIAGNOSTIC WORKUP

Routine laboratory tests include a CBC, sedimentation rate, urinalysis, chemistry panel, VDRL test, and culture of any material that can be obtained from an ulcer if present. An x-ray of the teeth and jaw may be necessary also. A therapeutic trial of antibiotics or antiviral therapy can be tried. If this is unsuccessful, a referral to an oral surgeon or dermatologist should be made.

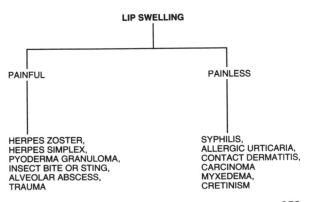

LIP SWELLING

PAINFUL

HERPES ZOSTER,
HERPES SIMPLEX,
PYODERMA GRANULOMA,
INSECT BITE OR STING,
ALVEOLAR ABSCESS,
TRAUMA

PAINLESS

SYPHILIS,
ALLERGIC URTICARIA,
CONTACT DERMATITIS,
CARCINOMA
MYXEDEMA
CRETINISM

LORDOSIS

This is often a *congenital* effusion or backward curvature of the spine causing the person to appear "high and mighty." However, it may be seen in untreated bilateral congenital dislocation of the hips, muscular dystrophy, tuberculosis, and spondylolisthesis. Lordosis is also seen in orthostatic albuminuria and chondrodystrophy.

An x-ray of the lumbosacral spine and hips will usually establish the diagnosis in cases of congenital dislocation of the hips and spondylolisthesis. A family history and muscle biopsy will assist in the diagnosis of muscular dystrophy.

LYMPHADENOPATHY

Ask the following questions:

1. Is there a history of drug ingestion? Many drugs can cause lymphadenopathy; the most notable is Dilantin, but the antibiotics, aspirin, iodides and certain antihypertensive drugs can cause lymphadenopathy also.
2. Is the lymphadenopathy focal or diffuse? If the adenopathy is focal, one should look for an infectious process in the area supplied by the respective lymph nodes. For example, if there is occipital node enlargement, one would look for ringworm, dermatitis of the scalp, furunculosis, pediculosis, and cellulitis. However, infectious mononucleosis and rubella may begin with enlargement of these nodes.
3. Is there fever? The presence of fever should make one think of infectious mononucleosis, brucellosis, dengue fever, toxoplasmosis, and Still's disease among other diseases.

DIAGNOSTIC WORKUP

Routine diagnostic tests include a CBC, sedimentation rate, nose and throat culture, and culture of material from any area supplied by the enlarged lymph nodes. In addition, a chemistry panel should be done and heterophile antibody titer, brucellin antibody titer, febrile agglutinins, and a VDRL test. A chest x-ray and flat plate of the abdomen may be helpful in diagnosing generalized lymphadenopathy.

X-ray of the long bones may identify metastatic carcinoma and x-ray of the hands may identify sarcoidosis. A bone marrow examination may identify leukemia. If an infectious process has been ruled out, biopsy of the local node may turn up metastatic carcinoma, Hodgkin's disease, and sarcoidosis. A tuberculin skin test should be done; a brucellergen skin test and Kveim test may also need to be done. A lymphangiogram may turn up a lymphosarcoma or multiple metastatic lymph nodes. Liver biopsy is also occasionally necessary. Imaging studies of the abdomen and pelvis and the mediastinum are occasionally necessary. Before ordering these, a consultation with a hematologist or infectious disease specialist would be prudent.

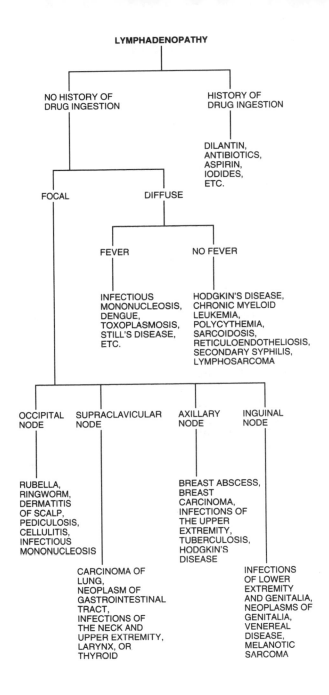

LYMPHADENOPATHY

NO HISTORY OF DRUG INGESTION

HISTORY OF DRUG INGESTION

DILANTIN, ANTIBIOTICS, ASPIRIN, IODIDES, ETC.

FOCAL

DIFFUSE

FEVER

NO FEVER

INFECTIOUS MONONUCLEOSIS, DENGUE, TOXOPLASMOSIS, STILL'S DISEASE, ETC.

HODGKIN'S DISEASE, CHRONIC MYELOID LEUKEMIA, POLYCYTHEMIA, SARCOIDOSIS, RETICULOENDOTHELIOSIS, SECONDARY SYPHILIS, LYMPHOSARCOMA

OCCIPITAL NODE

SUPRACLAVICULAR NODE

AXILLARY NODE

INGUINAL NODE

RUBELLA, RINGWORM, DERMATITIS OF SCALP, PEDICULOSIS, CELLULITIS, INFECTIOUS MONONUCLEOSIS

BREAST ABSCESS, BREAST CARCINOMA, INFECTIONS OF THE UPPER EXTREMITY, TUBERCULOSIS, HODGKIN'S DISEASE

CARCINOMA OF LUNG, NEOPLASM OF GASTROINTESTINAL TRACT, INFECTIONS OF THE NECK AND UPPER EXTREMITY, LARYNX, OR THYROID

INFECTIONS OF LOWER EXTREMITY AND GENITALIA, NEOPLASMS OF GENITALIA, VENEREAL DISEASE, MELANOTIC SARCOMA

Lymphadenopathy 357

MELENA

Ask the following questions:

1. Is it true or false melena? False melena may be induced by iron ingestion, bismuth ingestion, charcoal ingestion, red wine ingestion, and many other substances.
2. Is there a history of alcohol or drug ingestion? It is surprising how often the ingestion of alcohol is overlooked. Aspirin, caffeine, anticoagulants, and reserpine are among the other drugs that may cause melena.
3. Is there associated hematemesis? The presence of hematemesis should prompt a search for esophageal varices, peptic ulcer, gastritis, and many other conditions. For a more thorough discussion of this topic, one is referred to the section on hematemesis (page 264).
4. Is there abdominal pain? The presence of abdominal pain and heartburn should make one think of duodenal ulcer, esophagitis, gastritis, gastric ulcer, mesenteric embolism or thrombosis, and Meckel's diverticulum. On the other hand, the absence of abdominal pain would be more consistent with a blood dyscrasia or hereditary telangiectasia.

DIAGNOSTIC WORKUP

Routine laboratory tests include a CBC, sedimentation rate, urinalysis, chemistry panel, coagulation panel, VDRL test, and stool for occult blood. A stool for ovum and parasites may also need to be done. If these tests are inconclusive, an upper GI series and esophagram would be the next step. Perhaps a small bowel series should be added to the above studies.

If all of these tests are negative or still inconclusive, referral to a gastroenterologist should be made. He will probably perform panendoscopy and resolve the diagnostic dilemma. Occasionally a fluorescein string test may be useful. A radioactive scan following intravenous chromium or technetium-99 may show the site of bleeding in obscure cases. When bleeding continues despite therapy, mesenteric angiography or splenic venography may assist in the diagnosis. Exploratory laparotomy may be necessary in some cases. Needless to say a gastroenterologist should be consulted before untertaking this.

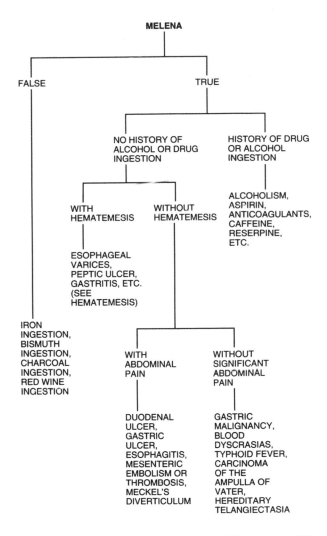

MEMORY LOSS

Ask the following questions:

1. Is there a history of trauma? A history of trauma would suggest concussion, intracranial hematoma, and posttraumatic epilepsy, among other conditions.
2. Is there a history of alcohol or drug ingestion? Chronic alcoholism is associated with Korsakoff's syndrome and Wernicke's encephalopathy. Drugs such as bromides, barbiturates, cocaine, and LSD may induce memory loss. Heavy metals such as lead may cause a chronic encephalopathy with memory loss.
3. Are there systemic signs and symptoms? If there is anemia and memory loss, one should consider pernicious anemia. Pellagra, beriberi, myxedema, lupus erythematosus, uremia, and liver failure may be associated with memory loss.
4. Are there other focal neurologic signs? Extrapyramidal symptoms may be found in Wilson's disease, Huntington's chorea, and Parkinson's disease. Long tract signs may be found in multiple sclerosis, Creutzfeldt-Jakob disease, general paresis, and normal pressure hydrocephalus. When there is memory loss without focal neurologic signs, Alzheimer's disease and Pick's disease should be considered, as well as malingering.

DIAGNOSTIC WORKUP

Routine laboratory tests include a CBC, sedimentation rate, urinalysis, chemistry panel, ANA, serum B_{12} and folic acid, and VDRL test. In the elderly, a chest x-ray should be done to look for a primary neoplasm.

If these studies are negative, the patient may be referred to a neurologist or a CT scan or MRI may be done. The neurology consultation is much less expensive. Ultimately, a spinal tap may need to be done to look for multiple sclerosis and central nervous system lues. A lumbar isotope cisternography may need to be done to rule out normal pressure hydrocephalus. A referral to a psychologist can be made for psychometric testing.

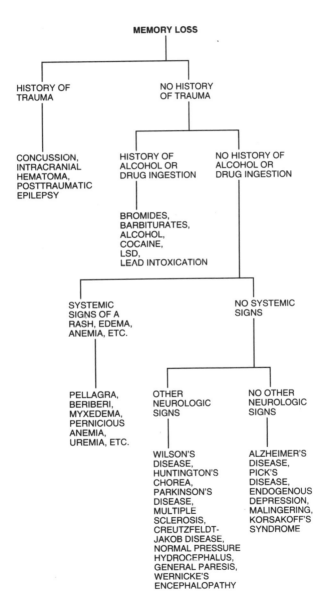

MEMORY LOSS

HISTORY OF TRAUMA

CONCUSSION, INTRACRANIAL HEMATOMA, POSTTRAUMATIC EPILEPSY

NO HISTORY OF TRAUMA

HISTORY OF ALCOHOL OR DRUG INGESTION

BROMIDES, BARBITURATES, ALCOHOL, COCAINE, LSD, LEAD INTOXICATION

NO HISTORY OF ALCOHOL OR DRUG INGESTION

SYSTEMIC SIGNS OF A RASH, EDEMA, ANEMIA, ETC.

PELLAGRA, BERIBERI, MYXEDEMA, PERNICIOUS ANEMIA, UREMIA, ETC.

NO SYSTEMIC SIGNS

OTHER NEUROLOGIC SIGNS

WILSON'S DISEASE, HUNTINGTON'S CHOREA, PARKINSON'S DISEASE, MULTIPLE SCLEROSIS, CREUTZFELDT-JAKOB DISEASE, NORMAL PRESSURE HYDROCEPHALUS, GENERAL PARESIS, WERNICKE'S ENCEPHALOPATHY

NO OTHER NEUROLOGIC SIGNS

ALZHEIMER'S DISEASE, PICK'S DISEASE, ENDOGENOUS DEPRESSION, MALINGERING, KORSAKOFF'S SYNDROME

Memory Loss   361

MENORRHAGIA

Ask the following questions:

1. Is there persistent or recurring abdominal or pelvic pain? The presence of pain with menorrhagia should make one suspect pelvic inflammatory disease, endometriosis, and ectopic pregnancy.
2. Are there abnormalities on the pelvic examination? The pelvic examination will usually be positive in cases of uterine fibroid, pregnancy, cervical polyp, pelvic inflammatory disease, and ectopic pregnancy. Endometriosis may not always be detected on pelvic examination.
3. Is there anemia or other systemic symptoms or signs? The clinician should remember that iron deficiency anemia, hypothyroidism, lupus erythematosus, and cirrhosis of the liver are just a few of the systemic conditions that may present with menorrhagia.

DIAGNOSTIC WORKUP

Routine studies include a CBC, sedimentation rate, urinalysis, pregnancy test, chemistry panel, antinuclear antibody titer, VDRL test, coagulation profile, thyroid profile, and flat plate of the abdomen. A Pap smear and vaginal smear and culture should be done.

If these tests are negative, referral to a gynecologist should be made before undertaking expensive tests such as pelvic ultrasound or CT scan of the abdomen and pelvis. Some clinicians will probably ignore this advice. A gynecologist will often be able to resolve the diagnostic dilemma with a good pelvic examination. Laparoscopy, culdocentesis, endometrial biopsy, and dilation and curettage are just a few of the diagnostic tools at his disposal.

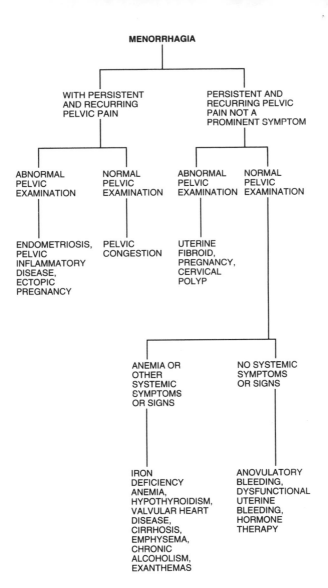

MENORRHAGIA

WITH PERSISTENT AND RECURRING PELVIC PAIN

PERSISTENT AND RECURRING PELVIC PAIN NOT A PROMINENT SYMPTOM

ABNORMAL PELVIC EXAMINATION

NORMAL PELVIC EXAMINATION

ABNORMAL PELVIC EXAMINATION

NORMAL PELVIC EXAMINATION

ENDOMETRIOSIS, PELVIC INFLAMMATORY DISEASE, ECTOPIC PREGNANCY

PELVIC CONGESTION

UTERINE FIBROID, PREGNANCY, CERVICAL POLYP

ANEMIA OR OTHER SYSTEMIC SYMPTOMS OR SIGNS

NO SYSTEMIC SYMPTOMS OR SIGNS

IRON DEFICIENCY ANEMIA, HYPOTHYROIDISM, VALVULAR HEART DISEASE, CIRRHOSIS, EMPHYSEMA, CHRONIC ALCOHOLISM, EXANTHEMAS

ANOVULATORY BLEEDING, DYSFUNCTIONAL UTERINE BLEEDING, HORMONE THERAPY

Menorrhagia   363

MENTAL RETARDATION

Ask the following questions:

1. Is there decreased hair and skin pigment? These findings would suggest phenylketonuria.
2. Are there abnormal secondary sex characteristics? These findings would suggest Klinefelter's syndrome, Turner's syndrome, and Laurence-Moon-Bardet-Biedl syndrome.
3. Are there abnormalities of the skull present? Findings of deformities or enlargement of the skull should suggest rickets, microcephaly, hypertelorism, oxycephaly, and hydrocephalus, among other things.
4. Is there hepatosplenomegaly? The findings of hepatosplenomegaly suggest galactosemia, Hurler's disease, and Gaucher's disease among other diagnostic possibilities.
5. Are there skin changes? Sturge-Weber syndrome, tuberous sclerosis, neurofibromatosis, and cretinism may present with skin changes. Kernicterus is associated with jaundice.
6. Are there other neurologic signs? Tay-Sachs disease, congenital syphilis, Arnold-Chiari malformation, and cerebral diplegia are just a few of the causes of mental retardation that may present with other neurologic signs.

DIAGNOSTIC WORKUP

Routine laboratory tests include a CBC, sedimentation rate, chemistry panel, serum galactose level, VDRL test, thyroid profile, and urine screen for carbohydrates, amino acids, and organic acids. Chromosomal analysis may detect Klinefelter's syndrome, Turner's syndrome, mongolism, and other disorders. If there are deformities of the skull present, a skull x-ray should be done.

An EEG, CT scan of the brain, and psychometric testing will often need to be done, but a referral to a neurologist should be made before ordering these expensive tests.

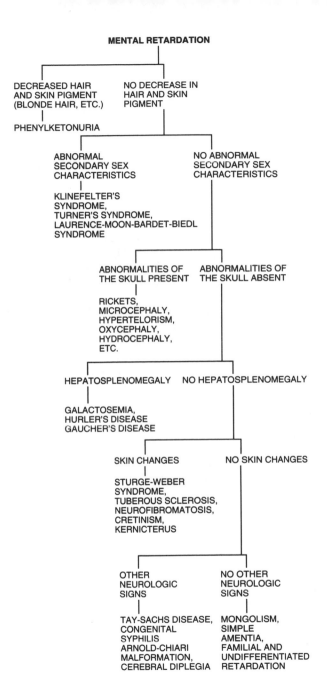

METEORISM

Ask the following questions:

1. Are there hyperactive bowel sounds? These findings should suggest intestinal obstruction, and in that case one would look for strangulated hernia, adhesions, volvulus, mesenteric embolism or thrombosis, and other disorders. Perhaps the problem is a fecal impaction.
2. Is there blood in the stool? Blood in the stool along with hyperactive bowel sounds would suggest a mesenteric embolism or thrombosis.
3. Are there systemic symptoms? The clinician should keep in mind that systemic diseases may present with meteorism. These include diabetes mellitus, lobar pneumonia, typhoid fever, acute pancreatitis, and steatorrhea.
4. Are there neurologic signs? Spinal cord trauma and transverse myelitis are among the many disorders that may present with meteorism.

DIAGNOSTIC WORKUP

Routine laboratory tests include a stat CBC, sedimentation rate, serum amylase and lipase, urinalysis, chemistry panel, stool for occult blood, culture, ovum and parasites, and quantitative fat. A chest x-ray and flat plate of the abdomen should also be done. If these tests are negative, referral to a gastroenterologist or general surgeon is in order before ordering CT scans, ultrasonography, or contrast radiography.

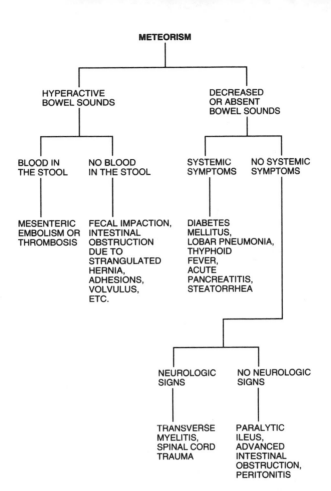

METEORISM

HYPERACTIVE BOWEL SOUNDS

DECREASED OR ABSENT BOWEL SOUNDS

BLOOD IN THE STOOL

NO BLOOD IN THE STOOL

SYSTEMIC SYMPTOMS

NO SYSTEMIC SYMPTOMS

MESENTERIC EMBOLISM OR THROMBOSIS

FECAL IMPACTION, INTESTINAL OBSTRUCTION DUE TO STRANGULATED HERNIA, ADHESIONS, VOLVULUS, ETC.

DIABETES MELLITUS, LOBAR PNEUMONIA, THYPHOID FEVER, ACUTE PANCREATITIS, STEATORRHEA

NEUROLOGIC SIGNS

NO NEUROLOGIC SIGNS

TRANSVERSE MYELITIS, SPINAL CORD TRAUMA

PARALYTIC ILEUS, ADVANCED INTESTINAL OBSTRUCTION, PERITONITIS

METRORRHAGIA

Ask the following questions:

1. Are there abnormalities found on the vaginal examination? An enlarged uterus suggests pregnancy, fibroids, retained secundina, hydatiform mole, choriocarcinoma, endometrial carcinoma, or endometrial polyp. An adnexal mass suggests a granulosa cell tumor, salpingitis, or ectopic pregnancy. Cervical lesions that cause metrorrhagia are cervicitis, carcinoma of the cervix, and cervical polyp. Vaginal lesions include vaginal carcinoma and senile vaginitis.
2. Is there a history of hormone therapy? If the patient has been taking estrogen or progesterone, withdrawal or breakthrough bleeding should be considered.
3. Is there pallor or other signs of anemia? Most types of anemia, but particularly iron deficiency anemia, are associated with metrorrhagia.
4. Is there a history of tremor, tachycardia, or edema? Both hyperthyroidism and hypothyroidism may be associated with metrorrhagia.

If all of these questions fail to turn up any positive answers, then dysfunctional uterine bleeding, collagen disease, and coagulation disorder should be strongly considered.

DIAGNOSTIC WORKUP

Routine studies include a CBC, sedimentation rate, urinalysis, pregnancy test, chemistry panel, antinuclear antibody test, coagulation profile, thyroid profile, and flat plate of the abdomen. A Pap smear and vaginal smear and culture should also be done.

If these are negative, referral to a gynecologist should be made before undertaking expensive diagnostic tests such as ultrasound or CT scans of the abdomen and pelvis. The gynecologist may be able to resolve the diagnostic dilemma with a good pelvic examination. If that is unsuccessful, he may perform laparoscopy or culdocentesis. A dilation and curettage or office endometrial biopsy are among the additional procedures at his disposal.

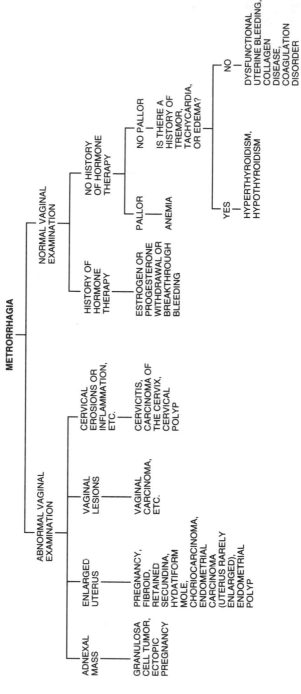

METRORRHAGIA

ABNORMAL VAGINAL EXAMINATION

ADNEXAL MASS — GRANULOSA CELL TUMOR, ECTOPIC PREGNANCY

ENLARGED UTERUS — PREGNANCY, FIBROID, RETAINED SECUNDINA, HYDATIFORM MOLE, CHORIOCARCINOMA, ENDOMETRIAL CARCINOMA (UTERUS RARELY ENLARGED), ENDOMETRIAL POLYP

VAGINAL LESIONS — VAGINAL CARCINOMA, ETC.

CERVICAL EROSIONS OR INFLAMMATION, ETC. — CERVICITIS, CARCINOMA OF THE CERVIX, CERVICAL POLYP

NORMAL VAGINAL EXAMINATION

HISTORY OF HORMONE THERAPY — ESTROGEN OR PROGESTERONE WITHDRAWAL OR BREAKTHROUGH BLEEDING

NO HISTORY OF HORMONE THERAPY

PALLOR — ANEMIA

NO PALLOR — IS THERE A HISTORY OF TREMOR, TACHYCARDIA, OR EDEMA?

YES — HYPERTHYROIDISM, HYPOTHYROIDISM

NO — DYSFUNCTIONAL UTERINE BLEEDING, COLLAGEN DISEASE, COAGULATION DISORDER

MONOPLEGIA

Ask the following questions:

1. Are there hyperactive or pathologic reflexes of the involved extremity? These findings suggest spinal cord tumor, parasagittal tumor, amyotrophic lateral sclerosis, anterior cerebral artery occlusion, spinal cord injury, transverse myelitis, and multiple sclerosis.
2. Are there decreased or absent reflexes of the involved extremity? These findings suggest a herniated disk, a cauda equina tumor or early cervical cord tumor, progressive muscular atrophy, brachial plexus neuropathy, sciatic neuritis, or peripheral neuropathy.
3. Is the onset acute or gradual? An acute onset would suggest a vascular lesion such as anterior cerebral artery occlusion, a spinal cord injury, transverse myelitis, and multiple sclerosis. A gradual onset suggests a space-occupying lesion such as spinal cord tumor, parasagittal tumor, and degenerative diseases such as amyotrophic lateral sclerosis.
4. Are there exacerbations or remissions? The presence of exacerbations or remissions should suggest multiple sclerosis, transient ischemic attack, and migraine.

DIAGNOSTIC WORKUP

Monoplegia of the upper extremities with hyperactive reflexes should suggest the need to order a CT scan or MRI of the brain and/or MRI of the cervical spine.

Monoplegia of the lower extremities with hyperactive reflexes or pathologic reflexes would suggest the need to order MRI of the thoracic spine. However, since an anterior spinal artery occlusion or parasagittal tumor may cause similar findings, a CT scan of the brain may be necessary. Rather than make this difficult choice yourself, a neurologist should be consulted. He may want to do a spinal fluid analysis or evoked potential studies as well. If he believes a vascular lesion is possible, then he may want to do a four-vessel angiography or simply a carotid scan.

The findings of monoplegia with hypoactive reflexes, especially of gradual onset, would suggest a radiculopathy, peripheral neuropathy, or plexopathy. In the lower extremities these findings would indicate the need for a CT scan or MRI of the lumbosacral spine. In the upper extremities these findings would suggest the need for MRI of the cervical spine.

A neuropathy workup is also indicated in monoplegia of the upper or lower extremity (page 425). Nerve conduction velocity studies and electromyographic studies of the involved extremities are extremely valuable also. The most cost-effective approach is to refer the patient to a neurologist at the outset.

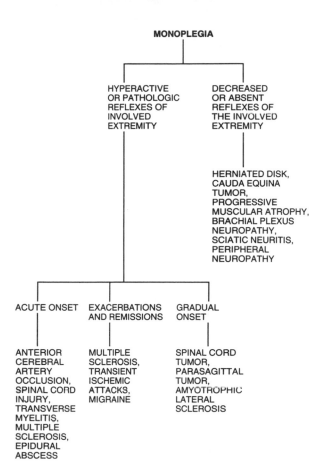

MONOPLEGIA

├── HYPERACTIVE OR PATHOLOGIC REFLEXES OF INVOLVED EXTREMITY

└── DECREASED OR ABSENT REFLEXES OF THE INVOLVED EXTREMITY

    HERNIATED DISK, CAUDA EQUINA TUMOR, PROGRESSIVE MUSCULAR ATROPHY, BRACHIAL PLEXUS NEUROPATHY, SCIATIC NEURITIS, PERIPHERAL NEUROPATHY

ACUTE ONSET

ANTERIOR CEREBRAL ARTERY OCCLUSION, SPINAL CORD INJURY, TRANSVERSE MYELITIS, MULTIPLE SCLEROSIS, EPIDURAL ABSCESS

EXACERBATIONS AND REMISSIONS

MULTIPLE SCLEROSIS, TRANSIENT ISCHEMIC ATTACKS, MIGRAINE

GRADUAL ONSET

SPINAL CORD TUMOR, PARASAGITTAL TUMOR, AMYOTROPHIC LATERAL SCLEROSIS

MOUTH PIGMENTATION

Ask the following questions:

1. Is there generalized pigmentation? The findings of generalized pigmentation would suggest Addison's disease, arsenic poisoning, and occasionally hemochromatosis. When there is no generalized pigmentation, one should suspect Peutz-Jeghers syndrome, chronic cachectic conditions, and acanthosis nigricans.
2. Is there hypotension or weight loss? These findings suggest Addison's disease and arsenic poisoning. If there is no hypotension or weight loss, then the mouth pigmentation and generalized pigmentation may be associated with African ancestry or Fabry's disease.

DIAGNOSTIC WORKUP

Routine laboratory workup includes a CBC, sedimentation rate, urinalysis, chemistry panel, and a VDRL test. If arsenic poisoning is suspected, hair analysis for arsenic should be done. If Addison's disease is suspected, a 24-hr urine collection for 17-hydroxysteroids and 17-ketosteroids should be done. The rapid ACTH test is a suitable alternative but usually more expensive. If Peutz-Jeghers syndrome or acanthosis nigricans is suspected, then a GI series with a small bowel follow-through and a barium enema may be necessary. Endoscopy procedures may also be useful in certain cases.

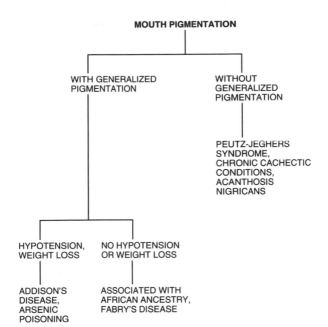

MOUTH PIGMENTATION

WITH GENERALIZED
PIGMENTATION

WITHOUT
GENERALIZED
PIGMENTATION

PEUTZ-JEGHERS
SYNDROME,
CHRONIC CACHECTIC
CONDITIONS,
ACANTHOSIS
NIGRICANS

HYPOTENSION,
WEIGHT LOSS

NO HYPOTENSION
OR WEIGHT LOSS

ADDISON'S
DISEASE,
ARSENIC
POISONING

ASSOCIATED WITH
AFRICAN ANCESTRY,
FABRY'S DISEASE

MUSCULAR ATROPHY

Ask the following questions:

1. Is it focal or diffuse? Focal muscular atrophy would suggest poliomyelitis, early spinal muscular atrophy, peripheral vascular disease, and sympathetic dystrophy. However, occasionally it is an indication of an early spinal cord tumor, herniated disk, or peroneal muscular atrophy. It can also be a sign of an entrapment syndrome of one of the peripheral nerves. Focal muscular atrophy with hyperactive reflexes suggests amyotrophic lateral sclerosis, multiple sclerosis, spinal cord tumors, or syringomyelia.
2. Are the reflexes hypoactive or hyperactive? Muscular atrophy with hypoactive reflexes suggests peripheral neuropathy, poliomyelitis, spinal muscular atrophy, myasthenia gravis, peripheral vascular disease, sympathetic dystrophy, herniated disk, early spinal cord tumor, and peroneal muscular atrophy. Muscular atrophy with hyperactive reflexes suggests multiple sclerosis, spinal cord tumors, syringomyelia, and amyotrophic lateral sclerosis.
3. Are there associated sensory changes? The finding of muscular atrophy with sensory changes suggests a peripheral neuropathy, Guillain-Barré syndrome, Friedreich's ataxia, multiple sclerosis, transverse myelitis, a herniated disk, spinal cord tumor, and peroneal muscular atrophy. It may also suggest syringomyelia.
4. Are the reflexes normal? The presence of normal reflexes suggests anorexia nervosa, tuberculosis, metastatic malignancy, and hyperthyroidism.

DIAGNOSTIC WORKUP

The basic workup includes a CBC, sedimentation rate, urinalysis, chemistry panel, antinuclear antibody titer, serum protein electrophoresis, and a

VDRL test. Additional muscle enzymes may be ordered such as serum aldolase and creatine phosphokinase. A 24-hr urine collection for creatinine and creatine may be done.

At this point it is best to consult a neurologist. He will probably order nerve conduction velocity studies and EMGs of the involved extremities. He also will be best qualified to determine the need for CT scans or MRIs of the brain or spine, as well as the particular study to order in each individual case. At times spinal fluid analysis and muscle biopsies may be necessary to solve the problem. Also, a Tensilon test or acetylcholine receptor antibody titer may be ordered in suspected myasthenia gravis.

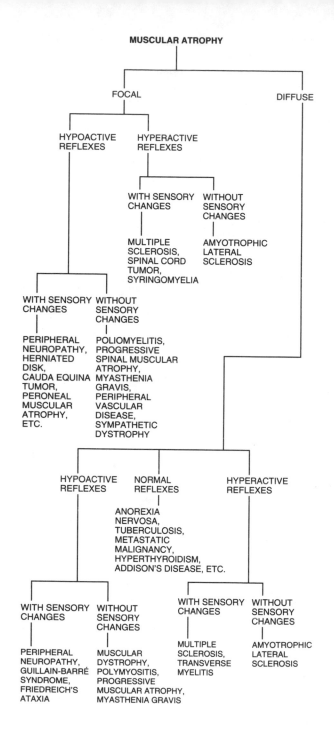

MUSCULOSKELETAL PAIN, GENERALIZED

Ask the following questions:

1. Is there fever? Musculoskeletal pain with fever suggests dengue fever, which is also called breakbone fever, poliomyelitis, Bornholm disease, acute trichinosis, epidemic myalgia, viral influenza, and meningitis, as well as almost any other febrile illness.
2. Is there paralysis? The presence of paralysis, especially if it is focal, would suggest poliomyelitis, but porphyria, polyneuritis, Guillain-Barré syndrome, dermatomyositis, and other collagen diseases may present with generalized musculoskeletal pain and paralysis. If there is diffuse pain without paralysis, one should consider trichinosis and chronic fibromyositis. Polymyalgia rheumatica may also present in this fashion.
3. Is it transient? Transient musculoskeletal pain may occur with fever, but it may also occur after injury, after fatigue and anxiety, and especially after extensive physical workouts.
4. Are there electrolyte abnormalities? One should always remember that electrolyte abnormalities such as hypokalemia, hyponatremia, and hypocalcemia will cause generalized musculoskeletal pain.

DIAGNOSTIC WORKUP

Routine studies include a CBC, sedimentation rate, urinalysis, chemistry panel including electrolytes, an antinuclear antibody (ANA) test, serum protein electrophoresis, febrile agglutinins, chest x-ray, and EKG.

If muscular disease is strongly suspected, then a 24-hr collection for urine creatine and creatinine should be done, as well as serial muscle enzymes.

Perhaps a *Trichinella* skin test or antibody titer will be helpful. An electromyogram and a nerve conduction velocity study may be helpful in both muscular disease and peripheral neuropathies.

A muscle biopsy may be necessary to diagnose dermatomyositis, trichinosis, cysticercosis, and various collagen diseases. Urine for porphyrins and porphobilinogen should be done in difficult diagnostic cases also.

Twenty-four hour urine quantitative potassium, sodium, or calcium will be helpful in the electrolyte disorders, as the serum electrolytes do not always reflect the decrease in intracellular electrolytes.

A spinal tap will help diagnose poliomyelitis, meningitis, and Guillain-Barré syndrome. It may be necessary to seek the help of a rheumatologist, a neurologist, or an infectious disease specialist.

MUSCULOSKELETAL PAIN, GENERALIZED

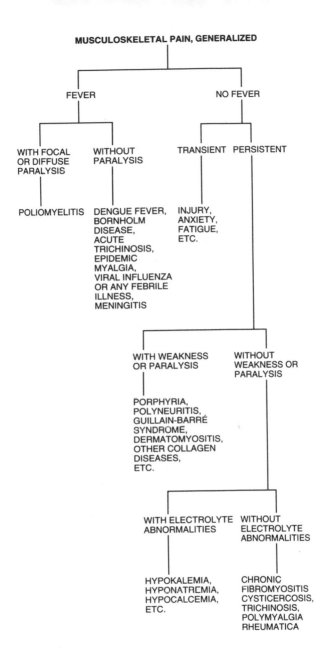

NAIL ABNORMALITIES

Ask the following questions:

1. Are the abnormalities focal or diffuse? Focal abnormalities include thickening, which is often due to fungus infections; inflammation, which is usually due to a paronychia, onychia, fungal infection, or syphilis; hemorrhages under the nail which may be due to trauma, subacute bacterial endocarditis, or trichinosis; pitting of the nail, which may be due to psoriasis; and atrophy or dystrophy of the nail, which may be due to peripheral vascular disease, epidermolysis bullosa, nail biting, peripheral neuropathy, and various other dermatoses. Diffuse abnormalities of the nail may include thickening due to syphilis, hyperthyroidism or hypothyroidism, clubbing, cyanotic heart disease, bronchiectasis, carcinoma of the lungs, and other disorders; yellow nails due to lymphedema or chest conditions; and spoon nails due to iron deficiency anemia.

   Diffuse spoon nails may be caused by iron deficiency anemia. Yellow nails may be due to lymphedema or chest conditions. Clubbing may be due to cyanotic heart disease, bronchiectasis, or carcinoma of the lung (see page 98). Thickening may result from syphilis, hyperthyroidism, or hypothyroidism. Hemorrhages may be due to trauma, subacute bacterial endocarditis, or trichinosis. Pitting may be due to psoriasis. Focal thickening may be due to fungus infections. Focal inflammation may be due to paronychia, onychia, or syphilis. Focal atrophy or dystrophy may be due to peripheral vascular disease, peripheral neuropathy, epidermolysis bullosa, nail biting, or other dermatoses.

DIAGNOSTIC WORKUP

Focal abnormalities of one nail warrant a culture and sensitivity of any scrapings or exudates from the area, as well as an x-ray of the digit or extremity. A CBC and sedimentation rate will help identify an infectious process. A glucose tolerance test will help identify diabetes mellitus. Careful assessment of the area for vascular insufficiency includes Doppler studies and possibly arteriography. A nerve conduction velocity study and EMG may be necessary if peripheral neuropathy is suspected. A skin or nail biopsy may be helpful.

Routine tests for diffuse nail changes include a CBC, sedimentation rate, chemistry panel, VDRL test, ANA, thyroid profile, chest x-ray, and EKG. Arterial blood gases and pulmonary function studies should be done if clubbing is suspected. Other tests for clubbing will be found on page 98. Serial blood cultures should be done if subacute bacterial endocarditis is suspected. *Trichinella* skin test or antibody titer should be done in cases where there are splintered nails with negative cultures for subacute bacterial endocarditis. Muscle or skin biopsy will be useful not only for trichinosis, but also for collagen disease. Nerve conduction velocity studies and EMGs will be helpful in diagnosing peripheral neuropathy.

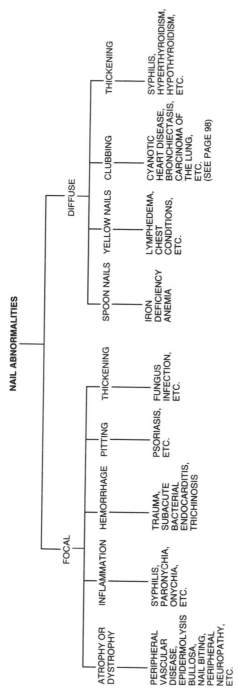

NAIL ABNORMALITIES

FOCAL

- **ATROPHY OR DYSTROPHY**
  - PERIPHERAL VASCULAR DISEASE, EPIDERMOLYSIS BULLOSA, NAIL BITING, PERIPHERAL NEUROPATHY, ETC.
- **INFLAMMATION**
  - SYPHILIS, PARONYCHIA, ONYCHIA, ETC.
- **HEMORRHAGE**
  - TRAUMA, SUBACUTE BACTERIAL ENDOCARDITIS, TRICHINOSIS
- **PITTING**
  - PSORIASIS, ETC.
- **THICKENING**
  - FUNGUS INFECTION, ETC.

DIFFUSE

- **SPOON NAILS**
  - IRON DEFICIENCY ANEMIA
- **YELLOW NAILS**
  - LYMPHEDEMA, CHEST CONDITIONS, ETC.
- **CLUBBING**
  - CYANOTIC HEART DISEASE, BRONCHIECTASIS, CARCINOMA OF THE LUNG, ETC. (SEE PAGE 98)
- **THICKENING**
  - SYPHILIS, HYPERTHYROIDISM, HYPOTHYROIDISM, ETC.

NASAL DISCHARGE

Ask the following questions:

1. Is it unilateral or bilateral? Unilateral nasal discharge, especially if it is purulent, suggests acute sinusitis, Wegener's granulomatosis, neoplasm, foreign body, and syphilis. If the discharge is clear or mucoid, it could be just simply chronic sinusitis. Bilateral nasal discharge suggests an upper respiratory infection, especially if it is an acute onset. If it is a chronic condition and it is mucoid or clear, allergic rhinitis, chronic sinusitis, or vasomotor rhinitis should be suspected. Rarely, cerebral spinal fluid rhinorrhea is the problem.

2. Is there fever? The presence of fever makes acute sinusitis most likely if the discharge is unilateral, but if it is bilateral one should suspect an acute viral upper respiratory infection. However, if there is significant pain associated with the fever, one should consider the possibility that there is an acute sinusitis.

3. Is it purulent, mucoid, or clear? The presence of a purulent discharge suggests acute sinusitis, chronic bacterial sinusitis, mucormycosis, Wegener's granulomatosis, neoplasm, foreign body, and syphilis. The presence of a mucoid discharge suggests allergic rhinitis or a chronic sinusitis. The presence of a clear discharge suggests cerebral spinal fluid rhinorrhea, and senile rhinorrhea, especially if the patient is older. If there is unilateral face pain, one should consider cluster headache or migraine.

4. Is there pain? The presence of pain with fever or purulent discharge certainly suggests acute sinusitis. However, when there is pain with a clear discharge, one should think of cluster headache or migraine.

5. Is there sneezing or an allergy history? The presence of sneezing or an allergic history should suggest allergic rhinitis and sinusitis. However, allergic rhinitis and sinusitis may also occur without sneezing or an allergic history.

DIAGNOSTIC WORKUP

Routine orders for the workup of a nasal discharge include a CBC, sedimentation rate, chemistry panel, VDRL test, smear and culture of the nasal discharge, and x-rays of the sinuses. If the discharge is chronic and mucoid or clear, one should do a nasal smear for eosinophils and serum IgE level to look for allergic rhinitis. A trial of therapy may be indicated in these cases also.

If there is still diagnostic confusion after the above tests have been done, referral to an ear, nose and throat specialist or an allergist is indicated. The specialist will perform nasopharyngoscopy and is in a better position to evaluate whether CT scans or bone scans are needed. Also, he can better evaluate when the patient should undergo allergy skin testing, inhalation testing, or radioallergosorbent tests (RAST).

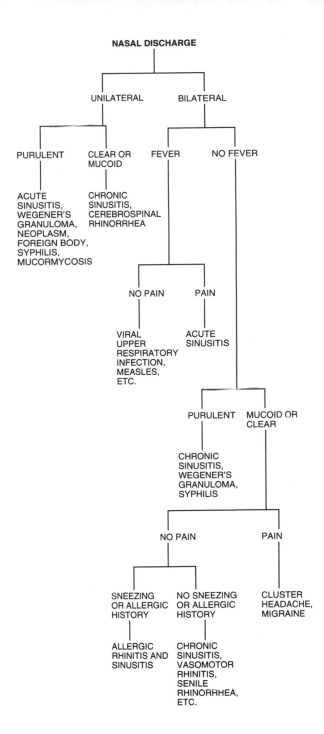

NASAL OBSTRUCTION

Ask the following questions:

1. Is it acute or chronic? The presence of acute
   nasal obstruction should suggest acute sinusitis,
   acute rhinitis, a viral upper respiratory infection
   (URI), allergic rhinitis, nasal diphtheria, cluster
   headache, migraine, foreign body, and trauma.
   The presence of chronic nasal obstruction, particularly if it is unilateral, would suggest sinusitis, foreign bodies, neoplasm, deviated septum,
   polyps, Wegener's granulomatosis, mucormycosis, and nasal gumma. If it is bilateral, it would
   suggest allergic rhinitis, vasomotor rhinitis, adenoid enlargement, rhinitis medicamentosa and
   ingestion of drugs such as reserpine.
2. Is it unilateral or bilateral? The presence of unilateral nasal obstruction suggests acute purulent
   sinusitis, foreign body, neoplasm, mucormycosis,
   Wegener's granulomatosis, polyps, and neoplasms. It also suggests a deviated septum. The
   presence of bilateral nasal obstruction suggests
   allergic rhinitis, acute viral upper respiratory infection, nasal diphtheria, rhinitis medicamentosa, adenoids, and vasomotor rhinitis.
3. Is there fever? The presence of fever with unilateral nasal obstruction would suggest acute sinusitis. The presence of fever with bilateral nasal
   obstruction would suggest acute rhinitis and
   acute viral upper respiratory infection. Nasal
   diphtheria may occasionally present with this
   picture, even in modern times.

DIAGNOSTIC WORKUP

Routine diagnostic studies include a CBC, sedimentation rate, chemistry panel, VDRL test, ANA, and a
nasal smear and culture for bacteria and fungi, and
x-rays of the sinuses. A nasal smear for eosinophils
and serum IgE antibodies should be done if allergy

is suspected. A trial of antibiotics or antihistamines may assist in the diagnosis.

If there is still confusion regarding the diagnosis at this point, a referral to an ear, nose and throat specialist or allergist would be indicated. The ear, nose and throat specialist may do a nasopharyngoscopy and is in a better position to determine when CT scans or bone scans are indicated. The allergist can best determine whether allergy skin testing, inhalation testing, or RAST studies would be indicated.

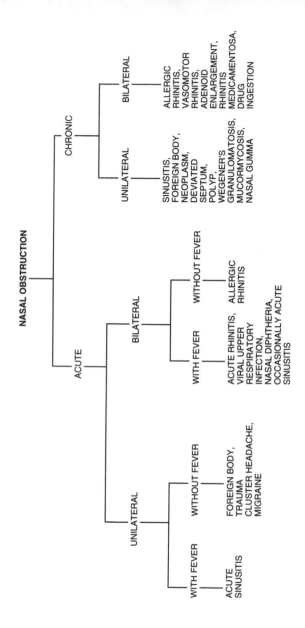

NASAL OBSTRUCTION

ACUTE

UNILATERAL

WITH FEVER
ACUTE SINUSITIS

WITHOUT FEVER
FOREIGN BODY, TRAUMA CLUSTER HEADACHE, MIGRAINE

BILATERAL

WITH FEVER
ACUTE RHINITIS, VIRAL UPPER RESPIRATORY INFECTION, NASAL DIPHTHERIA, OCCASIONALLY ACUTE SINUSITIS

WITHOUT FEVER
ALLERGIC RHINITIS

CHRONIC

UNILATERAL
SINUSITIS, FOREIGN BODY, NEOPLASM, DEVIATED SEPTUM, POLYP, WEGENER'S GRANULOMATOSIS, MUCORMYCOSIS, NASAL GUMMA

BILATERAL
ALLERGIC RHINITIS, VASOMOTOR RHINITIS, ADENOID ENLARGEMENT, RHINITIS MEDICAMENTOSA, DRUG INGESTION

NAUSEA AND VOMITING

Ask the following questions:

1. Is there a history of alcohol or drug ingestion? Alcohol and many drugs such as digitalis, aspirin, nonsteroidal anti-inflammatory agents, antihypertensives, and antibiotics may cause gastric irritation or gastritis.
2. Is there fever? Fever may point to a localized abdominal condition such as acute cholecystitis or acute appendicitis, as well as a systemic condition such as tuberculosis, brucellosis, yellow fever, and other febrile illnesses.
3. Is there abdominal pain? Abdominal pain suggests the possibility of acute cholecystitis, acute appendicitis, pyelonephritis, pancreatitis, renal calculus, and peritonitis.
4. Is there an abdominal mass? The presence of an abdominal mass suggests pyloric or intestinal obstruction, a pancreatic neoplasm, acute cholecystitis, Crohn's disease, perinephric abscess, diverticulitis, and other abscesses and neoplasms.
5. Is there vertigo? The clinician should remember that inner ear diseases such as Ménière's disease and labyrinthitis may be associated with vomiting and sometimes the vertigo is not mentioned by the patient.
6. Is there headache? Migraine, concussion, cerebral tumors or other space-occupying lesions, meningitis, and subarachnoid hemorrhage are associated with headaches, nausea, and vomiting.

DIAGNOSTIC WORKUP

The basic workup includes a CBC, sedimentation rate, urinalysis, urine drug screen, chemistry panel and electrolytes, serum amylase, arterial blood gases, stools for occult blood, chest x-ray, EKG, and flat plate of the abdomen. A pregnancy test should be routine in women of childbearing age. If there is fever, febrile agglutinins and a heterophile antibody titer should be done. If there is an abdominal mass, a gallbladder ultrasound and intravenous pyelogram may need to be done. Isotope scanning with iminodiacetic acid derivatives is extremely useful to detect acute cholecystitis. If there is chronic vomiting and abdominal pain, the diagnosis can often be made with an upper GI series, small bowel series, or barium enema.

When there is persistent vomiting with abdominal pain, an exploratory laparotomy may need to be considered. The presence of an abdominal mass merits consideration of a CT scan. However, before ordering expensive diagnostic tests, a general surgeon or gastroenterologist ought to be consulted. Laparoscopy, gastroscopy, esophagoscopy, duodenoscopy, and colonoscopy all need to be considered in the workup.

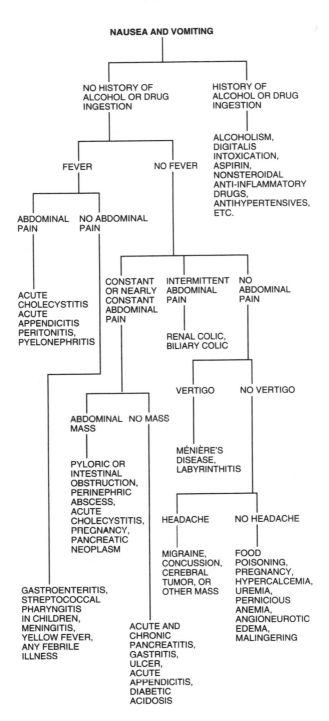

NAUSEA AND VOMITING

NO HISTORY OF ALCOHOL OR DRUG INGESTION

HISTORY OF ALCOHOL OR DRUG INGESTION

ALCOHOLISM, DIGITALIS INTOXICATION, ASPIRIN, NONSTEROIDAL ANTI-INFLAMMATORY DRUGS, ANTIHYPERTENSIVES, ETC.

FEVER

NO FEVER

ABDOMINAL PAIN

NO ABDOMINAL PAIN

ACUTE CHOLECYSTITIS ACUTE APPENDICITIS PERITONITIS, PYELONEPHRITIS

CONSTANT OR NEARLY CONSTANT ABDOMINAL PAIN

INTERMITTENT ABDOMINAL PAIN

NO ABDOMINAL PAIN

RENAL COLIC, BILIARY COLIC

VERTIGO

NO VERTIGO

ABDOMINAL MASS

NO MASS

MÉNIÈRE'S DISEASE, LABYRINTHITIS

PYLORIC OR INTESTINAL OBSTRUCTION, PERINEPHRIC ABSCESS, ACUTE CHOLECYSTITIS, PREGNANCY, PANCREATIC NEOPLASM

HEADACHE

NO HEADACHE

MIGRAINE, CONCUSSION, CEREBRAL TUMOR, OR OTHER MASS

FOOD POISONING, PREGNANCY, HYPERCALCEMIA, UREMIA, PERNICIOUS ANEMIA, ANGIONEUROTIC EDEMA, MALINGERING

GASTROENTERITIS, STREPTOCOCCAL PHARYNGITIS IN CHILDREN, MENINGITIS, YELLOW FEVER, ANY FEBRILE ILLNESS

ACUTE AND CHRONIC PANCREATITIS, GASTRITIS, ULCER, ACUTE APPENDICITIS, DIABETIC ACIDOSIS

Nausea and Vomiting   393

NECK PAIN

Ask the following questions:

1. Is there radiation of the pain to one or both upper extremities? The findings of radiation of the pain to one or both upper extremities would suggest a space-occupying lesion such as a herniated disk, spinal cord tumor, fracture, or cervical spondylosis.
2. Are there focal neurologic findings? The presence of focal neurologic findings make a space-occupying lesion even more likely and the conditions that should be considered are fracture, herniated disk, spinal cord tumor, and cervical spondylosis. One should not forget a Pancoast's tumor.
3. Is there nuchal rigidity? The findings of nuchal rigidity suggest meningitis or subarachnoid hemorrhage.

DIAGNOSTIC WORKUP

Routine tests include a CBC, sedimentation rate, urinalysis, chemistry panel, arthritis panel, and plain films of the cervical spine. If there are focal neurologic findings, MRI of the cervical spine, as well as electromyographic examinations, nerve conduction velocity studies, and dermatomal somatosensory evoked potential studies may need to be done.

It is wise to consult a neurologist or neurosurgeon before ordering these expensive tests. If there is nuchal rigidity, a CT scan of the brain should be done before performing a spinal tap unless there are clear-cut clinical findings of meningitis. If possible, a neurologist should be consulted first in these circumstances.

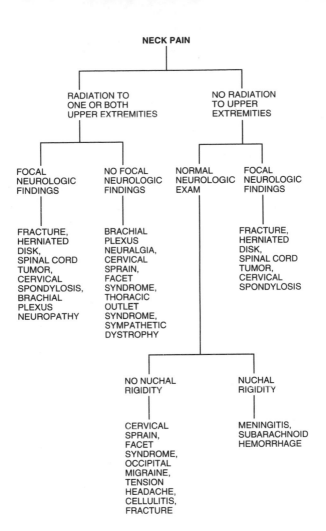

NECK PAIN

RADIATION TO ONE OR BOTH UPPER EXTREMITIES

NO RADIATION TO UPPER EXTREMITIES

FOCAL NEUROLOGIC FINDINGS

FRACTURE, HERNIATED DISK, SPINAL CORD TUMOR, CERVICAL SPONDYLOSIS, BRACHIAL PLEXUS NEUROPATHY

NO FOCAL NEUROLOGIC FINDINGS

BRACHIAL PLEXUS NEURALGIA, CERVICAL SPRAIN, FACET SYNDROME, THORACIC OUTLET SYNDROME, SYMPATHETIC DYSTROPHY

NORMAL NEUROLOGIC EXAM

FOCAL NEUROLOGIC FINDINGS

FRACTURE, HERNIATED DISK, SPINAL CORD TUMOR, CERVICAL SPONDYLOSIS

NO NUCHAL RIGIDITY

CERVICAL SPRAIN, FACET SYNDROME, OCCIPITAL MIGRAINE, TENSION HEADACHE, CELLULITIS, FRACTURE

NUCHAL RIGIDITY

MENINGITIS, SUBARACHNOID HEMORRHAGE

NECK STIFFNESS

Ask the following questions:

1. Is it acute or chronic? Acute stiffness of the neck should make one look for nuchal rigidity. If there is nuchal rigidity, then meningitis or subarachnoid hemorrhage would be high on the list of possibilities. If there is chronic neck stiffness, one should consider rheumatoid arthritis, cervical spondylosis, and idiopathic torticollis. With a history of trauma, the possibility of flexion-extension injury and fracture is more likely.
2. Is there nuchal rigidity or fever? The presence of nuchal rigidity or fever should make one think of meningitis, subarachnoid hemorrhage, or meningism due to some systemic infectious disease. Retropharyngeal abscess must also be considered.
3. Is it congenital or acquired? The presence of congenital stiffness of the neck should make one think of congenital torticollis or Klippel-Feil syndrome. Chronic acquired neck stiffness should make one think of cervical spondylosis, Parkinson's disease, idiopathic torticollis, rheumatoid arthritis, tuberculosis, fractures of the spine, flexion-extension injuries, and inflammation of the lymph nodes.
4. Are there x-ray changes? Plane films of the cervical spine will often reveal cervical spondylosis, fractures, and tuberculosis. However, one should not jump to the conclusion that this is the cause of the condition.

DIAGNOSTIC WORKUP

If there is nuchal rigidity and fever, a CT scan of the brain should be done to rule out a space-occupying lesion and then following that, a spinal tap for analysis, smear and culture.

If there is no nuchal rigidity or fever, plain films

of the cervical spine are a good place to start the diagnostic workup. A CBC, sedimentation rate, urinalysis, chemistry panel, and arthritis profile may also be helpful. If the stiffness is associated with pain radiating into the upper extremities, electromyography and nerve conduction velocity studies may be useful. If the stiffness persists, MRI of the cervical spine may be necessary. A bone scan may identify a subtle fracture or osteomyelitis. A neurologic specialist should be consulted before ordering expensive diagnostic tests.

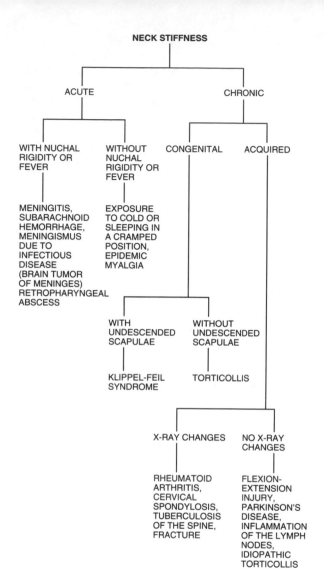

NECK STIFFNESS

ACUTE

CHRONIC

ACUTE:

WITH NUCHAL RIGIDITY OR FEVER
→ MENINGITIS, SUBARACHNOID HEMORRHAGE, MENINGISMUS DUE TO INFECTIOUS DISEASE (BRAIN TUMOR OF MENINGES) RETROPHARYNGEAL ABSCESS

WITHOUT NUCHAL RIGIDITY OR FEVER
→ EXPOSURE TO COLD OR SLEEPING IN A CRAMPED POSITION, EPIDEMIC MYALGIA

CHRONIC:

CONGENITAL

ACQUIRED

WITH UNDESCENDED SCAPULAE
→ KLIPPEL-FEIL SYNDROME

WITHOUT UNDESCENDED SCAPULAE
→ TORTICOLLIS

X-RAY CHANGES
→ RHEUMATOID ARTHRITIS, CERVICAL SPONDYLOSIS, TUBERCULOSIS OF THE SPINE, FRACTURE

NO X-RAY CHANGES
→ FLEXION-EXTENSION INJURY, PARKINSON'S DISEASE, INFLAMMATION OF THE LYMPH NODES, IDIOPATHIC TORTICOLLIS

NECK SWELLING

Ask the following questions:

1. Is it focal or diffuse? Focal masses or swellings may be thyroglossal cyst, branchial cleft cyst, aneurysm, an enlarged lymph node due to Hodgkin's disease, metastatic carcinoma, sarcoidosis, a cystic hygroma, carotid body tumor, Riedel's struma, and thyroid adenomas and carcinomas. Diffuse masses would be Graves' disease, subacute thyroiditis, superior vena cava syndrome, nontoxic goiter, venous distention of congestive heart failure or superior vena cava syndrome, and subcutaneous emphysema.
2. If the lesion is focal, is it in the midline or lateral to the midline? Midline masses are thyroglossal cysts, adenoma of the thyroid, Riedel's struma, and thyroid cyst. Lateral masses include a pharyngeal pouch, bronchial cyst, pulsion diverticulum, stone of Wharton's duct, Virchow's node, cervical rib, metastatic lymph nodes or Hodgkin's lymphoma, metastatic carcinoma, cystic hygroma, carotid body tumor, and some thyroid masses.
3. Is the swelling intermittent? The presence of an intermittent swelling suggests a pulsion diverticulum, venous distention of congestive heart failure, a bronchial cyst, a stone of Wharton's duct, and aneurysms.
4. Is there crepitus? Subcutaneous crepitus is present in subcutaneous emphysema.
5. Is the swelling associated with a tremor or tachycardia? The presence of tremor or tachycardia would make one think of Graves' disease and subacute thyroiditis.

DIAGNOSTIC WORKUP

Routine tests include a CBC, sedimentation rate, urinalysis, chemistry panel, thyroid profile, chest x-ray, and EKG.

Measurement of venous pressure and circulation time and pulmonary function studies will help differentiate congestive heart failure. A radioactive iodine uptake and scan will help differentiate thyroid tumors and enlargements. Ultrasound and needle aspiration will be needed in differentiating cystic adenomas. A lymph node biopsy will be useful in diagnosing sarcoidosis, lymphomas, and metastatic carcinoma. Esophagram will help detect Zenker's diverticulum. Angiography will be useful in diagnosing aortic aneurysms, innominate aneurysms, and subclavian aneurysms. A CT scan of the mediastinum will help diagnose superior vena cava syndrome.

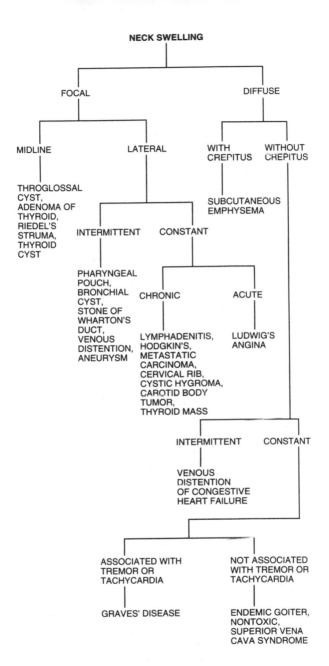

NECK SWELLING

- **FOCAL**
  - **MIDLINE**
    - THROGLOSSAL CYST, ADENOMA OF THYROID, RIEDEL'S STRUMA, THYROID CYST
  - **LATERAL**
    - **INTERMITTENT**
      - PHARYNGEAL POUCH, BRONCHIAL CYST, STONE OF WHARTON'S DUCT, VENOUS DISTENTION, ANEURYSM
    - **CONSTANT**
      - **CHRONIC**
        - LYMPHADENITIS, HODGKIN'S, METASTATIC CARCINOMA, CERVICAL RIB, CYSTIC HYGROMA, CAROTID BODY TUMOR, THYROID MASS
      - **ACUTE**
        - LUDWIG'S ANGINA
- **DIFFUSE**
  - **WITH CREPITUS**
    - SUBCUTANEOUS EMPHYSEMA
  - **WITHOUT CREPITUS**
    - **INTERMITTENT**
      - VENOUS DISTENTION OF CONGESTIVE HEART FAILURE
    - **CONSTANT**
      - **ASSOCIATED WITH TREMOR OR TACHYCARDIA**
        - GRAVES' DISEASE
      - **NOT ASSOCIATED WITH TREMOR OR TACHYCARDIA**
        - ENDEMIC GOITER, NONTOXIC, SUPERIOR VENA CAVA SYNDROME

Neck Swelling   401

NIGHTMARES

Ask the following questions:

1. Are they acute or chronic? The presence of acute nightmares should make one think of the possibility of infectious disease, acute situational maladjustment, or a head injury. Remember, there may be amnesia for the head injury. Chronic nightmares may be associated with drugs or alcohol use, epilepsy, and neuroses or psychoses.
2. Is there a history of trauma? Nightmares following trauma may be due to the acute anxiety associated with the trauma or actually a head injury.
3. Is there a history of drug or alcohol use? Acute alcoholic intoxication can create hallucinations and nightmares. Chronic alcoholism can lead to delirium tremens. Benzodiazepines and numerous other drugs may cause nightmares.
4. Is there a history of tongue biting or incontinence? These findings suggest grand mal epilepsy. Nightmares may result from complex partial seizures without tongue biting or incontinence.

DIAGNOSTIC WORKUP

A CBC, sedimentation rate, and chemistry panel will help rule out infectious diseases. A urine drug screen will help rule out the possibility of drug-induced nightmares. A wake and sleep EEG will help diagnose epilepsy. If epilepsy is strongly suspected, a therapeutic trial of anticonvulsants may be necessary. If the workup is negative, referral to a psychiatrist or psychologist is in order.

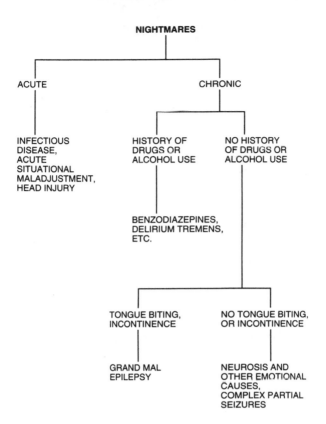

NIGHTMARES

ACUTE

INFECTIOUS
DISEASE,
ACUTE
SITUATIONAL
MALADJUSTMENT,
HEAD INJURY

CHRONIC

HISTORY OF
DRUGS OR
ALCOHOL USE

NO HISTORY
OF DRUGS OR
ALCOHOL USE

BENZODIAZEPINES,
DELIRIUM TREMENS,
ETC.

TONGUE BITING,
INCONTINENCE

NO TONGUE BITING,
OR INCONTINENCE

GRAND MAL
EPILEPSY

NEUROSIS AND
OTHER EMOTIONAL
CAUSES,
COMPLEX PARTIAL
SEIZURES

Nightmares   403

NOCTURIA

Ask the following questions:

1. Is there daytime frequency of urination also? If there is daytime frequency, the differential diagnosis of polyuria should be considered (page 449).
2. Is there associated pain or difficulty voiding? These findings would suggest cystitis, prostatitis, and urethritis.
3. Is there dyspnea, orthopnea, or peripheral edema? These findings would suggest congestive heart failure. If there is no dyspnea or edema, one should consider chronic nephritis.

DIAGNOSTIC WORKUP

Routine laboratory tests should include a CBC, sedimentation rate, urinalysis, chemistry panel, and urine culture and sensitivity. A quantitative 24-hr urine volume should be determined. If this is above normal, the differential diagnosis of polyuria should be considered and additional workup can be found on page 449.

Catheterization for residual urine will help determine if there is bladder neck obstruction. If congestive heart failure is suspected, a chest x-ray, EKG, and venous pressure and circulation time should be done. For further evaluation, a nephrologist or urologist may be consulted.

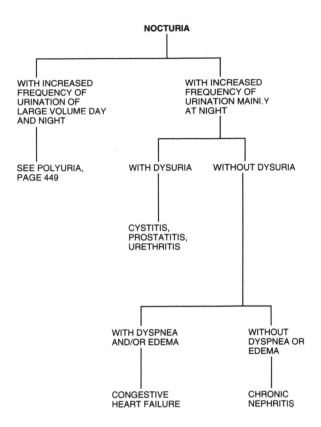

NOCTURIA

- WITH INCREASED FREQUENCY OF URINATION OF LARGE VOLUME DAY AND NIGHT
  - SEE POLYURIA, PAGE 449
- WITH INCREASED FREQUENCY OF URINATION MAINLY AT NIGHT
  - WITH DYSURIA
    - CYSTITIS, PROSTATITIS, URETHRITIS
  - WITHOUT DYSURIA
    - WITH DYSPNEA AND/OR EDEMA
      - CONGESTIVE HEART FAILURE
    - WITHOUT DYSPNEA OR EDEMA
      - CHRONIC NEPHRITIS

NOSE, REGURGITATION OF FOOD THROUGH

Ask the following questions:

1. Are there structural abnormalities on examination of the nasopharynx? Structural abnormalities of the palate indicate cleft palate, congenital short soft palate, trauma, tuberculosis, syphilis, carcinoma, leprosy, and post-tonsillectomy scarring.
2. Are the abnormalities congenital or acquired? Congenital abnormalities of the palate include cleft palate and congenital short soft palate. Acquired abnormalities of the palate include trauma, syphilis, tuberculosis, carcinoma, leprosy, and post-tonsillectomy scarring.
3. Is there paralysis of the soft palate? The finding of paralysis of the soft palate may suggest myasthenia gravis, poliomyelitis, Guillain-Barré syndrome, pseudobulbar palsy, brain tumor, basilar artery insufficiency, and syphilitic meningitis.
4. Is the paralysis of the soft palate intermittent or constant? Intermittent paralysis of the soft palate should suggest myasthenia gravis.
5. Are there associated hypoactive or hyperactive reflexes? The presence of hypoactive reflexes would suggest poliomyelitis or Guillain-Barré syndrome. The presence of hyperactive reflexes or sensory findings would suggest pseudobulbar palsy, a brain tumor, basilar artery insufficiency, and syphilitic meningitis among other conditions.

DIAGNOSTIC WORKUP

Routine laboratory tests include a CBC, sedimentation rate, urinalysis, chemistry panel, VDRL test, smear and culture from the lesions in the nasopharynx, and a tuberculin test. A chest x-ray also should be done if tuberculosis is suspected. A neurologic workup consists of MRI of the brain, electromyographic and nerve conduction velocity studies, spinal fluid analysis, acetylcholine receptor antibody titers, and Tensilon tests. It is best to consult an ear, nose and throat specialist or neurologic specialist before ordering expensive diagnostic tests.

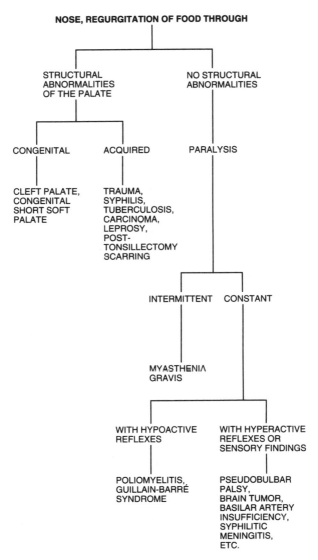

NOSE, REGURGITATION OF FOOD THROUGH

STRUCTURAL ABNORMALITIES OF THE PALATE

NO STRUCTURAL ABNORMALITIES

CONGENITAL

ACQUIRED

PARALYSIS

CLEFT PALATE, CONGENITAL SHORT SOFT PALATE

TRAUMA, SYPHILIS, TUBERCULOSIS, CARCINOMA, LEPROSY, POST-TONSILLECTOMY SCARRING

INTERMITTENT   CONSTANT

MYASTHENIA GRAVIS

WITH HYPOACTIVE REFLEXES

WITH HYPERACTIVE REFLEXES OR SENSORY FINDINGS

POLIOMYELITIS, GUILLAIN-BARRÉ SYNDROME

PSEUDOBULBAR PALSY, BRAIN TUMOR, BASILAR ARTERY INSUFFICIENCY, SYPHILITIC MENINGITIS, ETC.

NYSTAGMUS

Ask the following questions:

1. Is the nystagmus pendular? Pendular nystagmus without a fast or slow component suggests ocular nystagmus due to albinism, partial blindness, or other ocular disorders.
2. Is it intermittent or fatigable? Intermittent or fatigable nystagmus suggests otologic disorders such as acoustic neuroma, Ménière's disease, vestibular neuronitis, and acute labyrinthitis.
3. Is there associated tinnitus or deafness? The presence of nystagmus with tinnitus or deafness also suggests otologic disorders such as acoustic neuroma, Ménière's disease, or cholesteatoma. If there are long tract signs, then multiple sclerosis and brain stem tumors must be considered.
4. Is the nystagmus brought on by change of position? Nystagmus brought on by certain changes of position suggests benign positional vertigo. However, this also may be found in posttraumatic labyrinthitis and postconcussion syndrome.
5. Are there associated long tract signs? The presence of long tract signs suggests multiple sclerosis, basilar artery insufficiency, syringomyelia, and Friedreich's ataxia. Certain brain stem tumors may also be associated with long tract signs.

DIAGNOSTIC WORKUP

The basic diagnostic workup includes visual acuity, visual fields, audiogram, caloric testing, and x-rays of the skull, mastoids and petrous bones. If these are negative or indefinite, a CT scan or MRI of the brain will be necessary. A spinal fluid analysis will help diagnose central nervous system lues and multiple sclerosis. A brain stem evoked potential or visual evoked potential study may be needed to diagnose multiple sclerosis. The help of a neurologic specialist should be sought before ordering expensive diagnostic tests. Cisternography, tomography, and vertebral basilar angiography are occasionally necessary to establish the diagnosis.

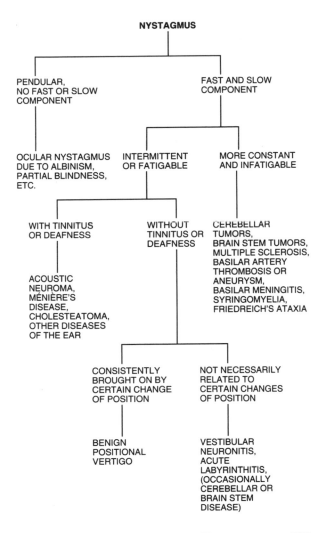

OBESITY, PATHOLOGIC

Ask the following questions:

1. Is there associated hyperphagia? If the patient recognizes that he or she has a ravenous appetite or eats more than is necessary, the possibility of an insulinoma or Fröhlich's syndrome should be considered.
2. Is the obesity centripetal? The presence of centripetal obesity, especially with moon facies, should suggest Cushing's syndrome.
3. Is the obesity mainly of the lower extremities? This finding would suggest lipodystrophy.
4. Is there mental retardation? The presence of mental retardation should suggest Laurence-Moon-Bardet-Biedl syndrome.
5. What is the sex of the patient? In male patients one should consider Klinefelter's syndrome and in female patients one should consider polycystic ovary.

DIAGNOSTIC WORKUP

Routine laboratory tests include a CBC, urinalysis, chemistry panel, 2-hr postprandial blood sugar, and thyroid profile. If an insulinoma is strongly suspected, a 24–36 hr fast, a 5-hr glucose tolerance test and tolbutamide tolerance test may be done. If Cushing's syndrome is suspected, a serum cortisol and cortisol suppression test should be done. Pelvic ultrasound will help diagnose polycystic ovaries. Chromosomal analysis will help diagnose Klinefelter's syndrome. Perhaps a psychiatrist should be consulted.

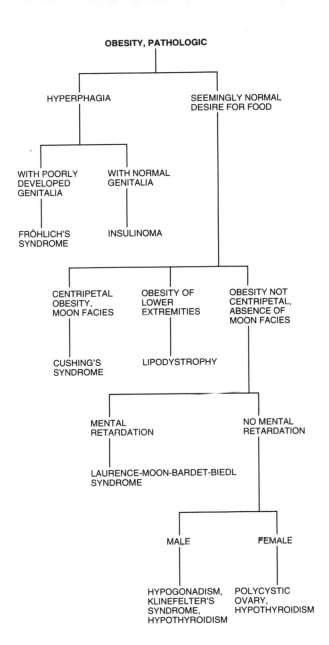

ODOR

Ask the following questions:

1. Is there coma or disturbances of consciousness? The presence of coma or disturbances of consciousness should suggest alcoholism, diabetic acidosis, uremia, and hepatic coma.
2. Is the odor sweet? The presence of a sweet odor to the breath should suggest diabetic acidosis, alcoholism, and maple syrup urine disease.
3. Is the odor unpleasant or foul? The presence of an unpleasant or foul odor should suggest uremia, hepatic coma, anaerobic infections in the mouth or nasopharynx, and isovaleric aciduria.

DIAGNOSTIC WORKUP

Routine laboratory work includes a CBC, urinalysis, chemistry panel, blood alcohol level, and tests for serum acetone and serum amino acids. Urine for chromatography may help pick up certain keto acids. A culture of the mouth, gums, and nasopharynx may be necessary to diagnose anaerobic infections.

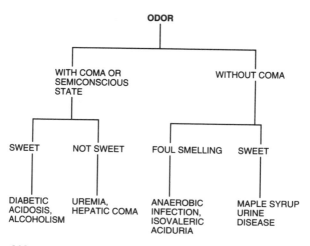

OPISTHOTONUS

Ask the following questions:

1. Is it acute? If it is acute, then strychnine poisoning, tetanus, and phenothiazine intoxication should be considered. Also, consider meningitis and uremia.
2. Is there a history of oral or intravenous drug use or a recent wound infection? If there is a recent wound infection, one should consider tetanus. If there is no recent wound infection, but a history of oral or intravenous drug use, tetanus and strychnine poisoning are both possibilities. Phenothiazine intoxication must also be considered.
3. Is the opisthotonus chronic or recurring? The presence of chronic or recurring opisthotonus should suggest epilepsy, stiff-man syndrome, and hysteria.
4. If it is chronic and recurring, is there incontinence or tongue biting? The presence of incontinence or tongue biting in a chronic recurring form of opisthotonus should suggest epilepsy.
5. Is there fever? If the opisthotonus is acute and there is a significant fever, one should consider meningitis. However, strychnine poisoning and tetanus may also induce fever in the later stages.

DIAGNOSTIC WORKUP

Routine studies include a CBC, sedimentation rate, urinalysis, chemistry panel including electrolytes, blood cultures, urine drug screen, and VDRL test. A spinal fluid analysis, smear and culture is indicated if meningitis is suspected. An EEG is indicated in the chronic recurring form.

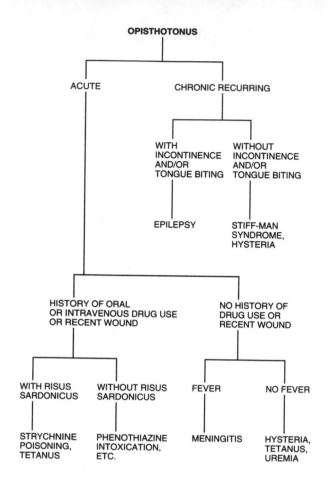

ORTHOPNEA

A patient with orthopnea is able to breathe without significant subjective difficulty in the sitting or upright position, but almost invariably develops shortness of breath in the recumbent position. This symptom is most characteristic of congestive heart failure, especially left ventricular failure. The differential diagnosis and workup are the same as for dyspnea (page 162).

PAIN IN THE PENIS

Ask the following questions:

1. Is the pain mostly during micturition? If the pain is mostly during micturition, one should consider the possibilities of urethritis, cystitis, bladder calculus, prostatitis, urethral stricture, carcinoma of the bladder, seminal vesiculitis, anal fissure, and hemorrhoids.
2. If the pain is during micturition, is it mostly at the end of micturition? If the pain in the penis is at the end of micturition, then chronic prostatitis, seminal vesiculitis, anal fissure, hemorrhoids, and bladder calculi should be suspected.
3. Is the pain mostly during an erection? If the pain is mostly during an erection, then Peyronie's disease should be considered.
4. Is the pain unrelated to micturition or erection? When the pain is not related to micturition or erection, then renal colic, epithelioma, appendicitis, anxiety, chancroid, and herpes simplex should be considered.
5. Is there a discharge? The presence of a urethral discharge should make one think of gonorrhea and nonspecific urethritis.

DIAGNOSTIC WORKUP

The most important diagnostic procedure is a urinalysis, urine culture and sensitivity, and smear and culture of any urethral discharge. It may be necessary to massage the prostate to obtain an adequate specimen! An intravenous pyelogram should be done if obstructive uropathy or bladder or renal calculi are suspected. If the above studies are negative, referral to a urologist should be made. He will probably do cystoscopy and retrograde pyelography among other diagnostic tests.

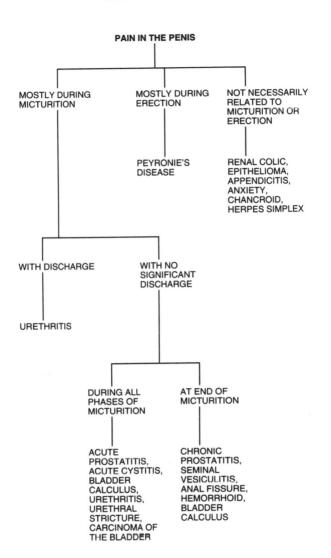

PAIN IN THE PENIS

MOSTLY DURING MICTURITION

MOSTLY DURING ERECTION

NOT NECESSARILY RELATED TO MICTURITION OR ERECTION

PEYRONIE'S DISEASE

RENAL COLIC, EPITHELIOMA, APPENDICITIS, ANXIETY, CHANCROID, HERPES SIMPLEX

WITH DISCHARGE

WITH NO SIGNIFICANT DISCHARGE

URETHRITIS

DURING ALL PHASES OF MICTURITION

AT END OF MICTURITION

ACUTE PROSTATITIS, ACUTE CYSTITIS, BLADDER CALCULUS, URETHRITIS, URETHRAL STRICTURE, CARCINOMA OF THE BLADDER

CHRONIC PROSTATITIS, SEMINAL VESICULITIS, ANAL FISSURE, HEMORRHOID, BLADDER CALCULUS

PALPITATIONS

Ask the following questions:

1. Are the palpitations constant or intermittent? Constant palpitations may signify tachycardia and that would suggest hyperthyroidism or overuse of caffeine and other drugs. Intermittent palpitations are more likely related to a cardiac arrhythmia, particularly extrasystoles. Also, constant palpitations may indicate a fever of unknown origin.
2. Are there associated symptoms? Palpitations with weight loss, increased appetite, and polyuria would suggest hyperthyroidism. Palpitations with shortness of breath and pitting edema would suggest congestive heart failure.
3. Are there positive physical findings? If there is cardiomegaly, one must think of the possibility of congestive heart failure or valvular heart disease. If one finds a cardiac murmur, it is more likely that there is valvular heart disease such as acute or chronic rheumatic fever. Cardiomegaly, murmur, and/or fever would suggest a bacterial endocarditis. Cardiomegaly without a murmur would suggest a myocardiopathy, congestive heart failure, and hypothyroidism. Palpitations with no cardiomegaly, but with hypertension would suggest pheochromocytoma, particularly if it is systolic hypertension, but it also can be found in hyperthyroidism. Persistent or intermittent palpitations with a totally normal physical examination suggest sensitivity to caffeine or the use of other drugs.

DIAGNOSTIC WORKUP

In the presence of tachycardia, weight loss, and increased appetite, it is obvious that a thyroid profile should be drawn. When there are palpitations and fever, a workup for an infectious disease, particularly rheumatic fever and bacterial endocarditis, is in order. Blood cultures, antistreptolysin-O titers, sedimentation rate, and echocardiography are useful. When the palpitations are intermittent, a pheochromocytoma should be considered and 24-hr urine collection for vanillylmandelic acid (VMA) or metanephrines should be ordered. In addition, 24-hr or 48-hr Holter monitoring is very useful in the diagnosis of intermittent palpitations. Arm-to-tongue circulation times as well as spirometry may diagnose early congestive heart failure.

PALPITATIONS

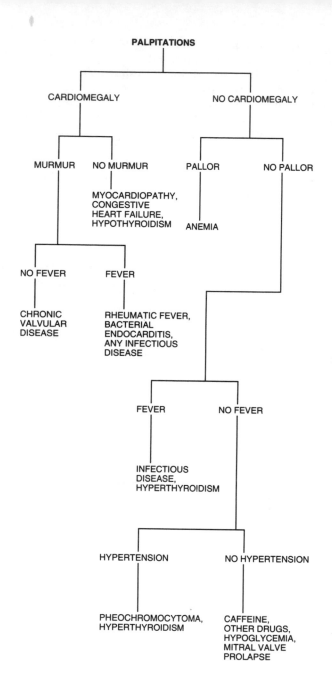

PAPILLEDEMA

Ask the following questions:

1. Is the onset acute or gradual? An acute onset would suggest optic neuritis, hypertensive encephalopathy, cerebral hemorrhage, extradural hematoma, brain abscess, dural sinus thrombosis, meningitis, and subarachnoid hemorrhage. On the other hand, a gradual onset would suggest a space-occupying lesion such as brain tumor, abscess, or subdural hematoma.
2. If the onset is acute, is there coma or focal neurologic signs? Findings of coma or focal neurologic signs should suggest cerebral hemorrhage, extradural hematoma, brain abscess, dural sinus thrombosis, meningitis, and subarachnoid hemorrhage. An acute onset without focal neurologic signs or coma would suggest hypertensive encephalopathy and optic neuritis.
3. If gradual, are there focal neurologic signs? Gradual onset of papilledema with focal neurologic signs suggests a brain tumor, abscess, or subdural hematoma.
4. Is there hypertension? The presence of hypertension and papilledema suggests hypertensive encephalopathy, acute glomerulonephritis, and certain collagen diseases. If there is no hypertension and no focal neurologic signs, then a diagnosis of pseudotumor cerebri or pseudopapilledema should be suspected.

DIAGNOSTIC WORKUP

Regardless of whether there are focal neurologic signs or hypertension, a CT scan or MRI should be done and a consultation with a neurologist should be made when papilledema is suspected.

If there is significant hypertension and the CT scan or MRI are negative, a hypertensive workup should be done (see page 303).

With a normal CT scan or MRI and no focal neurologic signs or hypertension, a spinal tap and visual field examination will assist in the diagnosis of pseudotumor cerebri. However, a blood lead level should be done to rule out lead poisoning. Also, the visual field exam may show optic neuritis when the clinical examination was inconclusive.

An ophthalmologist will help diagnose optic neuritis and pseudopapilledema.

PAPILLEDEMA

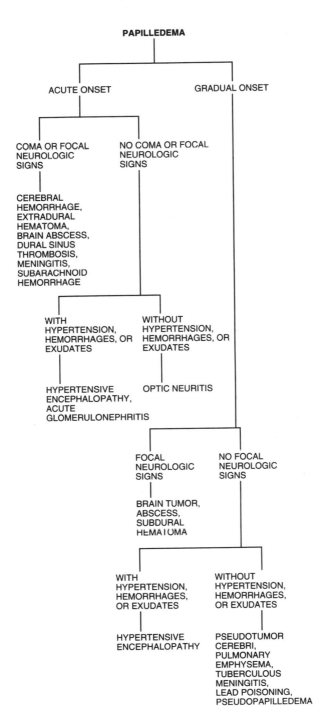

PARESTHESIAS OF THE LOWER EXTREMITY

Ask the following questions:

1. Are the pulses diminished? The presence of diminished pulses should suggest peripheral arteriosclerosis or Leriche's syndrome.

2. Is there associated pain in the involved extremity? The presence of pain in the involved extremity should suggest lumbar spondylosis, spinal stenosis, cauda equina tumor, spondylolisthesis, herniated disk, and pelvic tumors.

3. Is there a positive straight leg raising test and/or decreased Achilles reflex? These findings suggest a herniated disk of L4-L5 or L5-S1, lumbar spondylosis, spinal stenosis, a cauda equina tumor, or spondylolisthesis.

4. Is there a positive femoral stretch test or decreased knee jerk? These findings suggest a herniated disk of L3-L4 or L2-L3, or lumbar spondylosis.

5. Are there diffuse hyperactive reflexes? These findings suggest multiple sclerosis, pernicious anemia, degenerative diseases of the spinal cord such as syringomyelia, spinal cord tumor, or other space-occupying lesions. It may also suggest anterior spinal artery occlusion.

6. Are there diffuse hypoactive reflexes? The presence of diffuse hypoactive reflexes would suggest poliomyelitis, Guillain-Barré syndrome, cauda equina tumor, metastatic tumor of the lumbar spine, and occasionally pernicious anemia or peroneal neuropathy. Also, peripheral neuropathy will present with diffuse hypoactive reflexes.

7. Is there incontinence associated with the hypoactive reflexes? The presence of incontinence with the hypoactive reflexes may indicate poliomyelitis, cauda equina tumor, or metastatic tumors to the lumbar spine.

DIAGNOSTIC WORKUP

The basic diagnostic workup includes a CBC, sedimentation rate, urinalysis, chemistry panel, arthritis panel, VDRL test, and x-ray of the lumbosacral spine. A serum B_{12} and folic acid should be done if pernicious anemia is suspected. If these tests are negative, an orthopedic or neurologic specialist should be consulted. A CT scan of the lumbosacral spine, a nerve conduction velocity study, and an electromyogram may all be necessary in the workup. MRI is more expensive and often unnecessary.

Combined myelography and CT scan is often useful in evaluating the need for surgery. A bone scan may be helpful in diagnosing occult fractures metastases, or osteomyelitis.

If multiple sclerosis, Guillain-Barré syndrome, or central nervous system lues are suspected, a spinal tap may be done. Somatosensory evoked potentials are useful in diagnosing multiple sclerosis.

A neuropathy workup may be necessary. This involves a glucose tolerance test to rule out diabetes, urine tests for porphyrins and porphobilinogen to rule out porphyria, quantitative urine niacin, thiamine, pyridoxine, and other B vitamins after loading, an ANA and anti-dsDNA test to rule out collagen disease, serum protein electrophoresis and immunoelectrophoresis to diagnose various collagen diseases and macroglobulinemia, a lymph node biopsy and Kveim test for sarcoidosis, nerve conduction velocity studies and electromyography to establish the presence of a neuropathy, thyroid profile to rule out hypothyroidism or hyperthyroidism, human immunodeficiency virus (HIV) antibody titers, blood levels for heavy metals such as lead to rule out lead or arsenic neuropathy, and skin and muscle biopsies to rule out various collagen diseases. A trial of therapy is often necessary to rule out the nutritional neuropathies.

Lumbar puncture, as already mentioned, is useful in diagnosing Guillain-Barré syndrome. Nerve biopsy may be necessary when all the above procedures are negative.

Red blood cell transketolase activity is decreased in beriberi and the serum pyruvate and lactate levels are elevated.

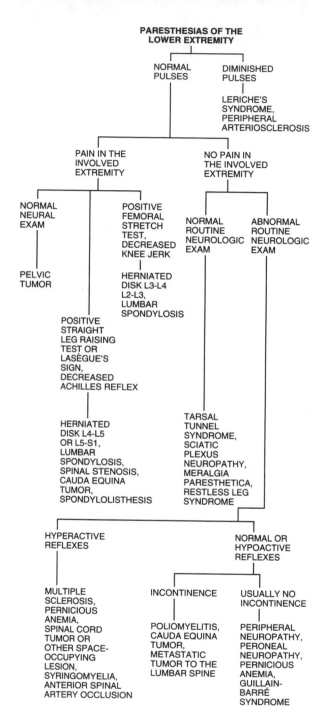

**PARESTHESIAS OF THE
LOWER EXTREMITY**

NORMAL
PULSES

DIMINISHED
PULSES

LERICHE'S
SYNDROME,
PERIPHERAL
ARTERIOSCLEROSIS

PAIN IN THE
INVOLVED
EXTREMITY

NO PAIN IN
THE INVOLVED
EXTREMITY

NORMAL
NEURAL
EXAM

POSITIVE
FEMORAL
STRETCH
TEST,
DECREASED
KNEE JERK

NORMAL
ROUTINE
NEUROLOGIC
EXAM

ABNORMAL
ROUTINE
NEUROLOGIC
EXAM

PELVIC
TUMOR

HERNIATED
DISK L3-L4
L2-L3,
LUMBAR
SPONDYLOSIS

POSITIVE
STRAIGHT
LEG RAISING
TEST OR
LASÈGUE'S
SIGN,
DECREASED
ACHILLES REFLEX

HERNIATED
DISK L4-L5
OR L5-S1,
LUMBAR
SPONDYLOSIS,
SPINAL STENOSIS,
CAUDA EQUINA
TUMOR,
SPONDYLOLISTHESIS

TARSAL
TUNNEL
SYNDROME,
SCIATIC
PLEXUS
NEUROPATHY,
MERALGIA
PARESTHETICA,
RESTLESS LEG
SYNDROME

HYPERACTIVE
REFLEXES

NORMAL OR
HYPOACTIVE
REFLEXES

MULTIPLE
SCLEROSIS,
PERNICIOUS
ANEMIA,
SPINAL CORD
TUMOR OR
OTHER SPACE-
OCCUPYING
LESION,
SYRINGOMYELIA,
ANTERIOR SPINAL
ARTERY OCCLUSION

INCONTINENCE

USUALLY NO
INCONTINENCE

POLIOMYELITIS,
CAUDA EQUINA
TUMOR,
METASTATIC
TUMOR TO THE
LUMBAR SPINE

PERIPHERAL
NEUROPATHY,
PERONEAL
NEUROPATHY,
PERNICIOUS
ANEMIA,
GUILLAIN-
BARRÉ
SYNDROME

PARESTHESIAS OF THE UPPER EXTREMITY

Ask the following questions:

1. Are there paresthesias of the face or cranial nerve signs? These findings would suggest a diagnosis of cerebral vascular disease, a space-occupying lesion of the brain, migraine, or multiple sclerosis.

2. Is there pain in the involved extremity? Pain in the involved extremity, particularly radicular pain, should suggest a herniated cervical disk, spinal cord tumor, or cervical spondylosis. However, many other conditions such as brachial plexus neuropathy, thoracic outlet syndrome, a cervical rib, Pancoast's tumor, Raynaud's syndrome, and sympathetic dystrophy should also be considered. Finally, the various entrapment syndromes should be considered, such as carpal tunnel syndrome and ulnar nerve entrapment at the elbow.

3. Are the Adson's tests positive? If the radial pulse diminishes in certain positions of the neck and shoulders, a thoracic outlet syndrome or cervical rib should be considered.

4. Is the Tinel's sign positive at the wrist or elbow? A positive Tinel's sign at the wrist would suggest a carpal tunnel syndrome and can be confirmed by positive Phalen's test. Positive Tinel's sign at the elbow would suggest ulnar entrapment syndrome. The ulnar nerve may also be entrapped in Guyon's canal and the median nerve may be trapped at the elbow in a pronator syndrome.

5. Is the cervical compression test positive? The presence of a positive cervical compression test or positive Sperling's test would suggest cervical spondylosis and herniated cervical disk.

6. Are there hyperactive reflexes? The presence of hyperactive reflexes in the upper or lower extremity would suggest a spinal cord tumor, multiple sclerosis, degenerative disease of the spinal

cord such as syringomyelia or amyotrophic lateral sclerosis, anterior spinal artery occlusion, and cervical spondylosis.

7. Are there normal or hypoactive reflexes noted? The presence of normal or hypoactive reflexes in the involved extremity should prompt the consideration of peripheral neuropathy, pernicious anemia, and brachial plexus neuropathy.

DIAGNOSTIC WORKUP

A CBC, sedimentation rate, urinalysis, chemistry panel, arthritis panel, and plain films of the cervical spine constitute the basic workup of paresthesias of the upper extremities. If these are negative, the next logical step is to consult a neurologist or neurosurgeon.

If there are paresthesias of the face or cranial nerve signs, MRI of the brain or CT scan of the brain will probably be the most logical test to order next. If not, MRI of the cervical spine will be useful. Nerve conduction velocity studies, electromyography, and dermatomal somatosensory evoked potentials complete the workup in most cases. However, somatosensory evoked potential studies and a spinal tap may be necessary to diagnose multiple sclerosis. If tabes dorsalis is suspected, a blood or spinal fluid fluorescent *Treponema pallidum* antibody test may be done.

PARESTHESIA OF THE UPPER EXTREMITY

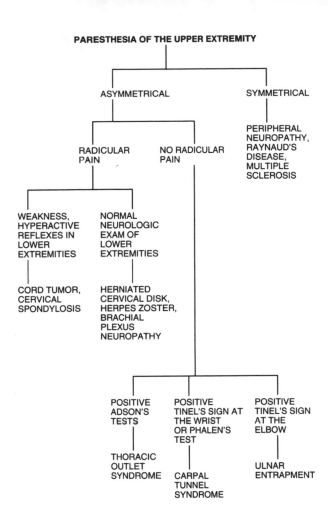

PATHOLOGIC REFLEXES

Ask the following questions:

1. Are the findings intermittent? If the pathologic reflexes come and go, then transient ischemic attacks, multiple sclerosis, migraine, epilepsy, and hypoglycemia should be considered in the differential diagnosis.
2. Are they unilateral or bilateral? Unilateral pathologic reflexes should signify either a brain tumor or vascular lesion. Bilateral pathologic reflexes should suggest an inflammatory or degenerative disease. However, multiple sclerosis may present with either unilateral or bilateral pathologic reflexes. Vascular lesions in the basilar circulation may also present with bilateral pathologic reflexes. It should be pointed out that there is no hard-and-fast rule.
3. Is there associated facial palsy or other cranial nerve signs? The presence of facial palsy or other cranial nerve signs should make one look for a lesion in the brain or brain stem.
4. Is there headache or papilledema? The presence of headache or papilledema should prompt the investigation for a space-occupying lesion of the brain or brain stem.
5. Is there hypertension or a possible source for an embolism? These findings would suggest a cerebral vascular accident such as cerebral hemorrhage or embolism.
6. Is the sensory examination normal? The findings of bilateral pathologic reflexes or unilateral pathologic reflexes with a normal sensory exam and no cranial nerve signs would suggest amyotrophic lateral sclerosis or primarily lateral sclerosis.

DIAGNOSTIC WORKUP

Routine studies include a CBC, sedimentation rate, urinalysis, chemistry panel, ANA assay, serum B_{12}

and folic acid, VDRL test, chest x-ray, and EKG. If there are cranial nerve signs, a CT scan or MRI of the brain will usually be necessary. However, it is wise to get a neurology consultation before undertaking these expensive tests. A spinal tap may be done if the imaging study is negative.

If vascular disease is suspected, carotid scans to rule out carotid stenosis or plaque and a search for an embolic source utilizing echocardiography and blood culture should be done. A cardiologist can assist in this search. Four-vessel cerebral angiography may be necessary. In fact, if a cerebral hemorrhage has been ruled out and there is no significant hypertension, a four-vessel cerebral angiographic study should probably be done. Evoked potential studies and HIV antibody titers should also be done. If there are no cranial nerve signs, MRI of the cervical spine or thoracic spine should be done depending on the level of the lesion. Myelography may also be helpful. Serum protein electrophoresis and immunoelectrophoresis all may be necessary in the workup.

PATHOLOGIC REFLEXES

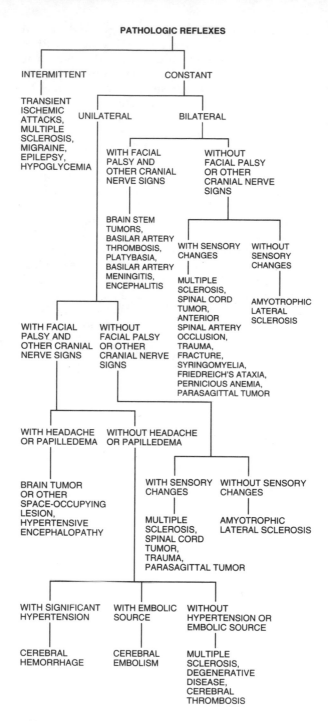

INTERMITTENT

TRANSIENT ISCHEMIC ATTACKS, MULTIPLE SCLEROSIS, MIGRAINE, EPILEPSY, HYPOGLYCEMIA

CONSTANT

UNILATERAL

BILATERAL

WITH FACIAL PALSY AND OTHER CRANIAL NERVE SIGNS

BRAIN STEM TUMORS, BASILAR ARTERY THROMBOSIS, PLATYBASIA, BASILAR ARTERY MENINGITIS, ENCEPHALITIS

WITHOUT FACIAL PALSY OR OTHER CRANIAL NERVE SIGNS

WITH SENSORY CHANGES

MULTIPLE SCLEROSIS, SPINAL CORD TUMOR, ANTERIOR SPINAL ARTERY OCCLUSION, TRAUMA, FRACTURE, SYRINGOMYELIA, FRIEDREICH'S ATAXIA, PERNICIOUS ANEMIA, PARASAGITTAL TUMOR

WITHOUT SENSORY CHANGES

AMYOTROPHIC LATERAL SCLEROSIS

WITH FACIAL PALSY AND OTHER CRANIAL NERVE SIGNS

WITHOUT FACIAL PALSY OR OTHER CRANIAL NERVE SIGNS

WITH HEADACHE OR PAPILLEDEMA

BRAIN TUMOR OR OTHER SPACE-OCCUPYING LESION, HYPERTENSIVE ENCEPHALOPATHY

WITHOUT HEADACHE OR PAPILLEDEMA

WITH SENSORY CHANGES

MULTIPLE SCLEROSIS, SPINAL CORD TUMOR, TRAUMA, PARASAGITTAL TUMOR

WITHOUT SENSORY CHANGES

AMYOTROPHIC LATERAL SCLEROSIS

WITH SIGNIFICANT HYPERTENSION

CEREBRAL HEMORRHAGE

WITH EMBOLIC SOURCE

CEREBRAL EMBOLISM

WITHOUT HYPERTENSION OR EMBOLIC SOURCE

MULTIPLE SCLEROSIS, DEGENERATIVE DISEASE, CEREBRAL THROMBOSIS

PELVIC MASS

Ask the following questions:

1. Is there abdominal pain? The presence of abdominal pain suggests pelvic inflammatory disease, ectopic pregnancy, and endometriosis, among other things. It should also suggest pelvic appendix.
2. Is there fever or vaginal discharge? The presence of fever or vaginal discharge would be most suggestive of pelvic inflammatory disease.
3. Is there a history of menorrhagia or metrorrhagia? The history of menorrhagia or metrorrhagia should suggest ectopic pregnancy, endometriosis, and threatened abortion, as well as retained secundina.
4. Is the pregnancy test positive? A positive pregnancy test is the key to a diagnosis of ectopic pregnancy when there is abdominal pain along with the abdominal mass. If there is no pain, the pregnancy test will help diagnose a normal pregnancy.

DIAGNOSTIC WORKUP

Routine diagnostic studies include a CBC, sedimentation rate, pregnancy test, urinalysis, urine culture, chemistry panel, VDRL test, and Pap smear. If there is a vaginal discharge, a smear and culture of the material should be made. If a distended bladder is suspected, a catheterization for residual urine must be done. Pelvic ultrasound or a CT scan will often be useful, but why not consult a gynecologist before ordering these more expensive tests? He may do a laparoscopy, a culdocentesis, and ultimately an exploratory laparotomy.

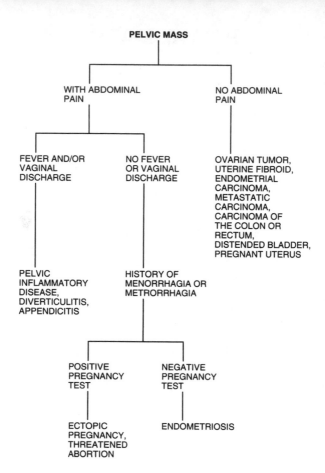

PELVIC MASS

WITH ABDOMINAL PAIN

NO ABDOMINAL PAIN

FEVER AND/OR VAGINAL DISCHARGE

NO FEVER OR VAGINAL DISCHARGE

OVARIAN TUMOR, UTERINE FIBROID, ENDOMETRIAL CARCINOMA, METASTATIC CARCINOMA, CARCINOMA OF THE COLON OR RECTUM, DISTENDED BLADDER, PREGNANT UTERUS

PELVIC INFLAMMATORY DISEASE, DIVERTICULITIS, APPENDICITIS

HISTORY OF MENORRHAGIA OR METRORRHAGIA

POSITIVE PREGNANCY TEST

NEGATIVE PREGNANCY TEST

ECTOPIC PREGNANCY, THREATENED ABORTION

ENDOMETRIOSIS

PELVIC PAIN

Ask the following questions:

1. Is there a pelvic mass? The presence of a pelvic mass would suggest salpingo-oophoritis, ectopic pregnancy, endometriosis, uterine fibroid, or an ovarian tumor that is twisting on its pedicle.
2. Is there fever or purulent vaginal discharge? The presence of fever or purulent vaginal discharge would suggest pelvic inflammatory disease, diverticulitis, and appendicitis.
3. Is there a history of metrorrhagia or menorrhagia? The history of metrorrhagia or menorrhagia would suggest ectopic pregnancy, threatened abortion, retained secundinae, uterine fibroids, and endometriosis.
4. Is there a positive pregnancy test? The presence of a positive pregnancy test would suggest an ectopic pregnancy or threatened abortion.
5. Is the pain related to the menstrual cycle? If the pain is related to the menstrual cycle, then Mittelschmerz should be considered.

DIAGNOSTIC WORKUP

Routine studies include a CBC, sedimentation rate, pregnancy test, urinalysis, urine culture, chemistry panel, VDRL test, and Pap smear. A vaginal smear and culture should also be done routinely.

The next step would logically be a pelvic ultrasound, but it is wise to consult a gynecologist before ordering expensive tests. The gynecologist may proceed with laparoscopy, culdocentesis, and ultimately an exploratory laparotomy. A CT scan of the abdomen and pelvis may also be necessary.

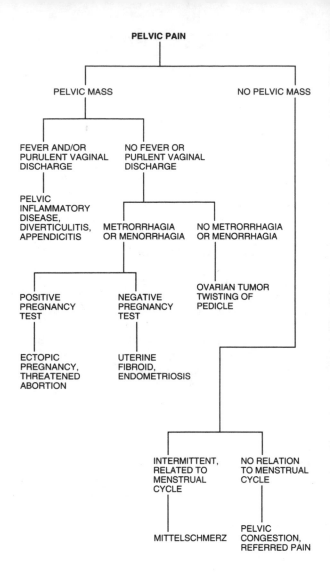

PENILE SORES

Ask the following questions:

1. Is it painful? The presence of a painful penile sore suggests chancroid, herpes simplex, herpes zoster, and balanitis. On the other hand, a painless penile sore should suggest chancre, lymphogranuloma venereum, epithelioma, granuloma inguinale, and papilloma.
2. Is there inguinal adenopathy? If there is inguinal adenopathy, lymphogranuloma venereum, epithelioma, and chancre should be suspected.

DIAGNOSTIC WORKUP

Routine studies include a smear and culture of material from the sore and a dark field examination. A VDRL test should be performed if syphilis is suspected. Many cases require a biopsy of the lesion or a biopsy of the lymph node.

A Frei test will help diagnose lymphogranuloma venereum. A Tzanek test, serologic test, and viral isolation will help diagnose herpes zoster and herpes simplex. There are also serologic tests for lymphogranuloma venereum if necessary. A Lygranum test may help diagnose lymphogranuloma inguinale. Difficult diagnostic problems should be referred to a urologist.

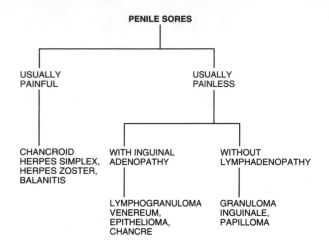

PENILE SORES

USUALLY PAINFUL

USUALLY PAINLESS

CHANCROID
HERPES SIMPLEX,
HERPES ZOSTER,
BALANITIS

WITH INGUINAL ADENOPATHY

WITHOUT LYMPHADENOPATHY

LYMPHOGRANULOMA VENEREUM,
EPITHELIOMA,
CHANCRE

GRANULOMA INGUINALE,
PAPILLOMA

PERINEUM PAIN

Ask the following questions:

1. Is there dysuria or a vaginal or urethral discharge? These findings suggest prostatitis, urethritis, cystitis, bladder calculus, bladder carcinoma, vaginitis, and abscesses of Cowper's glands.
2. Is there a rectal or anal mass or discharge? These findings suggest hemorrhoids, perirectal abscess, anal fissure, anal ulcer, rectal carcinoma, and condylomata lata.

DIAGNOSTIC WORKUP

Routine laboratory tests include a CBC, sedimentation rate, urinalysis and urine culture, and a smear and culture of any discharge that is available. If prostatitis is suspected, a serum prostatic specific antigen (PSA) should be done. An anoscopy and proctoscopy will help diagnose most rectal conditions. Pelvic ultrasound will be helpful in diagnosing endometriosis, ectopic pregnancy, and pelvic appendicitis. Referral to a gynecologist or urologist may be necessary in some cases.

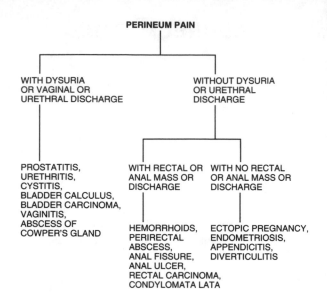

PERINEUM PAIN

WITH DYSURIA OR VAGINAL OR URETHRAL DISCHARGE

PROSTATITIS, URETHRITIS, CYSTITIS, BLADDER CALCULUS, BLADDER CARCINOMA, VAGINITIS, ABSCESS OF COWPER'S GLAND

WITHOUT DYSURIA OR URETHRAL DISCHARGE

WITH RECTAL OR ANAL MASS OR DISCHARGE

HEMORRHOIDS, PERIRECTAL ABSCESS, ANAL FISSURE, ANAL ULCER, RECTAL CARCINOMA, CONDYLOMATA LATA

WITH NO RECTAL OR ANAL MASS OR DISCHARGE

ECTOPIC PREGNANCY, ENDOMETRIOSIS, APPENDICITIS, DIVERTICULITIS

PERIORBITAL EDEMA

Ask the following questions:

1. Is there a periorbital or facial rash? The presence of a periorbital or facial rash should suggest contact dermatitis, angioneurotic edema, trichinosis, and herpes zoster. Remember, herpes zoster is usually unilateral.
2. Is there a generalized edema? The presence of generalized edema suggests myxedema, cirrhosis, acute and chronic glomerulonephritis, congestive heart failure, and other disorders.
3. Is there fever? The presence of fever suggests acute sinusitis, cavernous sinus thrombosis, orbital cellulitis, meningitis, and neurosyphilis.

DIAGNOSTIC WORKUP

Routine diagnostic studies include a CBC, sedimentation rate, urinalysis, chemistry panel, thyroid profile, chest x-ray, VDRL test, and x-ray of the sinuses and orbits. If there is fever, a nose and throat culture and blood culture should be done and antibiotics begun without delay. A CT scan of the brain and sinuses probably ought to be done in these cases, but why not get an ear, nose and throat or neurologic consultation first?

If there is generalized edema, the workup should proceed as outlined on page 172.

Trichinosis can be diagnosed by the skin test, serologic studies, or a muscle biopsy. Superior vena cava syndrome may be diagnosed by a chest x-ray in many cases, but a CT scan of the mediastinum may be necessary.

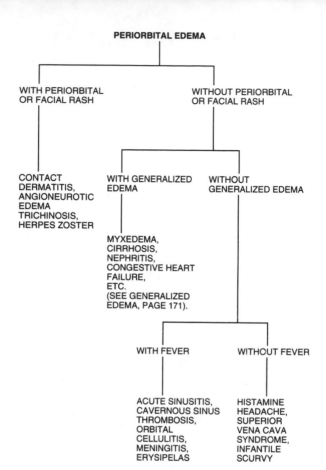

PERIORBITAL EDEMA

WITH PERIORBITAL OR FACIAL RASH

WITHOUT PERIORBITAL OR FACIAL RASH

CONTACT DERMATITIS, ANGIONEUROTIC EDEMA TRICHINOSIS, HERPES ZOSTER

WITH GENERALIZED EDEMA

WITHOUT GENERALIZED EDEMA

MYXEDEMA, CIRRHOSIS, NEPHRITIS, CONGESTIVE HEART FAILURE, ETC. (SEE GENERALIZED EDEMA, PAGE 171).

WITH FEVER

WITHOUT FEVER

ACUTE SINUSITIS, CAVERNOUS SINUS THROMBOSIS, ORBITAL CELLULITIS, MENINGITIS, ERYSIPELAS

HISTAMINE HEADACHE, SUPERIOR VENA CAVA SYNDROME, INFANTILE SCURVY

PERISTALSIS, VISIBLE

Visible peristalsis may be either gastric or intestinal, but it is invariably associated with vomiting and other signs of intestinal obstruction.

In infants with pyloric obstruction, the vomiting is projectile and the severe dehydration that follows along with the right upper quadrant mass (a hypertrophied pylorus) helps to make the diagnosis.

In adults with pyloric obstruction, the enlarged stomach with peristaltic waves going downward from left to right along with a succussion splash are useful diagnostic signs. A flat plate of the abdomen (demonstrating the dilated stomach) and significant electrolyte alteration of metabolic alkalosis and potassium depletion will help confirm the diagnosis, but an exploratory laparotomy will remove all doubt.

Intestinal peristalsis is also associated with vomiting. The peristalsis is transverse in small intestinal obstruction and vertical in large intestinal obstruction. The abdomen is markedly distended. Once again, a flat plate of the abdomen will confirm the diagnosis.

PHOTOPHOBIA

Ask the following questions:

1. Is there a history of exposure to drugs or toxins? Quinine, cocaine, atropine, and Presalin are just a few of the drugs that may cause photophobia.
2. Are there abnormalities on the eye examination? Almost any condition of the eye may cause photophobia and these include conjunctivitis, blepharitis, keratitis, iritis, corneal ulcers, and retinitis.
3. Are there abnormal tonometry readings? The eye may appear normal, but the tonometry may disclose glaucoma.
4. Is there nuchal rigidity? The presence of nuchal rigidity, especially with fever, would suggest meningitis. Without fever or with only a low-grade fever, the presence of nuchal rigidity should suggest subarachnoid hemorrhage.

DIAGNOSTIC WORKUP

A careful eye examination including tonometry and slit lamp examination should be done. A referral to an ophthalmologist may be necessary to accomplish this. If there is nuchal rigidity, a CT scan followed by a spinal tap should be done in conjunction with a neurologic consultation. If there is fever without nuchal rigidity, the workup can proceed as outlined on page 218. A histamine test may be helpful in diagnosing migraine.

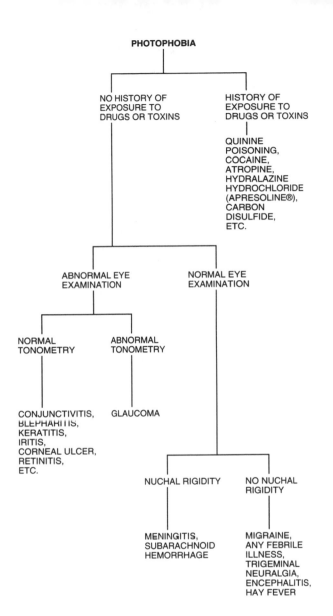

PNEUMATURIA

This condition is the passage of gas through the urethra. First, there may be a rectovesicular fistula. In these cases there is usually feces in the urine as well. The fistula results from ruptured diverticulitis, ruptured appendix, or a neoplasm that forms a pelvic abscess that gradually eats its way into the bladder.

Secondly, there may be a urinary tract infection with gas-producing organisms, usually *Escherichia coli*. The patients are usually elderly diabetic females.

Urinalysis shows pus and often blood in both types. The fistula may be diagnosed by an intravenous pyelogram, a barium enema, or cystoscopy. A urine culture may show *E. coli, Enterobacter aerogenes*, or yeasts in those cases without a communicating fistula. A course of antibiotic therapy will usually clear up the urinary tract infection and stop the pneumaturia. If it does not, the search should continue for a fistula.

POLYDIPSIA

Ask the following questions:

1. Is there a history of drug ingestion? Diuretics and arsenic poisoning are among the many causes of excessive thirst.
2. Is there associated polyphagia and weight loss? The presence of these symptoms would suggest diabetes mellitus and hyperthyroidism.
3. Is there massive polyuria? The presence of massive polyuria suggests diabetes insipidus or psychogenic polydipsia.
4. Is there mild polyuria? The presence of mild polyuria should suggest chronic renal failure, renal tubular acidosis, hyperparathyroidism, and febrile illnesses.

DIAGNOSTIC WORKUP

The basic workup includes a CBC, sedimentation rate, urinalysis, 24-hr urine volume, a serum and urine osmolality, a thyroid profile, and x-rays of the skull and long bones.

The diagnosis of hyperparathyroidism may be assisted by ordering a serum parathyroid hormone level. Also, a 24-hr urine collection for calcium may be done to help diagnose this condition. Microscopic examination of the urinary sediment will help diagnose renal disease, as will renal biopsies.

If pituitary diabetes insipidus is suspected, then a CT scan of the brain and blood tests for serum growth hormone, follicle-stimulating hormone (FSH), luteinizing hormone (LH), adrenocorticotropic hormone (ACTH), and thyroid-stimulating hormone (TSH) may be done. The Hickey-Hare test and monitoring intake and output before and after vasopressin (Pitressin®) will be useful in differentiating pituitary diabetes insipidus from nephrogenic diabetes insipidus. The concentrations of circulating vasopressin may be measured by immunoassay.

An endocrinologist should be consulted before ordering these expensive diagnostic tests.

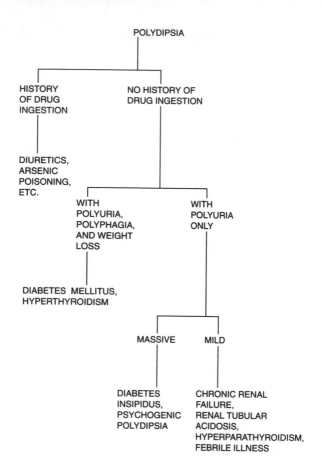

POLYDIPSIA

HISTORY OF DRUG INGESTION

NO HISTORY OF DRUG INGESTION

DIURETICS, ARSENIC POISONING, ETC.

WITH POLYURIA, POLYPHAGIA, AND WEIGHT LOSS

WITH POLYURIA ONLY

DIABETES MELLITUS, HYPERTHYROIDISM

MASSIVE

MILD

DIABETES INSIPIDUS, PSYCHOGENIC POLYDIPSIA

CHRONIC RENAL FAILURE, RENAL TUBULAR ACIDOSIS, HYPERPARATHYROIDISM, FEBRILE ILLNESS

448   Polydipsia

POLYURIA

Ask the following questions:

1. Is it transient? Migraine, asthma, and drugs such as diuretics may produce transient polyuria.
2. Is it massive? Massive polyuria is usually due to pituitary or nephrogenic diabetes insipidus and psychogenic polydipsia. It may also be due to diabetes mellitus.
3. Is there polyphagia and polydipsia? The presence of polyphagia and polydipsia suggests the possibility of diabetes mellitus and hyperthyroidism.
4. Is the polyuria mild? The presence of a mild polyuria suggests chronic nephritis, renal tubular acidosis, hyperparathyroidism, Fanconi's syndrome, and mild diabetes mellitus.
5. Is there glycosuria? The presence of glycosuria suggests diabetes mellitus, hyperthyroidism, and Fanconi's syndrome.

DIAGNOSTIC WORKUP

Routine tests include a CBC, sedimentation rate, urinalysis, urine culture and colony count, chemistry panel, thyroid panel, and x-rays of the skull and long bones. The 24-hr intake and output should be measured. A serum and urine osmolality will be helpful, as would a spot urine sodium.

If pituitary diabetes insipidus is suspected, a CT scan of the brain and tests for pituitary hormones should be done. The intake and output before and after Pitressin may be measured.

If renal disease is suspected, the urinary sediment should be examined microscopically and renal biopsy may be necessary. An endocrinologist and nephrologist should be consulted before undertaking expensive diagnostic tests.

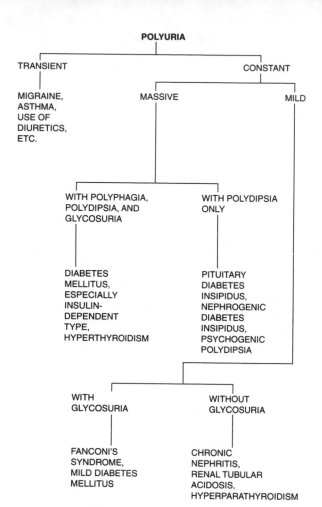

POPLITEAL SWELLING

Ask the following questions:

1. Is it soft or firm? A soft popliteal swelling may be an abscess, varicose vein, Baker's cyst, popliteal aneurysm, or swollen bursa. A firm popliteal swelling may be an osteosarcoma, periostitis, giant cell tumor, exostoses, lymphadenitis, lipoma, or fibroma.
2. If the mass is firm, is it connected to the bone? Masses that are connected to the bone are more likely exostoses, osteosarcomas, periostitis, or giant cell tumors. They may also be a subperiosteal hematoma.
3. Is there fever? The presence of fever with a popliteal swelling would suggest an acute abscess.
4. Is it reducible? If the popliteal swelling is reducible, a varicose vein is most likely.
5. Is there associated arthritis of the knee joint? The presence of associated arthritis of the knee joint suggests a Baker's cyst.
6. Is it pulsatile? If the mass is pulsatile, a popliteal aneurysm should be suspected.

DIAGNOSTIC WORKUP

Routine tests include a CBC, sedimentation rate, and x-ray of the knee. If these are negative, MRI or a CT scan of the knee may be ordered and aspiration of the mass may be undertaken if the mass is not pulsatile or there is no bruit over the mass. However, it is more cost-effective to seek an orthopedic consultation before ordering these tests or undertaking aspiration of the swelling. If the mass is pulsatile, ultrasonography or angiography may be performed. If osteomyelitis is suspected, a bone scan will be helpful.

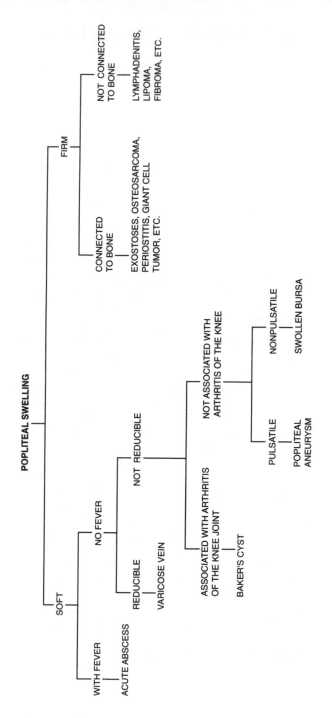

POPLITEAL SWELLING

FIRM
- CONNECTED TO BONE
  - EXOSTOSES, OSTEOSARCOMA, PERIOSTITIS, GIANT CELL TUMOR, ETC.
- NOT CONNECTED TO BONE
  - LYMPHADENITIS, LIPOMA, FIBROMA, ETC.

SOFT
- WITH FEVER
  - ACUTE ABSCESS
- NO FEVER
  - REDUCIBLE
    - VARICOSE VEIN
  - NOT REDUCIBLE
    - ASSOCIATED WITH ARTHRITIS OF THE KNEE JOINT
      - BAKER'S CYST
    - NOT ASSOCIATED WITH ARTHRITIS OF THE KNEE
      - PULSATILE
        - POPLITEAL ANEURYSM
      - NONPULSATILE
        - SWOLLEN BURSA

PRECOCIOUS PUBERTY

Ask the following questions:

1. Is there a history of anabolic steroid ingestion? Children may take birth control pills early in life and young boys may want to take anabolic steroids to increase their muscular mass.
2. Is there headache, papilledema, or other neurologic signs? These findings would suggest a brain tumor and a pinealoma is one that should be excluded.
3. Is there unilateral hyperpigmentation? This finding suggests McCune-Albright syndrome.
4. Is there a testicular mass? The presence of a testicular mass would suggest Leydig cell tumor or hyperplasia.
5. Is there an adnexal mass? The presence of an adnexal mass would suggest a granulosa cell tumor or arrhenoblastoma.
6. Is there an adrenal mass? The presence of an adrenal mass would suggest adrenocortical hyperplasia or tumor.
7. Is there masculinization? This finding would suggest an arrhenoblastoma.
8. Is there no mass detected on physical examination? The absence of any mass would suggest constitutional precocious puberty.

DIAGNOSTIC WORKUP

Routine diagnostic studies include a CBC, sedimentation rate, urinalysis, chemistry panel, VDRL test, rapid ACTH test, serum testosterone, dihydrotestosterone, and dehydroepiandosterone, and a flat plate of the abdomen. If a brain tumor is suspected, a CT scan of the brain may be done. If an adrenal tumor is suspected, a CT scan of the abdomen and pelvis may be performed. Pelvic ultrasound or a CT scan of the pelvis may identify an ovarian tumor. Ultrasound may help evaluate a testicular mass. It is best to consult an endocrinologist, urologist, or gynecologist before ordering these expensive diagnostic tests.

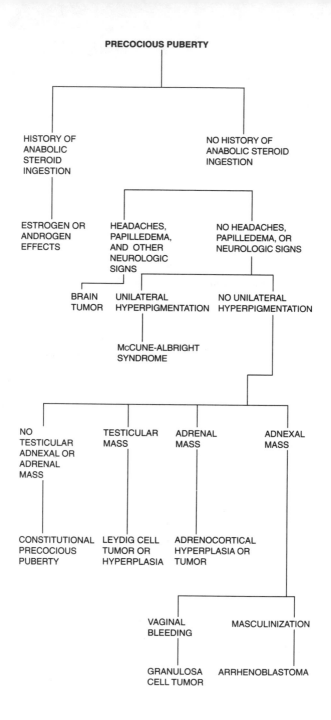

PRECORDIAL THRILL

Since a thrill is essentially a murmur that is bold enough to be felt by the hand placed on the precordium, the differential diagnosis of this sign is the same as for murmurs (page 82). Conditions more often associated with a thrill are ventricular septal defect, pulmonic stenosis, and the combination of the two that is found with tetralogy of Fallot. The diagnostic workup is the same as for murmurs.

PREMENSTRUAL TENSION

This is the emotional tension, insomnia, depression, and irritability associated with the premenstrual week. Somatic sensations associated with this syndrome are bloating, cramping, tenderness of the breasts, swelling of the hands and feet, and temporary weight gain. The regular association of these symptoms with a certain period of the menstrual cycle makes the diagnosis almost a certainty.

PRIAPISM

Ask the following questions:

1. Is there paraplegia or other neurologic signs? Neurologic findings would suggest spinal cord trauma, tumor or inflammation, multiple sclerosis, and several other disorders.
2. Is there splenomegaly or lymphadenopathy? These findings would suggest leukemia and other blood dyscrasias.
3. Is there a negro ancestry? This finding would suggest sickle cell anemia.
4. Are there abnormalities on urologic examination? Urethral tumors, traumatic hematomas of the penis, thrombosis of the corpora cavernosa and prostatism may cause priapism.

DIAGNOSTIC WORKUP

The basic workup includes a CBC, sedimentation rate, urinalysis, urine culture and colony count, sickle cell preparation, coagulation profile, chemistry panel, and serum protein electrophoresis. A urologist should also be consulted.

If there are neurologic signs, MRI of the brain or appropriate level of the spinal cord should probably be done. However, a neurologist should be consulted before ordering these expensive tests. A spinal tap will be helpful in diagnosing multiple sclerosis and central nervous system syphilis.

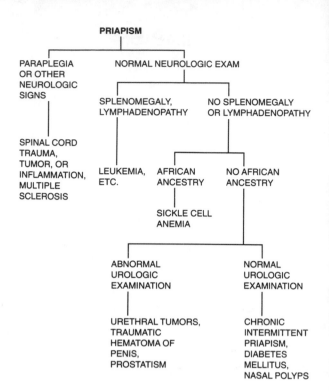

PRIAPISM

PARAPLEGIA OR OTHER NEUROLOGIC SIGNS

SPINAL CORD TRAUMA, TUMOR, OR INFLAMMATION, MULTIPLE SCLEROSIS

NORMAL NEUROLOGIC EXAM

SPLENOMEGALY, LYMPHADENOPATHY

NO SPLENOMEGALY OR LYMPHADENOPATHY

LEUKEMIA, ETC.

AFRICAN ANCESTRY

SICKLE CELL ANEMIA

NO AFRICAN ANCESTRY

ABNORMAL UROLOGIC EXAMINATION

URETHRAL TUMORS, TRAUMATIC HEMATOMA OF PENIS, PROSTATISM

NORMAL UROLOGIC EXAMINATION

CHRONIC INTERMITTENT PRIAPISM, DIABETES MELLITUS, NASAL POLYPS

PRURITUS ANI

Itching at the anus is almost always due to anal or rectal conditions and the most likely is hemorrhoids. If there is frequent passage of bright red blood in the stool along with a painful bowel movement, an anal fissure should be sought for. If there is a chronic discharge, one should look for an anal fissure or rectal prolapse. In children pinworms must be looked for. Finally, contact dermatitis and candidiasis are always possible. If candidiasis is the cause, a search for diabetes mellitus should be made.

DIAGNOSTIC WORKUP

If the physical examination is normal, examination with an anoscope is essential. Sigmoidoscopy should also be done, but is not adequate to detect hemorrhoids, anal fissures, and fistulae. If these are negative, a trial of antifungal creams (Lotrimin, etc.) should be given before other expensive diagnostic tests are ordered. A Scotch tape test and stool for ovum and parasites are useful especially in children.

PRURITUS, GENERALIZED

Ask the following questions:

1. Is the pruritus associated with a generalized rash? Almost every generalized rash may be associated with pruritus, but the most common ones are urticaria, dermatitis herpetiformis, eczema, scabies, and pemphigus.
2. Is there hepatomegaly or jaundice? The presence of hepatomegaly or jaundice should make one think of obstructive jaundice, hepatitis, metastatic carcinoma to the liver, and biliary cirrhosis. However, almost any form of liver disease may be associated with pruritus.
3. Is there polyuria, polydipsia, and polyphagia? These findings would suggest diabetes mellitus, hyperthyroidism, and pregnancy.
4. Is there an unusual odor? The presence of an unusual odor should bring to mind the possibility of uremia, liver failure, or diabetic acidosis.
5. Is there plethoric facies? The presence of plethoric facies suggests polycythemia vera.

DIAGNOSTIC WORKUP

If there is an associated skin rash, microscopic examination of a potassium hydroxide preparation of curetted burrows will be helpful. Additional examinations include Wood's lamp evaluation, a patch test, and skin biopsies. Routine laboratory tests for the various systemic diseases that may cause pruritus include a CBC, sedimentation rate, urinalysis, chemistry panel, ANA assay, thyroid profile, and serum protein electrophoresis. A bone marrow examination and lymph node biopsy may be useful. A dermatologist, hematologist, or endocrinologist may help solve the diagnostic dilemma. Further workup may include plain films of the chest and abdomen and CT scans of the abdomen and pelvis. A bone scan may be useful in diagnosing metastatic carcinoma.

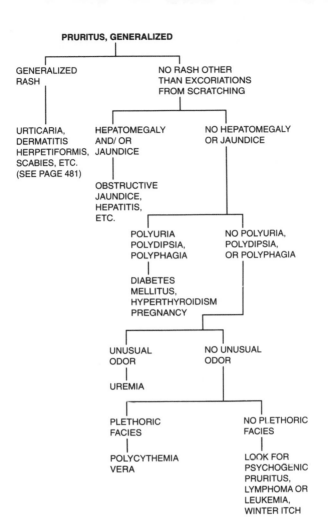

PRURITUS, GENERALIZED

GENERALIZED RASH

URTICARIA, DERMATITIS HERPETIFORMIS, SCABIES, ETC. (SEE PAGE 481)

NO RASH OTHER THAN EXCORIATIONS FROM SCRATCHING

HEPATOMEGALY AND/ OR JAUNDICE

OBSTRUCTIVE JAUNDICE, HEPATITIS, ETC.

NO HEPATOMEGALY OR JAUNDICE

POLYURIA POLYDIPSIA, POLYPHAGIA

DIABETES MELLITUS, HYPERTHYROIDISM PREGNANCY

NO POLYURIA, POLYDIPSIA, OR POLYPHAGIA

UNUSUAL ODOR

UREMIA

NO UNUSUAL ODOR

PLETHORIC FACIES

POLYCYTHEMIA VERA

NO PLETHORIC FACIES

LOOK FOR PSYCHOGENIC PRURITUS, LYMPHOMA OR LEUKEMIA, WINTER ITCH

Pruritus, Generalized   461

PRURITUS, VULVAE

Ask the following questions:

1. Is there a vaginal discharge? The presence of a vaginal discharge should suggest candidiasis, trichomoniasis vaginitis, and bacterial vaginitis.
2. Is there a rash? The presence of a rash would suggest eczema, herpes simplex, folliculitis, scabies, and tinea infections.
3. Are there vulval or vaginal lesions? The presence of a lesion in the vulva or vagina would suggest kraurosis vulvae, leukoplakia or vulval carcinoma, condylomata lata, and condylomata acuminata.

DIAGNOSTIC WORKUP

If there is a discharge, microscopic examination of a potassium hydroxide preparation and saline preparation is necessary. A smear and culture of the discharge should be done for bacteria and fungi. Scrapings of the burrows for scabies may be useful. Skin biopsy may help diagnose the cause of a rash. Lesions should be biopsied also. If senile vaginitis is suspected, then serum FSH and estradiol and a Pap smear may help determine if there is estrogen deficiency. A gynecologist should be consulted in all difficult diagnostic problems.

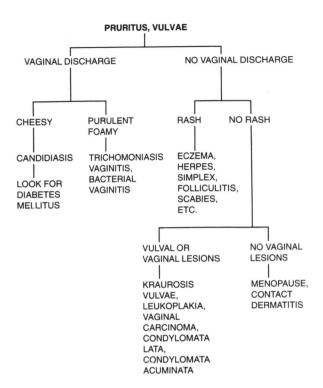

PTOSIS

Ask the following questions:

1. Are there abnormalities on the eye examination? Pseudoptosis occurs when there is inflammation of the eyelid, cornea, or other ocular structures. Periorbital edema, conjunctivitis, and trachoma are among the many disorders to consider.
2. Is it intermittent? Intermittent ptosis would suggest myasthenia gravis, ophthalmoplegic migraine, and transient ischemic attacks.
3. Is it partial? The presence of partial ptosis should suggest Horner's syndrome, especially if there is a constricted pupil. However, myotonic dystrophy, myasthenia gravis, and progressive muscular atrophy are just three of the disorders that may present with partial ptosis.
4. Is there a dilated pupil? The presence of a dilated pupil, especially with a unilateral ptosis suggests a ruptured cerebral aneurysm. However, if the dilated pupil is associated with many other neurologic signs, then there are many other conditions to consider.
5. Is there a constricted pupil? The presence of a constricted pupil with unilateral complete ptosis would suggest diabetic neuropathy. However, if there is bilateral complete ptosis, then chronic progressive external ophthalmoplegia and myasthenia gravis should be considered.
6. Are there other cranial nerves involved? The presence of other cranial nerve signs should suggest cavernous sinus thrombosis, cerebral aneurysm, tuberculous meningitis, syphilitic meningitis, Wernicke's encephalopathy, diphtheria, and subdural hematoma.
7. Are there hyperactive reflexes? The presence of hyperactive reflexes would suggest syringomyelia, platybasia, brain stem tumors, vertebral basilar occlusion or insufficiency, multiple sclerosis, epidemic encephalitis, and general paresis.

8. Are there hypoactive reflexes? The presence of hypoactive reflexes would suggest myotonic dystrophy, tabes dorsalis, and progressive muscular atrophy.

DIAGNOSTIC WORKUP

If there are local conditions responsible for the ptosis, then a smear and culture of the exudate and slit lamp examination or tonometry can be done or the patient should be referred to an ophthalmologist. If a neurologic disease is suspected, a neurologist should be consulted, especially if the onset is acute.

Routine diagnostic tests include a CBC, sedimentation rate, urinalysis, chemistry panel, glucose tolerance test, ANA, VDRL test, and x-rays of the skull and sinuses. A CT scan or MRI of the brain must be done in most cases. If myasthenia gravis is suspected, a Tensilon test and acetylcholine receptor antibody titer can be done.

If encephalitis, meningitis, central nervous system lues, or multiple sclerosis are suspected, a spinal tap may be useful. Intravenous thiamine is administered in Wernicke's encephalopathy. If Horner's syndrome is suspected, the workup may be found on page 292. If muscular dystrophy is suspected, a 24-hr urine collection for creatinine and creatine and a muscle biopsy may be done. Cerebral angiography will be necessary to diagnose most cerebral aneurysms and cerebral vascular disease, including transient ischemic attacks.

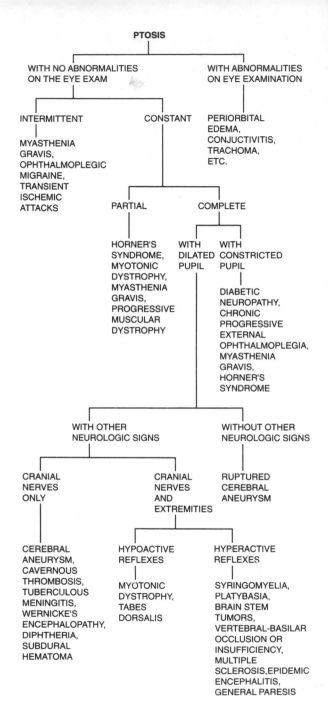

PTOSIS

WITH NO ABNORMALITIES ON THE EYE EXAM

WITH ABNORMALITIES ON EYE EXAMINATION

INTERMITTENT

MYASTHENIA GRAVIS, OPHTHALMOPLEGIC MIGRAINE, TRANSIENT ISCHEMIC ATTACKS

CONSTANT

PERIORBITAL EDEMA, CONJUCTIVITIS, TRACHOMA, ETC.

PARTIAL

HORNER'S SYNDROME, MYOTONIC DYSTROPHY, MYASTHENIA GRAVIS, PROGRESSIVE MUSCULAR DYSTROPHY

COMPLETE

WITH DILATED PUPIL

WITH CONSTRICTED PUPIL

DIABETIC NEUROPATHY, CHRONIC PROGRESSIVE EXTERNAL OPHTHALMOPLEGIA, MYASTHENIA GRAVIS, HORNER'S SYNDROME

WITH OTHER NEUROLOGIC SIGNS

WITHOUT OTHER NEUROLOGIC SIGNS

CRANIAL NERVES ONLY

CRANIAL NERVES AND EXTREMITIES

RUPTURED CEREBRAL ANEURYSM

CEREBRAL ANEURYSM, CAVERNOUS THROMBOSIS, TUBERCULOUS MENINGITIS, WERNICKE'S ENCEPHALOPATHY, DIPHTHERIA, SUBDURAL HEMATOMA

HYPOACTIVE REFLEXES

MYOTONIC DYSTROPHY, TABES DORSALIS

HYPERACTIVE REFLEXES

SYRINGOMYELIA, PLATYBASIA, BRAIN STEM TUMORS, VERTEBRAL-BASILAR OCCLUSION OR INSUFFICIENCY, MULTIPLE SCLEROSIS, EPIDEMIC ENCEPHALITIS, GENERAL PARESIS

PTYALISM

Ask the following questions:

1. Is there a history of drug ingestion? Mercury, iodides, and mouthwash are some of the substances that may cause ptyalism.
2. Is the oral examination abnormal? Peritonsillar
   abscess, carious tooth, ulcerating tumor, herpes
   simplex, aphthous stomatitis, and ill-fitting dental plates are all conditions that may cause ptyalism. In addition, fracture and dislocation of the
   jaw may cause ptyalism.
3. Is it intermittent? The presence of intermittent
   ptyalism should suggest myasthenia gravis.
4. Are there abnormalities on the neurologic examination? The presence of abnormalities on the
   neurologic examination should suggest pseudobulbar palsy, bulbar palsy, parkinsonism, dementia, idiocy, rabies, and facial palsies.
5. Is there atrophy of the tongue? Atrophy of the
   tongue will differentiate bulbar palsy from
   pseudobulbar palsy.

DIAGNOSTIC WORKUP

If there are abnormalities on the examination of the
mouth, a referral to a dentist or oral surgeon should
be considered. However, many of these conditions
can be treated by the family physician. If there are
neurologic abnormalities, a referral to a neurologist
should be considered before ordering a CT scan or
MRI of the brain and other expensive diagnostic
tests. In addition to imaging studies, the basic
workup of ptyalism might include a spinal tap,
nerve conduction velocity studies, electromyography, Tensilon tests, and evoked potential studies. A
neurologist is in a better position to determine
which of these studies is appropriate in any given
case.

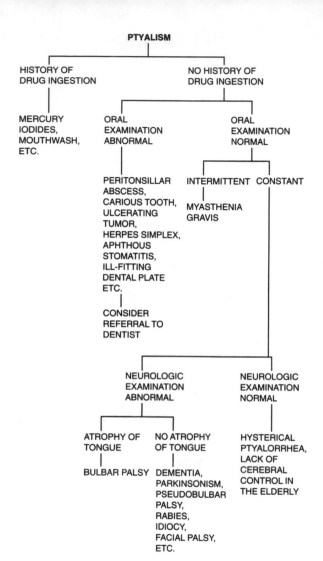

PTYALISM

HISTORY OF DRUG INGESTION
- MERCURY IODIDES, MOUTHWASH, ETC.

NO HISTORY OF DRUG INGESTION

ORAL EXAMINATION ABNORMAL
- PERITONSILLAR ABSCESS, CARIOUS TOOTH, ULCERATING TUMOR, HERPES SIMPLEX, APHTHOUS STOMATITIS, ILL-FITTING DENTAL PLATE ETC.
- CONSIDER REFERRAL TO DENTIST

ORAL EXAMINATION NORMAL

INTERMITTENT
- MYASTHENIA GRAVIS

CONSTANT

NEUROLOGIC EXAMINATION ABNORMAL

ATROPHY OF TONGUE
- BULBAR PALSY

NO ATROPHY OF TONGUE
- DEMENTIA, PARKINSONISM, PSEUDOBULBAR PALSY, RABIES, IDIOCY, FACIAL PALSY, ETC.

NEUROLOGIC EXAMINATION NORMAL
- HYSTERICAL PTYALORRHEA, LACK OF CEREBRAL CONTROL IN THE ELDERLY

PULSATILE SWELLING

A pulsatile swelling anywhere is an aneurysm until proven otherwise. However, frequently there is simply a benign or malignant tumor over a large artery that gives the false impression that the mass is an aneurysm when it is not. In the abdomen, a normal abdominal aorta may be mistaken for an aortic aneurysm, especially in thin patients. In the neck, normal carotid, brachial, or innominate arteries may pulsate vigorously when there is aortic regurgitation. *Eggshell cracking* along with the pulsation in a mass should suggest an osteosarcoma. A pulsating mass in the right upper quadrant is most likely the enlarged liver due to tricuspid regurgitation or stenosis. The presence of dependent edema and ascites will support the diagnosis. A pulsating tumor of the orbit is most likely a carotid-cavernous fistula.

DIAGNOSTIC WORKUP

In cases of suspected abdominal aortic aneurysms, abdominal ultrasound will help differentiate the normal aorta or a tumor from a true aneurysm. When in doubt, CT scan or aortography should be done. It will be necessary before surgery anyway.

All other cases of pulsatile masses suggesting an aneurysm should receive angiography of the artery or arteries supplying the area.

PULSE IRREGULARITY

Ask the following questions:

1. Is the rate normal, rapid, or slow? A rapid rate would suggest supraventricular tachycardia, ventricular tachycardia, atrial flutter and fibrillation. A slow rate would suggest atrioventricular (AV) nodal rhythm, third degree AV block, sinoatrial block, Wenckebach phenomena, and sick sinus syndrome. A normal rate would suggest atrial and ventricular premature contractions, AV dissociation, bigeminal rhythm, and controlled flutter or fibrillation.
2. If the rate is rapid, is it regular or irregular? A rapid regular rate would suggest supraventricular tachycardia or ventricular tachycardia, while a rapid irregular rate would suggest atrial flutter or fibrillation.
3. If the rate is slow, is it regular or irregular? A slow regular rhythm would suggest AV nodal rhythm, third degree AV block, or sinoatrial block. A slow irregular rhythm would suggest Wenckebach phenomena or sick sinus syndrome.

DIAGNOSTIC WORKUP

Some physicians will want to refer the patient with a pulse irregularity to a cardiologist at the outset. Other clinicians would rather investigate the patient further.

Routine tests orders include CBC, sedimentation rate, urinalysis, chemistry panel, serial cardiac enzymes, thyroid profile, antinuclear antibody test, EKG, and chest x-ray with lateral and anterior oblique views. If there is fever, an antistreptolysin-O titer or streptozyme test should be done to rule out rheumatic fever and blood cultures should be done to rule out bacterial endocarditis. If the electrocardiogram is normal and the symptoms are intermittent, 24-hr Holter monitoring should be done.

The patient also can be hospitalized for a few days for telemetry. Echocardiography will disclose valvular disease and myocardiopathies. His' bundle studies may be necessary in some cases. Also, angiography and catheterization studies should be considered in difficult cases. Before expensive tests are ordered, it is wise to consult a cardiologist.

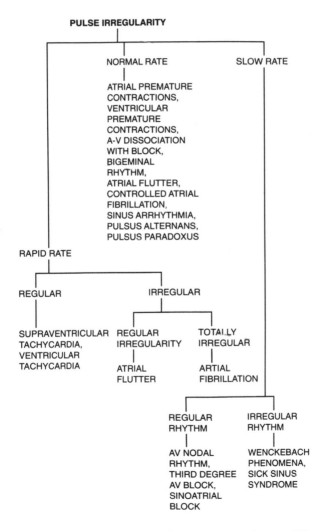

PULSES, UNEQUAL

Ask the following questions:

1. Is it acute? Acute reduction of the pulse of an extremity may be due to an arterial embolism, dissecting aneurysm, or fracture of the limb.
2. Does it involve the upper extremities only? The upper extremities are involved selectively in the subclavian steal syndrome, Takayasu's disease, a few cases of coarctation of the aorta, congenital anomalies, thoracic outlet syndrome, aneurysm of the arch of the aorta, and supravalvular aortic stenosis.
3. Is there a history of transient ischemic attacks? The presence of transient ischemic attacks should suggest subclavian steal syndrome and Takayasu's disease.
4. Is there hypertension? The presence of hypertension should suggest coarctation of the aorta.
5. Does it involve the lower extremities only? Involvement of the lower extremities only would suggest peripheral arteriosclerosis, Buerger's disease, arteriovenous fistula, and Leriche's syndrome.
6. Are both the proximal and distal pulses in the lower extremities diminished? These findings would suggest a Leriche's syndrome.
7. Does it involve the upper and lower extremities? Involvement of both the upper and lower extremities would suggest coarctation of the aorta and dissecting aneurysm.

DIAGNOSTIC WORKUP

If the onset is acute, angiography must be done without delay. With a history of trauma, plain films of the involved extremity are essential to rule out fracture. If the onset is gradual, then Doppler studies may be done before angiography. However, angiography will ultimately be necessary in most cases. It is well to consult a cardiovascular surgeon at the outset. If an arterial embolism is suspected, the source for the embolism must be looked for. Serial electrocardiograms and serial cardiac enzymes may disclose an acute myocardial infarction with a mural thrombus. An EKG may disclose auricular fibrillation. Blood cultures may disclose subacute bacterial endocarditis.

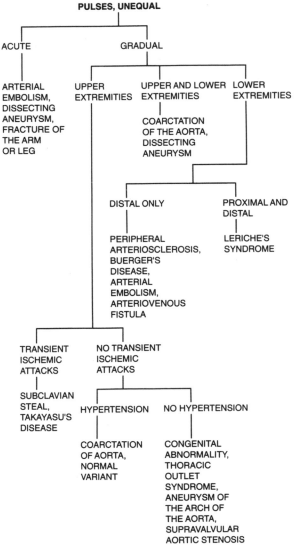

PUPIL ABNORMALITIES

Ask the following questions:

1. Are both pupils dilated? The presence of dilated pupils in an otherwise normal subject would suggest drug intoxication such as phenobarbital, marijuana, and PCP. However, the patient may not know that he had a concussion recently. Also, glaucoma may cause dilatation of both pupils.
2. Are both pupils constricted? The presence of constricted pupils would suggest narcotic intoxication.
3. Is one pupil dilated? The presence of a dilated pupil should suggest oculomotor nerve palsy such as may be due to a ruptured aneurysm or intracranial hematoma. However, if the pupil reacts to light and accommodation, then a local condition such as iritis, glaucoma, anisocoria, or irritation of the cervical sympathetic nerves must be considered. If the pupil reacts to accommodation, but not to light, then central nervous system syphilis must be suspected. If there is no reaction to light or accommodation, blindness must be considered due to optic nerve lesions.
4. If one pupil is dilated, does it react to light and accommodation? This finding would suggest a local condition such as iritis, glaucoma, anisocoria, or irritation of the cervical sympathetic nerves.
5. Is one pupil constricted? The presence of a constricted pupil would suggest Horner's syndrome.
6. Is there ptosis? The presence of ptosis with a constricted pupil would suggest Horner's syndrome. If there is no ptosis with the constricted pupil, then a brain stem lesion such as syringomyelia, tumor, abscess, or encephalitis must be considered.
7. Is there blindness? The presence of blindness with a dilated pupil would suggest optic nerve lesions.

DIAGNOSTIC WORKUP

Patients with bilateral dilated or constricted pupils should have a urine drug screen and possibly a blood test for alcohol level. If there is fever or a history of trauma with dilated or constricted pupils or other pupillary abnormalities, a neurologist or neurosurgeon should be consulted immediately before ordering expensive diagnostic tests.

Primary eye conditions can be excluded by tonometry, slit lamp examination, or ophthalmology consultation. Intracranial neoplasms and aneurysms must be excluded by CT scans, MRIs and possibly angiography. A spinal tap will help diagnose central nervous system lues or multiple sclerosis. Visual evoked potentials will help diagnose multiple sclerosis. The workup for Horner's syndrome can be found on page 292.

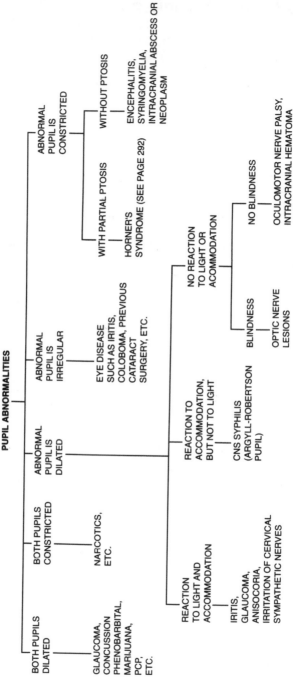

PUPIL ABNORMALITIES

BOTH PUPILS DILATED
— GLAUCOMA, CONCUSSION PHENOBARBITAL, MARIJUANA, PCP, ETC.

BOTH PUPILS CONSTRICTED
— NARCOTICS, ETC.

ABNORMAL PUPIL IS DILATED
— REACTION TO LIGHT AND ACCOMMODATION
  — IRITIS, GLAUCOMA, ANISOCORIA, IRRITATION OF CERVICAL SYMPATHETIC NERVES
— REACTION TO ACCOMMODATION, BUT NOT TO LIGHT
  — CNS SYPHILIS (ARGYLL-ROBERTSON PUPIL)
— NO REACTION TO LIGHT OR ACCOMMODATION
  — BLINDNESS
    — OPTIC NERVE LESIONS
  — NO BLINDNESS
    — OCULOMOTOR NERVE PALSY, INTRACRANIAL HEMATOMA

ABNORMAL PUPIL IS IRREGULAR
— EYE DISEASE SUCH AS IRITIS, COLOBOMA, PREVIOUS CATARACT SURGERY, ETC.

ABNORMAL PUPIL IS CONSTRICTED
— WITH PARTIAL PTOSIS
  — HORNER'S SYNDROME (SEE PAGE 292)
— WITHOUT PTOSIS
  — ENCEPHALITIS, SYRINGOMYELIA, INTRACRANIAL ABSCESS OR NEOPLASM

PURPURA AND ABNORMAL BLEEDING

Ask the following questions:

1. Is there a petechial rash? The presence of a petechial rash suggests either a thrombocytopenic purpura which may be idiopathic or secondary to leukemia, aplastic anemia, collagen disease, or drugs. In addition, petechiae may suggest platelet dysfunction, in which case the platelet count will be normal, or vasculitis such as from collagen diseases, hereditary telangiectasia, scurvy, or drugs.
2. Is there ecchymosis or bruises? The presence of ecchymosis or bruises would suggest hemophilia, Christmas disease, or other major coagulation defects, but may also be related to platelet disorders or disseminated intravascular coagulation.
3. If there is a petechial rash, is the platelet count normal? The presence of a normal platelet count would suggest either thrombocytopathy or vasculitis.
4. Is there significant mucosal bleeding? The presence of mucosal bleeding along with ecchymosis and bruises suggests platelet disorders or disseminated intravascular coagulation.

DIAGNOSTIC WORKUP

Routine diagnostic studies include a CBC, platelet count, sedimentation rate, blood smear for red cell morphology, urinalysis, chemistry panel, coagulation profile, rheumatoid arthritis factor, antinuclear antibody test, serum protein electrophoresis, VDRL test, EKG, chest x-ray, and flat plate of the abdomen. The coagulation profile should include a platelet count, a bleeding time, a coagulation time, a partial thromboplastin time, and a prothrombin time.

If there is fever, blood cultures should be done. A bone marrow examination and bone marrow culture may be useful. If disseminated intravascular coagulation is suspected, a fibrinogen assay and estimation of fibrin degradation products should be done. Platelet function may be assessed by clot retraction tests. Spleen and liver scans and bone scans may be needed. A CT scan of the abdomen and pelvis may also be necessary. Skin, muscle, and even kidney biopsies are often done to complete the workup.

It can be seen from the above array of diagnostic tests that a hematologist should be consulted at the outset.

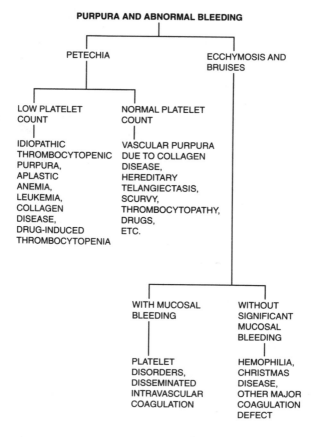

PURPURA AND ABNORMAL BLEEDING

PETECHIA

ECCHYMOSIS AND BRUISES

LOW PLATELET COUNT

IDIOPATHIC THROMBOCYTOPENIC PURPURA, APLASTIC ANEMIA, LEUKEMIA, COLLAGEN DISEASE, DRUG-INDUCED THROMBOCYTOPENIA

NORMAL PLATELET COUNT

VASCULAR PURPURA DUE TO COLLAGEN DISEASE, HEREDITARY TELANGIECTASIS, SCURVY, THROMBOCYTOPATHY, DRUGS, ETC.

WITH MUCOSAL BLEEDING

PLATELET DISORDERS, DISSEMINATED INTRAVASCULAR COAGULATION

WITHOUT SIGNIFICANT MUCOSAL BLEEDING

HEMOPHILIA, CHRISTMAS DISEASE, OTHER MAJOR COAGULATION DEFECT

RALES

Ask the following questions:

1. Are they crepitant, sibilant or sonorous? Crepitant rales signify congestive heart failure, pneumonia, tuberculosis, pulmonary embolism, adult respiratory distress syndrome, and aspiration pneumonitis. Carcinoma of the lung may also present with crepitant rales. Sibilant or sonorous rales, on the other hand, signify bronchiectasis, asthma, emphysema, pneumoconiosis, and foreign body. Carcinoma of the lung is more likely to be associated with sibilant and sonorous rales than crepitant rales.
2. Are they focal or diffuse? Focal crepitant rales may signify pulmonary embolism, lobar pneumonia, or tuberculosis, while diffuse crepitant rales are more likely to be associated with congestive heart failure, adult respiratory distress syndrome, and aspiration pneumonitis. Focal sibilant and sonorous rales are more likely to be associated with foreign bodies, bronchiectasis, and carcinoma of the lung, while diffuse sibilant and sonorous rales are more likely to be associated with asthma, emphysema, or pneumoconiosis.
3. Is there associated chest pain? The presence of crepitant rales with chest pain suggests pulmonary embolism, but it may also be associated with congestive heart failure secondary to an acute myocardial infarction.
4. Is there cardiomegaly? The presence of cardiomegaly suggests congestive heart failure or pericardial effusion.

DIAGNOSTIC WORKUP

Routine diagnostic studies include a CBC, sedimentation rate, urinalysis, chemistry panel, antinuclear antibody titer, VDRL test, chest x-ray, EKG, and pulmonary function test. If sputum can be obtained, a smear and culture of the sputum should be done. Sputum for eosinophils may also be necessary if asthma is suspected.

If congestive heart failure is suspected, a venous pressure and circulation time should be done. If pulmonary embolism is suspected, a ventilation-perfusion scan and possibly pulmonary angiography may be necessary. Arterial blood gases are also helpful. If tuberculosis is suspected, then the appropriate skin tests and acid-fast bacilli culture and guinea pig inoculation may be required. Skin tests and cultures for the various fungi may be useful. Bronchoscopy and biopsy will be helpful in diagnosing carcinoma of the lung. A consultation with a pulmonologist, if not already done, is certainly necessary at this point.

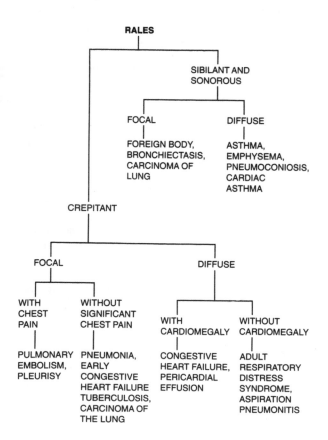

RASH—DISTRIBUTION

Ask the following questions:

1. Is it focal or diffuse? Focal rashes suggest the dermatophytoses, scabies, actinic dermatitis, herpes zoster, warts, contact dermatitis, erythema nodosum, actinic dermatosis, dyshidrosis, skin tumors, nummular eczema, stasis dermatitis, pyoderma, acne vulgaris, herpes simplex, impetigo, and tuberous sclerosis. Diffuse rashes suggest xanthoma, erythema multiforme, psoriasis, lichen planus, eczema, drug eruptions, dermatitis herpetiformis, secondary syphilis, exfoliative dermatitis, and pemphigus. A diffuse rash also may be due to pityriasis rosea and tinea versicolor.

2. If diffuse, is it primarily the extremities that are involved? A diffuse rash that involves primarily the extremities would suggest smallpox and erythema multiforme, eczema, milium, lichen planus, and psoriasis.

3. If diffuse, does it involve primarily the face and trunk? A diffuse rash that involves primarily the face and trunk suggests chickenpox, typhoid fever, German measles, pityriasis rosea, tinea versicolor, and pemphigus.

4. If focal, does it primarily involve the extremities? A focal rash that involves primarily the extremities suggests dermatophytosis, erythema nodosum, contact dermatitis, warts, discoid lupus, actinic dermatosis, scabies, dyshidrosis, skin tumors, nummular eczema, stasis dermatitis, and pyoderma.

5. If focal, is it primarily involving the face and head? A rash that involves primarily the face and head should suggest acne vulgaris, acne rosacea, seborrheic dermatitis, herpes simplex, actinic dermatosis, carcinoma, impetigo, contact dermatitis, Sturge-Weber syndrome, tuberous sclerosis, and tinea capitis.

6. Is it equally distributed to the trunk and extremities? A rash that is equally distributed to the trunk and extremities would suggest herpes

zoster, neurofibromatosis, scarlet fever, drug eruptions, dermatitis herpetiformis, secondary syphilis, measles, and exfoliative dermatitis.

DIAGNOSTIC WORKUP

If there are any exudates, a smear and culture for fungi and routine bacteria should be done. Skin scrapings may be examined microscopically with a saline or potassium hydroxide preparation to rule out scabies and fungi. A Wood's lamp examination is very useful in diagnosing various fungi. All isolated lesions should be biopsied.

Diffuse rashes require routine CBC, sedimentation rate, urinalysis, chemistry panel, antinuclear antibody test, and VDRL test. If there is fever, blood cultures should probably be done. Skin biopsies in consultation with a dermatologist should be done in a timely fashion. Patch testing and intradermal skin testing should be done when appropriate. A dark field examination may be necessary. GI series and barium enemas may be necessary to look for GI neoplasms, Crohn's disease, and ulcerative colitis.

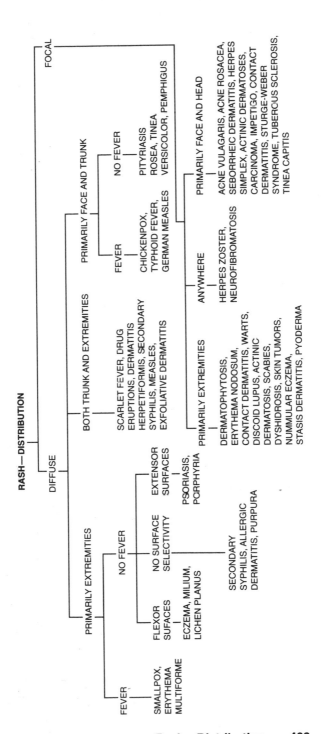

RASH—DISTRIBUTION

DIFFUSE

PRIMARILY EXTREMITIES

FEVER
SMALLPOX, ERYTHEMA MULTIFORME

NO FEVER

FLEXOR SUFACES
ECZEMA, MILIUM, LICHEN PLANUS

NO SURFACE SELECTIVITY
SECONDARY SYPHILIS, ALLERGIC DERMATITIS, PURPURA

EXTENSOR SURFACES
PSORIASIS, PORPHYRIA

BOTH TRUNK AND EXTREMITIES
SCARLET FEVER, DRUG ERUPTIONS, DERMATITIS HERPETIFORMIS, SECONDARY SYPHILIS, MEASLES, EXFOLIATIVE DERMATITIS

PRIMARILY FACE AND TRUNK

FEVER
CHICKENPOX, TYPHOID FEVER, GERMAN MEASLES

NO FEVER
PITYRIASIS ROSEA, TINEA VERSICOLOR, PEMPHIGUS

FOCAL

PRIMARILY EXTREMITIES
DERMATOPHYTOSIS, ERYTHEMA NODOSUM, CONTACT DERMATITIS, WARTS, DISCOID LUPUS, ACTINIC DERMATOSIS, SCABIES, DYSHIDROSIS, SKIN TUMORS, NUMMULAR ECZEMA, STASIS DERMATITIS, PYODERMA

ANYWHERE
HERPES ZOSTER, NEUROFIBROMATOSIS

PRIMARILY FACE AND HEAD
ACNE VULGARIS, ACNE ROSACEA, SEBORRHEIC DERMATITIS, HERPES SIMPLEX, ACTINIC DERMATOSES, CARCINOMA, IMPETIGO, CONTACT DERMATITIS, STURGE-WEBER SYNDROME, TUBEROUS SCLEROSIS, TINEA CAPITIS

Rash—Distribution   483

RASH—MORPHOLOGY

Ask the following questions:

1. Is the rash macular or papular? A macular or papular rash would suggest scarlet fever, measles, erythema multiforme, exfoliative dermatitis, pityriasis rosea, eczema, contact dermatitis, secondary syphilis, drug eruption, and actinic dermatoses.
2. Is the rash pustular? A pustular rash suggests staphylococcus, scabies, secondary syphilis, acne, folliculitis, and dermatophytosis.
3. Is the rash vesicular or bullous? A bullous or vesicular rash would suggest chickenpox, smallpox, dermatitis herpetiformis, contact dermatitis, pemphigus, herpes zoster, bullous impetigo, herpes simplex, dyshidrosis, and nummular eczema.
4. Is the rash scaly? A scaly rash suggests ichthyosis, psoriasis, lichen planus, neurodermatitis, dermatophytosis, exfoliative dermatitis, and drug eruptions.
5. Are there ulcers? The presence of ulcers in the lesions would suggest basal cell carcinoma, syphilis, lupus erythematosus, diabetic ulcers, ischemic ulcers, pyoderma gangrenosum, and ecthyma.
6. Is there fever? The presence of fever suggests scarlet fever, measles, erythema multiforme, exfoliative dermatitis, serum sickness, chickenpox, and smallpox.

DIAGNOSTIC WORKUP

This can be found under Rash—Distribution (page 482).

RASH — MORPHOLOGY

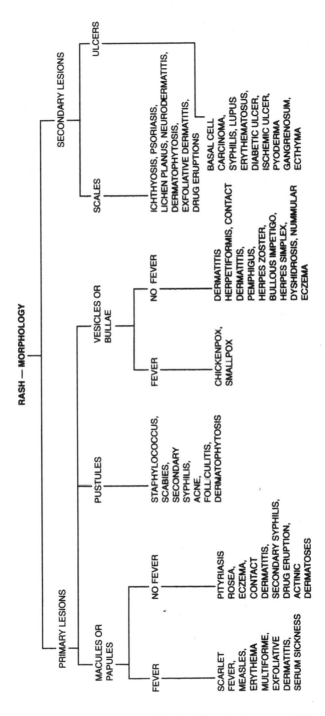

PRIMARY LESIONS

MACULES OR PAPULES

FEVER

SCARLET FEVER, MEASLES, ERYTHEMA MULTIFORME, EXFOLIATIVE DERMATITIS, SERUM SICKNESS

NO FEVER

PITYRIASIS ROSEA, ECZEMA, CONTACT DERMATITIS, SECONDARY SYPHILIS, DRUG ERUPTION, ACTINIC DERMATOSES

PUSTULES

STAPHYLOCOCCUS, SCABIES, SECONDARY SYPHILIS, ACNE, FOLLICULITIS, DERMATOPHYTOSIS

VESICLES OR BULLAE

FEVER

CHICKENPOX, SMALLPOX

NO FEVER

DERMATITIS HERPETIFORMIS, CONTACT DERMATITIS, PEMPHIGUS, HERPES ZOSTER, BULLOUS IMPETIGO, HERPES SIMPLEX, DYSHIDROSIS, NUMMULAR ECZEMA

SECONDARY LESIONS

SCALES

ICHTHYOSIS, PSORIASIS, LICHEN PLANUS, NEURODERMATITIS, DERMATOPHYTOSIS, EXFOLIATIVE DERMATITIS, DRUG ERUPTIONS

ULCERS

BASAL CELL CARCINOMA, SYPHILIS, LUPUS ERYTHEMATOSUS, DIABETIC ULCER, ISCHEMIC ULCER, PYODERMA GANGRENOSUM, ECTHYMA

Rash—Morphology   485

RAYNAUD'S PHENOMENA

Ask the following questions:

1. Is there a history of drug ingestion? Ergotamine, methysergide, and β-adrenergic receptor blockers are just a few of the drugs that may cause Raynaud's phenomena.
2. Is there involvement of only one upper extremity? When there is involvement of only one upper extremity, thoracic outlet syndrome, especially cervical rib, arteriosclerosis of the subclavian artery, and embolism should be considered.
3. Is there thickening of the skin? Thickening of the skin should bring to mind scleroderma.
4. Is there hypertension? The presence of hypertension might suggest periarteritis nodosa and other collagen diseases, polycythemia vera, macroglobulinemia, cold agglutinins, and sickle cell anemia.
5. Are there abnormalities of the blood cells, red cell mass, or serum proteins? These findings would suggest polycythemia vera, macroglobulinemia, cold agglutinins, and sickle cell anemia.

DIAGNOSTIC WORKUP

Routine diagnostic studies include a CBC, sedimentation rate, urinalysis, chemistry panel, serum protein electrophoresis, antinuclear antibody titer, chest x-ray, and EKG.

If macroglobulinemia is suspected, a Sia water test and serum immunoelectrophoresis may be done. If cold agglutinins are suspected, a test for cold agglutinins may be done. A sickle cell preparation may be necessary if the patient is black. Collagen diseases may be further evaluated by skin and muscle biopsy and esophageal manometry.

Raynaud's phenomena may be demonstrated by immersing the hands in water at a temperature of

10–15°C. Whole body exposure to cold is an even better way of demonstrating the actual Raynaud's phenomena.

Doppler studies and arteriography will rule out subclavian artery occlusions. A rheumatology or neurology consultation may be helpful.

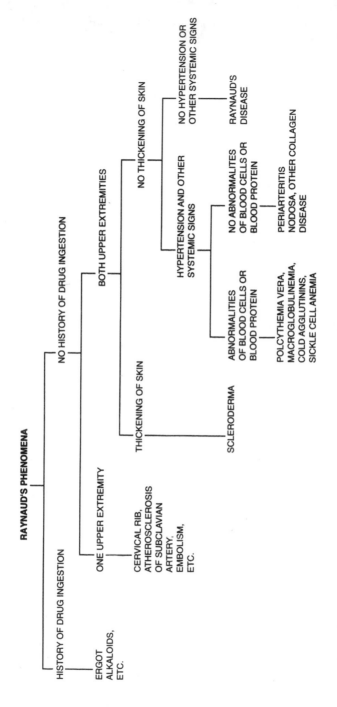

RAYNAUD'S PHENOMENA

- HISTORY OF DRUG INGESTION
  - ERGOT ALKALOIDS, ETC.
- NO HISTORY OF DRUG INGESTION
  - ONE UPPER EXTREMITY
    - CERVICAL RIB, ATHEROSCLEROSIS OF SUBCLAVIAN ARTERY, EMBOLISM, ETC.
  - BOTH UPPER EXTREMITIES
    - THICKENING OF SKIN
      - SCLERODERMA
    - NO THICKENING OF SKIN
      - HYPERTENSION AND OTHER SYSTEMIC SIGNS
        - ABNORMALITIES OF BLOOD CELLS OR BLOOD PROTEIN
          - POLCYTHEMIA VERA, MACROGLOBULINEMIA, COLD AGGLUTININS, SICKLE CELL ANEMIA
        - NO ABNORMALITES OF BLOOD CELLS OR BLOOD PROTEIN
          - PERIARTERITIS NODOSA, OTHER COLLAGEN DISEASE
      - NO HYPERTENSION OR OTHER SYSTEMIC SIGNS
        - RAYNAUD'S DISEASE

RECTAL BLEEDING

Ask the following questions:

1. Is it severe? The presence of severe rectal bleeding would suggest ulcerative colitis, amebic dysentery, bacillary dysentery, intussusception, mesenteric thrombosis or embolism, diverticulitis, ischemic colitis, and coagulation disorders.
2. Is there diarrhea and/or mucus? The presence of diarrhea with or without mucus would suggest ulcerative colitis, amebic dysentery, or bacillary dysentery.
3. Are there signs of intestinal obstruction? The presence of signs of intestinal obstruction would suggest intussusception, mesenteric thrombosis, or embolism.
4. If the bleeding is mild, is the bleeding mixed well with the stools? Rectal bleeding that is mixed well with the stools suggests carcinoma of the colon, ulcerative colitis, Crohn's disease, Meckel's diverticulum, diverticulitis, and coagulation disorder.
5. Are there painful bowel movements? The presence of painful bowel movements, especially with bright red bleeding would suggest anal fissure or thrombosed hemorrhoid.
6. Is there a rectal mass? The presence of a rectal mass would suggest a polyp, carcinoma, or internal hemorrhoids.

DIAGNOSTIC WORKUP

Most cases can be diagnosed by anoscopy, sigmoidoscopy, and a barium enema. A stool culture and examination for ovum and parasites should also be done. If the diagnosis is uncertain after these studies, referral to a gastroenterologist should be done for colonoscopy and other diagnostic studies that he is more capable of selecting.

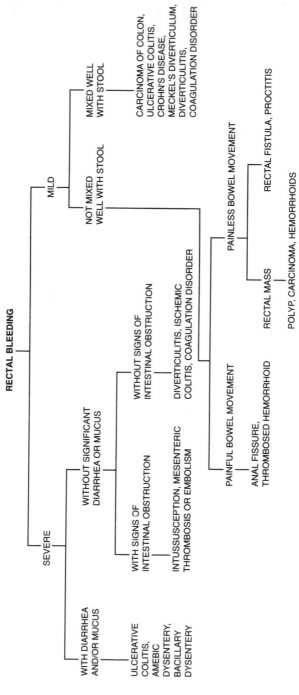

RECTAL BLEEDING

SEVERE

- **WITH DIARRHEA AND/OR MUCUS**
  - ULCERATIVE COLITIS, AMEBIC DYSENTERY, BACILLARY DYSENTERY

- **WITHOUT SIGNIFICANT DIARRHEA OR MUCUS**
  - **WITH SIGNS OF INTESTINAL OBSTRUCTION**
    - INTUSSUSCEPTION, MESENTERIC THROMBOSIS OR EMBOLISM
  - **WITHOUT SIGNS OF INTESTINAL OBSTRUCTION**
    - DIVERTICULITIS, ISCHEMIC COLITIS, COAGULATION DISORDER

MILD

- **NOT MIXED WELL WITH STOOL**
  - **PAINFUL BOWEL MOVEMENT**
    - ANAL FISSURE, THROMBOSED HEMORRHOID
  - **PAINLESS BOWEL MOVEMENT**
    - **RECTAL MASS**
      - POLYP, CARCINOMA, HEMORRHOIDS
    - **RECTAL FISTULA, PROCTITIS**

- **MIXED WELL WITH STOOL**
  - CARCINOMA OF COLON, ULCERATIVE COLITIS, CROHN'S DISEASE, MECKEL'S DIVERTICULUM, DIVERTICULITIS, COAGULATION DISORDER

RECTAL DISCHARGE

Ask the following questions:

1. Is it mucopurulent or feculent? A mucopurulent discharge suggests an anal fistula, perirectal abscess, proctitis, anal ulcer, or rectal prolapse. A feculent discharge suggests anal incontinence, internal hemorrhoids, chronic anal fissure, or ulcer.
2. Is it painful? Painful discharge suggests a perirectal abscess, proctitis, anal ulcer, or rectal prolapse.
3. Is there an abnormal neurologic examination? An abnormal neurologic examination suggests that there is anal incontinence from an upper or lower motor neuron lesion. This may be due to spinal cord trauma, multiple sclerosis, spinal cord tumor, transverse myelitis, and many other disorders.

DIAGNOSTIC WORKUP

Routine laboratory tests include a CBC, sedimentation rate, urinalysis, chemistry panel, and smear and culture of the discharge. A Frei test may be necessary to rule out lymphogranuloma venereum. Sigmoidoscopy, colonoscopy, and a barium enema may be needed in selected cases. A proctologist or gastroenterologist should be consulted in difficult diagnostic problems. If there are abnormalities on the neurologic examination, a neurologist should be consulted.

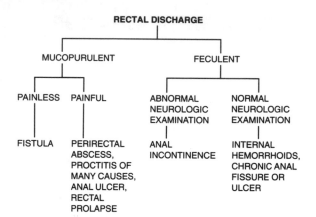

RECTAL MASS

Ask the following questions:

1. Is it painful? A painful rectal mass should suggest perirectal abscess, thrombosed hemorrhoid, anal ulcer, ruptured ectopic pregnancy, tuboovarian abscess, and pelvic appendix.
2. Is it soft or cystic? The presence of a soft or cystic mass would suggest internal hemorrhoids, polyps, intussusception, villous tumor, granular proctitis, ovarian cyst, and blood or pus in the cul-de-sac.
3. Is it hard? The presence of a hard lesion would suggest a fecal impaction, foreign body, retroverted uterus, enlarged prostate, malignant deposits in the pouch of Douglas, stricture, and carcinoma.
4. Is there associated bleeding? The presence of bleeding should make one suspect carcinoma above all else, but may be due to internal hemorrhoids, polyps, intussusception, villous tumors, or granular proctitis.

DIAGNOSTIC WORKUP

Routine laboratory tests include a CBC, sedimentation rate, and urinalysis. A smear and culture should be made of any rectal or vaginal discharge. Most cases will be diagnosed by anoscopy and proctoscopy. A pelvic ultrasound and CT scan of the abdomen and pelvis may be useful in evaluating ectopic pregnancy and other gynecologic disorders. Ultrasound of the prostate may also be done to evaluate a prostatic mass. A gynecologist, proctologist, or urologist should be consulted in difficult cases.

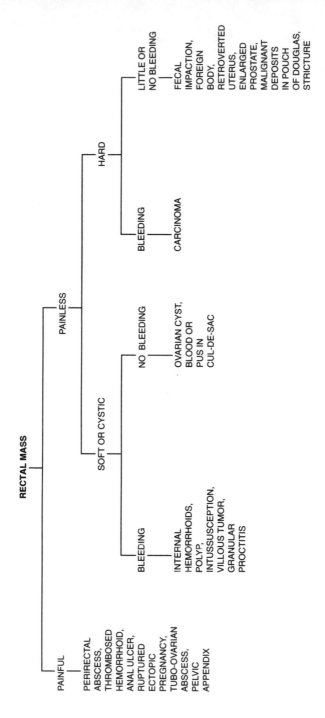

RECTAL MASS

PAINFUL

PERIRECTAL ABSCESS, THROMBOSED HEMORRHOID, ANAL ULCER, RUPTURED ECTOPIC PREGNANCY, TUBO-OVARIAN ABSCESS, PELVIC APPENDIX

PAINLESS

SOFT OR CYSTIC

BLEEDING

INTERNAL HEMORRHOIDS, POLYP, INTUSSUSCEPTION, VILLOUS TUMOR, GRANULAR PROCTITIS

NO BLEEDING

OVARIAN CYST, BLOOD OR PUS IN CUL-DE-SAC

HARD

BLEEDING

CARCINOMA

LITTLE OR NO BLEEDING

FECAL IMPACTION, FOREIGN BODY, RETROVERTED UTERUS, ENLARGED PROSTATE, MALIGNANT DEPOSITS IN POUCH OF DOUGLAS, STRICTURE

RECTAL PAIN

Ask the following questions:

1. Is there bleeding? The presence of bleeding with pain suggests an anal fissure, hemorrhoids, carcinoma, rectal prolapse, and intussusception.
2. Is there a mass? The presence of rectal pain along with a mass would suggest internal and external hemorrhoids, rectal carcinoma, and perirectal or ischiorectal abscesses. However, in females, masses in the cul-de-sac such as an acute salpingitis, ectopic pregnancy, or endometriosis will cause rectal pain. In males, prostatic abscess, foreign bodies, and seminal vesiculitis may cause rectal pain.
3. Is there a purulent discharge? Fistula in ano, perirectal abscess, ischiorectal abscess, and submucous abscess may cause a purulent discharge.

DIAGNOSTIC WORKUP

Routine diagnostic studies include a CBC, sedimentation rate, urinalysis, chemistry panel, VDRL, anoscopy, sigmoidoscopy, and barium enema. In females a pregnancy test and vaginal smear and culture should be done. Ultimately, culdocentesis, pelvic ultrasound, and laparoscopy may be necessary, but a gynecologist should be consulted before considering these tests. In males, prostatic massage may yield a urethral discharge for smear and culture. An intravenous pyelogram or cystoscopy with retrograde pyelography may also be helpful.

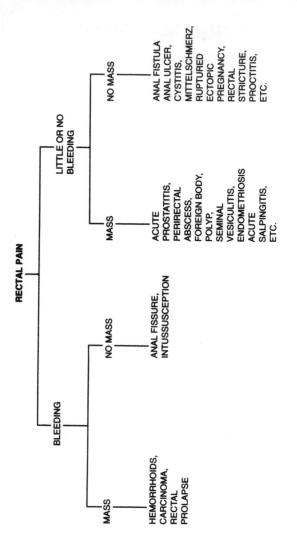

RECTAL PAIN

BLEEDING

   MASS

HEMORRHOIDS,
CARCINOMA,
RECTAL
PROLAPSE

   NO MASS

ANAL FISSURE,
INTUSSUSCEPTION

LITTLE OR NO
BLEEDING

   MASS

ACUTE
PROSTATITIS,
PERIRECTAL
ABSCESS,
FOREIGN BODY,
POLYP,
SEMINAL
VESICULITIS,
ENDOMETRIOSIS
ACUTE
SALPINGITIS,
ETC.

   NO MASS

ANAL FISTULA
ANAL ULCER,
CYSTITIS,
MITTELSCHMERZ,
RUPTURED
ECTOPIC
PREGNANCY,
RECTAL
STRICTURE,
PROCTITIS,
ETC.

REGURGITATION, ESOPHAGEAL

Ask the following questions:

1. Is there dysphagia? The presence of difficulty swallowing should suggest carcinoma of the esophagus, esophageal strictures, esophageal diverticulum, achalasia, aortic aneurysm, and other mediastinal masses.
2. Is there significant weight loss? The presence of significant weight loss suggests carcinoma of the esophagus and esophageal stricture. It is also found in the late stages of achalasia.
3. Is there heartburn? Several of the conditions associated with esophageal regurgitation may be accompanied by heartburn, but reflux esophagitis and gastric ulcer are the most common.

DIAGNOSTIC WORKUP

Most disorders will be diagnosed by an upper GI series with an esophagram and esophagoscopy with a biopsy. A Bernstein test, esophageal pH monitoring, and esophageal manometry may be useful in diagnosing reflux esophagitis. A CBC, serum iron, ferritin, and iron binding capacity will help diagnose Plummer-Vinson syndrome. An ANA titer and skin biopsy will help diagnose scleroderma. A CT scan of the mediastinum will help diagnose most mediastinal masses and angiography will be useful in diagnosing an aortic aneurysm.

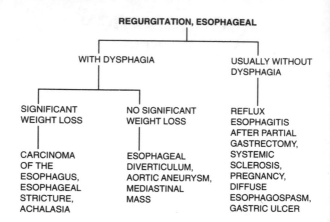

REGURGITATION, ESOPHAGEAL

WITH DYSPHAGIA

USUALLY WITHOUT DYSPHAGIA

SIGNIFICANT WEIGHT LOSS

NO SIGNIFICANT WEIGHT LOSS

REFLUX ESOPHAGITIS AFTER PARTIAL GASTRECTOMY, SYSTEMIC SCLEROSIS, PREGNANCY, DIFFUSE ESOPHAGOSPASM, GASTRIC ULCER

CARCINOMA OF THE ESOPHAGUS, ESOPHAGEAL STRICTURE, ACHALASIA

ESOPHAGEAL DIVERTICULUM, AORTIC ANEURYSM, MEDIASTINAL MASS

RESPIRATION ABNORMALITIES

Ask the following questions:

1. Is the respiration rapid? The presence of rapid respiration indicates dyspnea (page 162) and may be caused by shock, congestive heart failure, asthma, emphysema, and other disorders.
2. Is the respiration slow? The presence of slow respiration should suggest diabetes mellitus, alcoholic stupor, uremia, opium poisoning, cerebral concussion, and metabolic acidosis from other causes.
3. Are the breaths irregular or alternating fast and slow? This would suggest Cheyne-Stokes respiration or Biot's breathing and the causes to consider are coma, congestive heart failure, uremia, tuberculosis, bacterial meningitis, typhoid fever, chorea, and many other conditions.
4. Are the breaths deep or shallow? The presence of deep respiration should suggest metabolic acidosis such as due to diabetes mellitus, renal failure, alcoholic stupor, or respiratory alkalosis from salicylate intoxication. The presence of shallow respiration would suggest uremia, opium poisoning, and concussion.

DIAGNOSTIC WORKUP

The basic workup includes a CBC, sedimentation rate, urinalysis, chemistry panel, EKG, chest x-ray, urine drug screen, blood alcohol level, arterial blood gases, and pulmonary function tests. If there is fever, then blood cultures, febrile agglutinins, tuberculin and other skin tests may be ordered. If there is coma, further diagnostic workup may be found on page 100. If there is dyspnea, further diagnostic workup may be found on page 162.

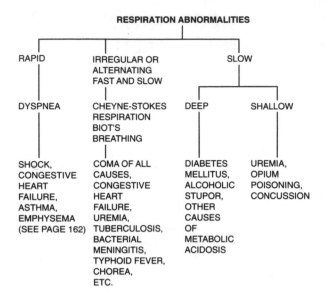

RESPIRATION ABNORMALITIES

RAPID

DYSPNEA

SHOCK,
CONGESTIVE
HEART
FAILURE,
ASTHMA,
EMPHYSEMA
(SEE PAGE 162)

IRREGULAR OR
ALTERNATING
FAST AND SLOW

CHEYNE-STOKES
RESPIRATION
BIOT'S
BREATHING

COMA OF ALL
CAUSES,
CONGESTIVE
HEART
FAILURE,
UREMIA,
TUBERCULOSIS,
BACTERIAL
MENINGITIS,
TYPHOID FEVER,
CHOREA,
ETC.

SLOW

DEEP

DIABETES
MELLITUS,
ALCOHOLIC
STUPOR,
OTHER
CAUSES
OF
METABOLIC
ACIDOSIS

SHALLOW

UREMIA,
OPIUM
POISONING,
CONCUSSION

RESTLESS LEG SYNDROME

Ask the following questions:

1. Is there a history of drug use? Many drugs, including barbiturates and benzodiazepines, may cause a restless leg syndrome.
2. Are there abnormalities on neurologic examination? Various forms of peripheral neuropathy and multiple sclerosis may be associated with restless leg syndrome. Parkinson's disease may also be associated with the restless leg syndrome.
3. Is there pallor? Various types of anemia may be associated with restless leg syndrome also.

DIAGNOSTIC WORKUP

Routine tests include a CBC, sedimentation rate, urinalysis, urine drug screen, chemistry panel, glucose tolerance test, and nerve conduction velocity studies. Somatosensory evoked potential studies may be useful in detecting multiple sclerosis. Doppler studies may detect peripheral vascular disease. A pregnancy test should be done on a woman of child-bearing age. A therapeutic trial of a combination of dopa and carbidopa may be useful.

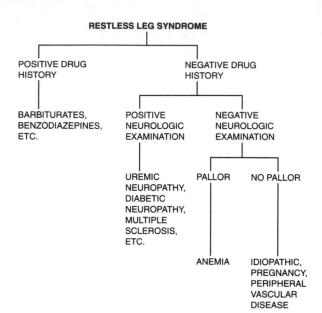

RESTLESS LEG SYNDROME

POSITIVE DRUG HISTORY

BARBITURATES, BENZODIAZEPINES, ETC.

NEGATIVE DRUG HISTORY

POSITIVE NEUROLOGIC EXAMINATION

UREMIC NEUROPATHY, DIABETIC NEUROPATHY, MULTIPLE SCLEROSIS, ETC.

NEGATIVE NEUROLOGIC EXAMINATION

PALLOR

NO PALLOR

ANEMIA

IDIOPATHIC, PREGNANCY, PERIPHERAL VASCULAR DISEASE

RISUS SARDONICUS

Ask the following questions:

1. Is there a history of recent wound infection or intravenous drug use? The presence of these findings should suggest tetanus.
2. Is there a history of psychosis or suicidal ideation? The presence of these findings should suggest strychnine poisoning and cataplexy.

DIAGNOSTIC WORKUP

Routine diagnostic studies include a CBC, sedimentation rate, urinalysis, urine drug screen, chemistry panel, blood cultures, chest x-ray, and EKG. A careful search for a puncture wound or evidence of frequent intravenous injections should be done and cultures of any exudate obtained. If tetanus has been ruled out, a psychiatrist should be consulted.

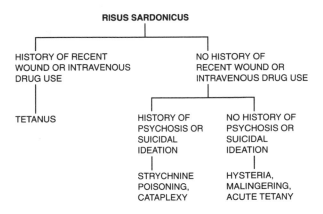

SCALP TENDERNESS

The cause of scalp tenderness is usually obvious when there is dermatitis or inflammatory disorders of the skin such as herpes zoster, pediculosis, tinea capitis, infected sebaceous cyst, and impetigo.

The tenderness is more subtle in temporal arteritis unless there is associated homolateral blindness or obvious enlargement of the superficial temporal artery. Tenderness in the occipital area is usually due to occipital major or minor entrapment by the posterior cervical muscles. This is common after flexion-extension injuries of the cervical spine or cervical spondylosis. Referred tenderness from trigeminal neuralgia, sinusitis, otitis media, mastoiditis, and disorders of the teeth may occur. When a patient presents with scalp tenderness, especially at the top of the head, and the physical examination is normal, the diagnosis of psychoneurosis should be entertained.

DIAGNOSTIC WORKUP

When there are obvious skin lesions, cultures, potassium hydroxide preparations or biopsies will usually establish the diagnosis. A skull x-ray should be done to exclude fracture, rickets, syphilitic periostitis, and primary and secondary tumors of the cranium. A sedimentation rate should be done to exclude temporal arteritis, especially in the elderly. If the physical examination and diagnostic workup are normal and the patient persists with the complaint, a referral to a psychiatrist is in order.

SCOLIOSIS

Ask the following questions:

1. Is there a history of trauma? Patients with scoliosis and a history of trauma should be suspected of having a thoracic or lumbosacral sprain, fracture, or herniated disk.
2. Is the neurologic examination abnormal? Abnormal neurologic findings should suggest poliomyelitis, muscular dystrophy, multiple sclerosis, syringomyelia, Friedreich's ataxia, and many other disorders.
3. If the neurologic examination is abnormal, are there motor findings only or both sensory and motor findings? Abnormal motor findings would suggest poliomyelitis or muscular dystrophy, while abnormal sensory and motor findings would suggest multiple sclerosis, syringomyelia, and Friedreich's ataxia, among other disorders.
4. Does x-ray show bone disease? Diseases of the bone that may cause scoliosis are Paget's disease, osteoporosis, destructive disease of the vertebrae such as tuberculosis, osteogenesis imperfecta, rickets, congenital hemivertebra, and Klippel-Feil syndrome.
5. If x-ray shows bone disease, is the patient a child or an adult? Children with scoliosis and bone disease may have rickets, osteogenesis imperfecta, congenital hemivertebra, and Klippel-Feil syndrome. Adults with x-ray changes of bone diseases may have Paget's disease, osteoporosis, destructive disease of the vertebrae, and other disorders.
6. Is one leg shorter than the other? A short leg would suggest congenital or acquired short-leg syndrome.

DIAGNOSTIC WORKUP

Routine diagnostic workup may include a CBC, sedimentation rate, urinalysis, chemistry panel, arthritis panel with ANA and HLA B27 antigen, tuberculin test, and a spinal survey including both recumbent and upright views. A bone survey may need to be done also. A bone scan may be necessary to detect subtle bone disease. If these tests are negative, the patient should be referred to an orthopedic surgeon. Electromyographic examinations, nerve conduction velocity studies, CT scans, and MRIs may be necessary. Remember, scoliosis is rarely the cause of back pain unless the spinal angulation exceeds 40 degrees.

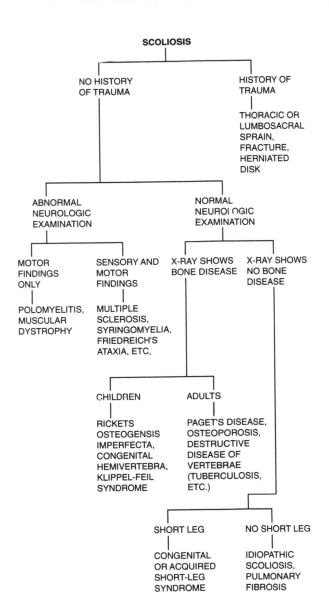

SCOLIOSIS

NO HISTORY
OF TRAUMA

HISTORY OF
TRAUMA

THORACIC OR
LUMBOSACRAL
SPRAIN,
FRACTURE,
HERNIATED
DISK

ABNORMAL
NEUROLOGIC
EXAMINATION

NORMAL
NEUROLOGIC
EXAMINATION

MOTOR
FINDINGS
ONLY

POLOMYELITIS,
MUSCULAR
DYSTROPHY

SENSORY AND
MOTOR
FINDINGS

MULTIPLE
SCLEROSIS,
SYRINGOMYELIA,
FRIEDREICH'S
ATAXIA, ETC,

X-RAY SHOWS
BONE DISEASE

X-RAY SHOWS
NO BONE
DISEASE

CHILDREN

RICKETS
OSTEOGENSIS
IMPERFECTA,
CONGENITAL
HEMIVERTEBRA,
KLIPPEL-FEIL
SYNDROME

ADULTS

PAGET'S DISEASE,
OSTEOPOROSIS,
DESTRUCTIVE
DISEASE OF
VERTEBRAE
(TUBERCULOSIS,
ETC.)

SHORT LEG

CONGENITAL
OR ACQUIRED
SHORT-LEG
SYNDROME

NO SHORT LEG

IDIOPATHIC
SCOLIOSIS,
PULMONARY
FIBROSIS

Scoliosis   507

SCOTOMA

Ask the following questions:

1. Is it transient? If the scotomas are transient, then migraine, transient ischemic attacks, and retrobulbar neuritis should be suspected.
2. Are there abnormalities on the eye examination other than the optic nerve? On a careful eye examination the clinician may find corneal opacities, muscae volitantes, cataracts, choroiditis, glaucoma, retinitis, retinal hemorrhage, and detached retina.
3. Are there other neurologic signs? The presence of other neurologic signs may suggest multiple sclerosis, carotid artery thrombosis or insufficiency, basilar artery thrombosis or insufficiency, and pseudotumor cerebri among other disorders.

DIAGNOSTIC WORKUP

This should include a careful eye examination with slit lamp, tonometry, and visual field examinations. If the initial findings suggest an ocular disorder, then referral to an ophthalmologist should be made. If the neurologic examination is abnormal, the patient should be referred to a neurologist, rather than ordering expensive tests such as a CT scan, MRI scan, visual evoked potentials, angiography, and spinal fluid examinations.

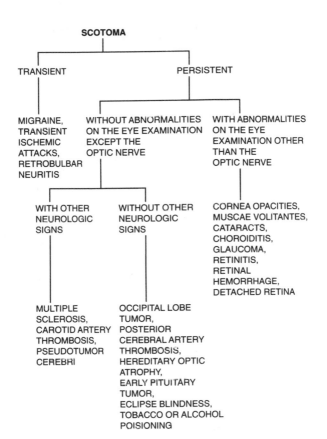

SCOTOMA

TRANSIENT

PERSISTENT

MIGRAINE,
TRANSIENT
ISCHEMIC
ATTACKS,
RETROBULBAR
NEURITIS

WITHOUT ABNORMALITIES
ON THE EYE EXAMINATION
EXCEPT THE
OPTIC NERVE

WITH ABNORMALITIES
ON THE EYE
EXAMINATION OTHER
THAN THE
OPTIC NERVE

WITH OTHER
NEUROLOGIC
SIGNS

WITHOUT OTHER
NEUROLOGIC
SIGNS

CORNEA OPACITIES,
MUSCAE VOLITANTES,
CATARACTS,
CHOROIDITIS,
GLAUCOMA,
RETINITIS,
RETINAL
HEMORRHAGE,
DETACHED RETINA

MULTIPLE
SCLEROSIS,
CAROTID ARTERY
THROMBOSIS,
PSEUDOTUMOR
CEREBRI

OCCIPITAL LOBE
TUMOR,
POSTERIOR
CEREBRAL ARTERY
THROMBOSIS,
HEREDITARY OPTIC
ATROPHY,
EARLY PITUITARY
TUMOR,
ECLIPSE BLINDNESS,
TOBACCO OR ALCOHOL
POISIONING

SCROTAL SWELLING

Ask the following questions:

1. Is it diffuse or focal? Diffuse scrotal swelling would suggest congestive heart failure, nephrosis, uremia, and cirrhosis, as well as focal disease such as filariasis or bilateral hydrocele. Focal scrotal swelling would suggest a hernia, hydrocele, torsion of the testicle, abscesses, epididymitis, orchitis, varicoceles, and testicular tumors.
2. If it is diffuse, is there ascites or generalized edema? The presence of diffuse edema of the scrotum with ascites or generalized edema would suggest congestive heart failure, nephrosis, uremia, or cirrhosis.
3. If it is focal, is it painful? The presence of painful scrotal swelling would suggest an incarcerated or strangulated inguinal hernia, torsion of the testicle, a hematoma, orchitis, epididymitis, furuncle, or periurethral abscess.
4. Does it transilluminate? If the mass transilluminates, it is very likely a hydrocele of the testicle or a spermatocele.
5. Is it reducible? If the mass is reducible, it is most likely an inguinal hernia or a varicocele.

DIAGNOSTIC WORKUP

Routine laboratory tests include a CBC, sedimentation rate, urinalysis, urine culture, and urethral smear. If prostatic disease is suspected, a prostatic specific antigen should be ordered. If intestinal obstruction is suspected, a flat plate of the abdomen and lateral decubiti should be ordered. A radionuclide testicular scan with technetium-99m is useful in differentiating between testicular torsion and epididymitis. Scrotal ultrasound may be done to evaluate any kind of testicular or scrotal mass. However, it is much less costly to refer the patient to a urologist.

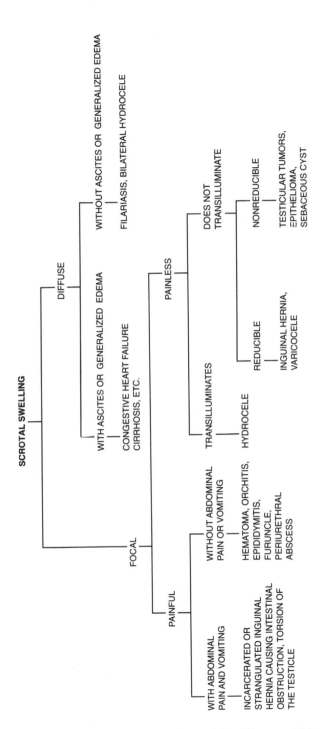

SENSORY LOSS

Ask the following questions:

1. Is it intermittent? The presence of intermittent sensory changes would suggest a transient ischemic attack, migraine, and epilepsy.
2. Is there loss of vibratory and position sense only? The findings of loss of vibratory and position sense only, particularly if it involves all four extremities, would suggest pernicious anemia. If the loss of vibratory and position sense is on one side of the body only, then a parietal lobe tumor should be suspected. Diffuse loss of vibratory and position sense only may also be seen in multiple sclerosis, cervical spondylosis, and Friedreich's ataxia.
3. Is there loss of pain or temperature only? The presence of loss of pain and temperature on one side of the body is more likely to occur with posterior inferior cerebellar artery occlusions. Rarely, syringomyelia may cause loss of pain and temperature only in the lower extremities if the syringomyelia is in the thoracic cord and in the upper extremities if it is in the cervical cord. Anterior spinal artery occlusions may cause loss of pain and temperature in the lower extremities. Multiple sclerosis can occasionally cause loss of pain and temperature in a diffuse manner.
4. Is there loss of all modalities together? If all modalities are lost together on one-half of the body, then one should consider thalamic syndrome due to vascular occlusion of the thalamogeniculate artery or its branches. Loss of all modalities in the lower extremities and up to a certain sensory level would probably be due to spinal cord trauma, a space-occupying lesion, or transverse myelitis. However, this condition can also be seen with multiple sclerosis. Loss of all modalities together in the upper extremity may be found in brachial plexus neuropathy or injuries. It may be found with malingering

as well. Loss of all modalities in a glove and stocking distribution would suggest peripheral neuropathy. Loss of all modalities in a dermatomal distribution would suggest radiculopathy due to herniated disk, tumor, or arthritic spurs. Platybasia and foramen magnum tumors may cause selective loss of vibratory and position sense in one or more extremities or loss of sensation to all modalities in one or more extremities.

DIAGNOSTIC WORKUP

Routine diagnostic studies include a CBC, sedimentation rate, urinalysis, chemistry panel, ANA, serum protein electrophoresis, VDRL test, chest x-ray, and x-ray of the spine. Findings of a clear-cut sensory loss are a good reason to consult a neurologist at this point. When one is not available, further workup depends on what part of the body is affected.

If only the lower extremities are involved, a CT scan or MRI of the lumbar or thoracic spine may be done. Electromyography and nerve conduction velocity studies of the lower extremities will complement the diagnostic evaluation.

If the upper and lower extremities both are involved, then an MRI of the cervical spine would be the best procedure to perform. A CT scan of the cervical spine is not nearly as precise. Electromyographic examination of the upper and possibly the lower extremities should be done in these cases. Nerve conduction velocity studies may need to be done also.

If the face is involved along with the extremities, a CT scan or MRI of the brain should be done. Skull x-rays are not very useful unless a fracture of the skull is suspected.

Carotid scans and four-vessel angiography are very useful in evaluating cerebral vascular disease. If peripheral neuropathy is suspected, a neuropathy workup (see page 425) should be done. If multiple sclerosis is suspected, a spinal tap and somatosensory evoked potential studies or visual evoked potential studies will assist in the diagnosis. A spinal tap will also be useful in diagnosing central nervous

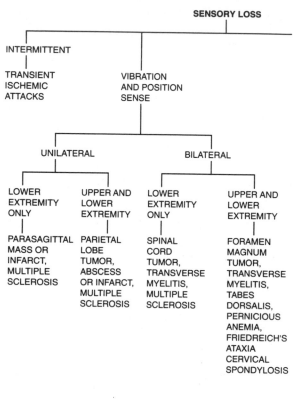

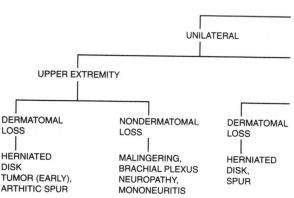

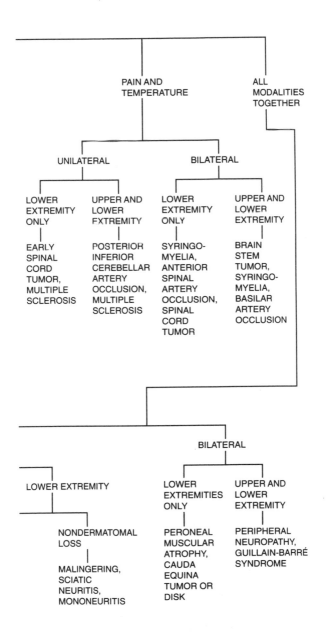

system lues. If pernicious anemia is suspected, then a serum B_{12} and folic acid and possibly a Schilling test should be done. Guillain-Barré syndrome is diagnosed by a spinal fluid examination which will show a markedly elevated spinal fluid protein in the face of a normal cell count.

Entrapment syndromes such as carpal tunnel syndrome, ulnar nerve entrapment, or tarsal tunnel syndrome are diagnosed by nerve conduction velocity studies.

A wake and sleep EEG may diagnose complex partial seizures or parietal lobe seizures. Sometimes combined myelography and CT scan are better than MRI studies in selected cases.

SHOULDER PAIN

Ask the following questions:

1. Is there significant radiation of pain down the arm? The presence of significant radiation of pain down the arm would suggest thoracic outlet syndrome, herpes zoster, herniated cervical disk, spinal cord tumor, brachial plexus neuritis, myocardial infarction, sympathetic dystrophy, Pancoast's tumor, and aortic aneurysm.
2. Is the radiation down the arm transient? The presence of transient radiation of pain down the arm would suggest coronary insufficiency.
3. Are there hypoactive reflexes or significant dermatomal loss of sensation in the involved extremity? These findings would suggest spinal cord tumor, herniated cervical disk, and brachial plexus neuritis, among other disorders.
4. Is there pain on active motion only? Pain on active motion only is more frequently found in subacromial bursitis, calcific tendinitis, and torn rotator cuff.
5. Is there pain on both active and passive motion? This finding would suggest osteoarthritis, rheumatoid arthritis, gout, dislocation of the shoulder, adhesive capsulitis, shoulder hand syndrome, aseptic bone necrosis, and osteomyelitis.
6. Is there normal range of motion of the shoulder and normal neurologic examination? These findings would suggest that the pain is referred from gallbladder disease, pancreatitis, ruptured peptic ulcer, pleurisy, or tuberculosis.
7. Are there diminished pulses in the involved extremity? These findings would suggest occlusion of the subclavian artery, or thoracic outlet syndrome, dissecting aneurysm.

DIAGNOSTIC WORKUP

Routine diagnostic studies include a CBC, sedimentation rate, urinalysis, chemistry panel, arthritis

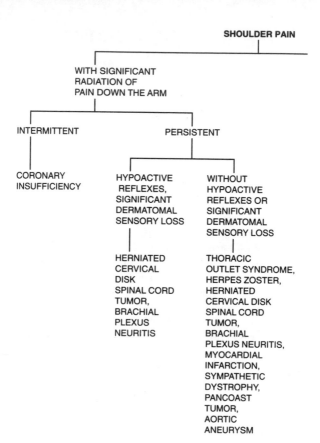

SHOULDER PAIN

WITH SIGNIFICANT RADIATION OF PAIN DOWN THE ARM

INTERMITTENT

PERSISTENT

CORONARY INSUFFICIENCY

HYPOACTIVE REFLEXES, SIGNIFICANT DERMATOMAL SENSORY LOSS

WITHOUT HYPOACTIVE REFLEXES OR SIGNIFICANT DERMATOMAL SENSORY LOSS

HERNIATED CERVICAL DISK SPINAL CORD TUMOR, BRACHIAL PLEXUS NEURITIS

THORACIC OUTLET SYNDROME, HERPES ZOSTER, HERNIATED CERVICAL DISK SPINAL CORD TUMOR, BRACHIAL PLEXUS NEURITIS, MYOCARDIAL INFARCTION, SYMPATHETIC DYSTROPHY, PANCOAST TUMOR, AORTIC ANEURYSM

panel including ANA, x-ray of the shoulder, chest x-ray, and EKG. If there are abnormal neurologic findings, electromyography, nerve conduction velocity studies, and MRI of the cervical spine may need to be done. A neurologist should be consulted before ordering these expensive diagnostic tests.

If there are focal trigger points in the bursa or shoulder joints, a therapeutic trial of lidocaine hydrochloride (Xylocaine®) and corticosteroid injections should be done if the x-rays of the shoulder

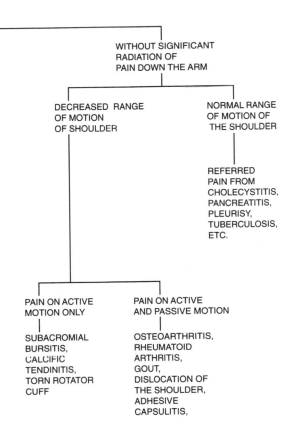

WITHOUT SIGNIFICANT
RADIATION OF
PAIN DOWN THE ARM

DECREASED RANGE
OF MOTION
OF SHOULDER

NORMAL RANGE
OF MOTION OF
THE SHOULDER

REFERRED
PAIN FROM
CHOLECYSTITIS,
PANCREATITIS,
PLEURISY,
TUBERCULOSIS,
ETC.

PAIN ON ACTIVE
MOTION ONLY

SUBACROMIAL
BURSITIS,
CALCIFIC
TENDINITIS,
TORN ROTATOR
CUFF

PAIN ON ACTIVE
AND PASSIVE MOTION

OSTEOARTHRITIS,
RHEUMATOID
ARTHRITIS,
GOUT,
DISLOCATION OF
THE SHOULDER,
ADHESIVE
CAPSULITIS,

are negative or show only calcific tendinitis. If there are abnormalities of the brachial or radial pulses, then angiography may need to be done. When there is intermittent pain down the arm, an exercise tolerance test may need to be ordered. However, it may be wise to refer the patient to a cardiologist before ordering this test. A gastroenterologist may need to be consulted to rule out cholecystitis, pancreatitis, and peptic ulcer disease.

SKIN THICKENING

Thickening of the skin is most commonly seen in myxedema and scleroderma. The association of Raynaud's phenomena will help distinguish scleroderma. Thickening of the skin of the lower legs may also be seen in lymphedema, carcinoid syndrome, and vascular insufficiency. Localized thickening in the pretibial area may be seen in hyperthyroidism. Thickening of the skin of the face is seen in Chagas' disease and porphyria cutanea tarda.

DIAGNOSTIC WORKUP

In cases of diffuse thickening of the skin, a thyroid profile with T3, T4, and thyroid-stimulating hormone (TSH) should be done. This should also identify hypothyroidism. A positive ANA test with a speckled pattern will help identify scleroderma, but a skin biopsy should also be done. Esophageal motility studies will be helpful in early diagnosis. A skin biopsy will help identify many of the other conditions mentioned above. Urine for porphyrins will help identify porphyria.

SLEEP APNEA

Ask the following questions:

1. Is there excessive snoring? Excessive snoring would indicate obstructive sleep apnea from large tonsils, deviated nasal septum, cleft palate, other abnormalities, and obesity.
2. Is there obesity? Over 60% of patients with sleep apnea have obesity, and Pickwickian syndrome should be considered in these patients, as well as idiopathic obesity.
3. Are there abnormalities of the neurologic examination? The presence of neurologic abnormalities should make one think of poliomyelitis, Shy-Drager syndrome, brain stem tumors, and other neurologic disorders.

DIAGNOSTIC WORKUP

The most important diagnostic test is an all-night polygraphic recording (polysomnography). This will differentiate between obstructive and nonobstructive sleep apnea. If obstructive sleep apnea is suspected, a referral should be made to an ear, nose and throat specialist. If there are abnormalities on the neurologic examination, then a neurologic consultation should be sought. If idiopathic nonobstructive sleep apnea is suspected, the patient should be referred to a pulmonologist. A therapeutic trial of continuous positive airway pressure may be done. Some cases should have evaluation for a pituitary tumor, a thyroid profile, and a trial of tricyclic drugs and progesterone.

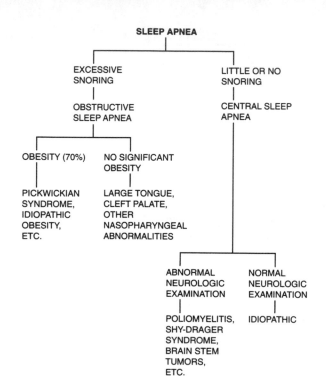

SLEEPWALKING

Occasional sleepwalking is normal in children and of no pathologic significance. It is reported in at least 15% of normal children. When it is frequent it is a sign of significant emotional disturbances, and a referral to a psychiatrist is in order. Before you do, a wake and sleep EEG, preferably with nasopharyngeal electrodes, should be done to exclude partial complex seizures (psychomotor epilepsy).

SNEEZING

Acute sneezing is often seen in the early stage of the common cold and can be found in almost all upper respiratory infections. It is also seen in measles and other infectious disease.

Chronic sneezing is another matter. When environmental irritants such as tobacco (especially snuff), ammonia, and other irritant gases have been eliminated, it is almost invariably caused by allergy. The only exception is prolonged repetitive sneezing, which is usually psychological.

DIAGNOSTIC WORKUP

The diagnostic workup is the same as for nasal discharge (page 386). Patients with prolonged repetitive sneezing and a negative workup for allergy should be referred to a psychiatrist.

SNORING

Ask the following questions:

1. Are there abnormalities on the ear, nose and throat examination? A careful ear, nose and throat examination may disclose hypertrophic tonsils and adenoids, deviated septum, bifid uvula, large floppy palate, and hypertrophic turbinates, among other conditions.
2. Are there abnormalities on the neurologic examination? A careful neurologic examination may disclose bulbar palsy, pseudobulbar palsy, myasthenia gravis, and cerebral vascular disease, among other conditions.

DIAGNOSTIC WORKUP

A sleep diary should be kept by the patient and his spouse. A tape recording during sleep will be helpful. Polysomnography is the most important diagnostic test. It will often confirm the diagnosis of obstructive sleep apnea. If there are ear, nose and throat abnormalities, a referral to an ear, nose and throat specialist should be made. If there are neurologic abnormalities, a referral to a neurologist should be made. A therapeutic trial of continuous positive airway pressure may be useful (see page 521).

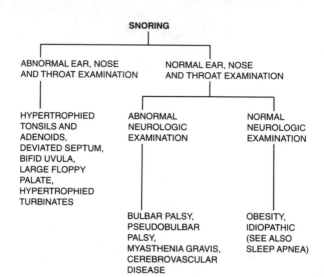

SNORING

ABNORMAL EAR, NOSE
AND THROAT EXAMINATION

NORMAL EAR, NOSE
AND THROAT EXAMINATION

HYPERTROPHIED
TONSILS AND
ADENOIDS,
DEVIATED SEPTUM,
BIFID UVULA,
LARGE FLOPPY
PALATE,
HYPERTROPHIED
TURBINATES

ABNORMAL
NEUROLOGIC
EXAMINATION

NORMAL
NEUROLOGIC
EXAMINATION

BULBAR PALSY,
PSEUDOBULBAR
PALSY,
MYASTHENIA GRAVIS,
CEREBROVASCULAR
DISEASE

OBESITY,
IDIOPATHIC
(SEE ALSO
SLEEP APNEA)

SORE THROAT

Ask the following questions:

1. Are there exudates? This is a key question when evaluating a sore throat. Most cases of sore throat with exudates will be found to have streptococcal pharyngitis. Without exudates one could still have a streptococcal sore throat, but it is less likely.
2. Is there a temperature elevation? A significant elevation of the temperature with or without exudates is also characteristic of streptococcal pharyngitis.
3. Are there enlarged lymph nodes? If the lymph nodes are enlarged in the peritonsillar area, this is often a sign of streptococcal sore throat, but it certainly is not diagnostic. Interestingly enough, 90% of patients with infectious mononucleosis have posterior cervical adenopathy.
4. Are there systemic symptoms and signs? Patients who present with exudative tonsillitis and splenomegaly certainly should be considered to have infectious mononucleosis until proven otherwise. Also, an exudative tonsillitis along with a fever and heart murmur should make one consider rheumatic fever. Systemic symptoms such as dry cough, runny nose, and generalized malaise or fatigue should make one think of a viral upper respiratory infection.

DIAGNOSTIC WORKUP

In a sore throat with typical exudates very suggestive of streptococcal pharyngitis, a throat culture may be all one needs before starting definitive antibiotic therapy. In the more difficult cases, screening for streptococcal antigens (streptozyme test and antistreptolysin-O [ASO] titer) might be indicated. An ASO titer is particularly important when one suspects rheumatic fever. If the patient's streptococcal sore throat persists, a Monospot test and a culture for gonorrhea should be done. While there are hardly any false-negative Monospot tests, there are 10% false positives and that should be kept in mind. A blood smear for atypical lymphocytes may be helpful, as well as a heterophile antibody titer in those cases.

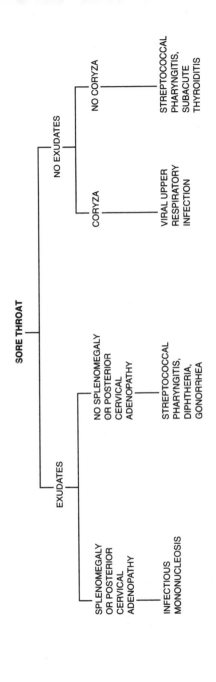

Sore Throat   529

SPASTICITY

Spasticity may arise from pyramidal tract lesions anywhere from the spinal cord to the cerebral cortex. Consequently, the differential diagnosis and workup of this type of spasticity is the same as for hemiplegia (page 274). Spasticity may also be due to extrapyramidal disorders such as parkinsonism. The differential diagnosis and workup of this type of spasticity may be found under Tremor (page 576).

In the stiff-man syndrome, there is persistent muscle rigidity, often painful, gradually increasing over months or years. The cause is unknown, but a hereditary form is known to occur.

SPEECH ABNORMALITIES

These are a group of speech abnormalities that do not fit into the category of aphasia (page 38) or dysarthria (page 153). These are almost always psychogenic in origin. *Stammering speech* is found in emotionally high-strung people and is probably due to psychological trauma in childhood. It is common in left-handed children who were forced to use the right hand. *Lalling speech* is typified by difficulty with consonants. It is more common in mental retardation, but can be normal. *Idioglossia* is a substitution of consonants, making the speech very difficult to understand. It may be associated with high-tone deafness. *Perseveration* means the repetition of a word or sentence. When a patient repeats a word or sentence that he or she just heard, it is called *echolalia*. Both of the last two conditions occur in schizophrenia, but perseveration may occur in organic brain syndrome, especially Korsakoff's psychosis. *Mutism* is often due to schizophrenia or hysteria, but occasionally it is due to total motor aphasia.

SPLENOMEGALY, ACUTE OR SUBACUTE

Ask the following questions:

1. Is there fever? The presence of fever should suggest infectious mononucleosis, infectious hepatitis, leptospirosis, acute leukemia, lymphoma, malaria, and bacterial endocarditis, among other things.
2. Is there a rash? The presence of a rash should suggest thrombocytopenic purpura, acute leukemia, typhoid fever, septicemia, and lupus erythematosus.
3. Is there jaundice? The presence of jaundice should suggest infectious hepatitis, leptospirosis, malaria, hereditary spherocytosis and other hemolytic anemias, and portal vein thrombosis secondary to chronic liver disease.
4. Is there lymphadenopathy? The presence of lymphadenopathy should suggest infectious mononucleosis, acute lymphatic leukemia, lymphoma, brucellosis, and reticuloendotheliosis.
5. Is there a history of trauma? The presence of a history of trauma would suggest a traumatic rupture of the spleen.

DIAGNOSTIC WORKUP

Routine tests include a CBC, platelet count, sedimentation rate, chemistry panel, febrile agglutinins, serum haptoglobins, antinuclear antibody test, Monospot test, serum protein electrophoresis, a tuberculin test, chest x-ray, EKG, and flat plate of the abdomen.

If there is jaundice, a hepatitis profile, red cell fragility test, and blood smear for parasites should be done. If there is fever, serial blood cultures, leptospirosis antibody titer, and smear for malarial parasites should be done. If there is a petechial rash, a coagulation profile should be done. Lymph node biopsies and bone marrow examinations may be necessary. A CT scan of the abdomen and radionuclide scan for liver and spleen size and ratio should be done. The assistance of a hematologist or infectious disease expert should be sought. A surgeon may need to be consulted for an exploratory laparotomy.

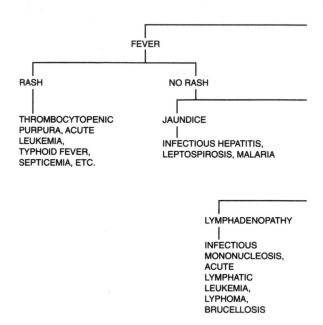

FEVER

RASH

THROMBOCYTOPENIC
PURPURA, ACUTE
LEUKEMIA,
TYPHOID FEVER,
SEPTICEMIA, ETC.

NO RASH

JAUNDICE

INFECTIOUS HEPATITIS,
LEPTOSPIROSIS, MALARIA

LYMPHADENOPATHY

INFECTIOUS
MONONUCLEOSIS,
ACUTE
LYMPHATIC
LEUKEMIA,
LYPHOMA,
BRUCELLOSIS

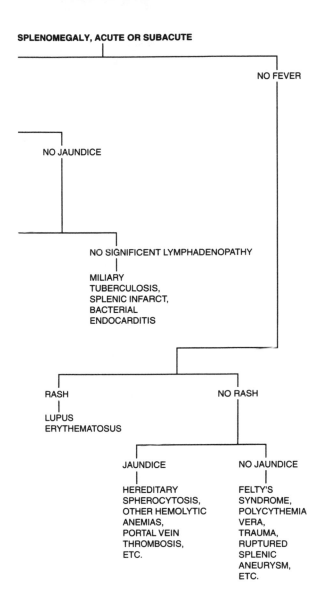

SPLENOMEGALY, ACUTE OR SUBACUTE

NO FEVER

NO JAUNDICE

NO SIGNIFICANT LYMPHADENOPATHY

MILIARY
TUBERCULOSIS,
SPLENIC INFARCT,
BACTERIAL
ENDOCARDITIS

RASH

LUPUS
ERYTHEMATOSUS

NO RASH

JAUNDICE

HEREDITARY
SPHEROCYTOSIS,
OTHER HEMOLYTIC
ANEMIAS,
PORTAL VEIN
THROMBOSIS,
ETC.

NO JAUNDICE

FELTY'S
SYNDROME,
POLYCYTHEMIA
VERA,
TRAUMA,
RUPTURED
SPLENIC
ANEURYSM,
ETC.

Splenomegaly, Acute or Subacute   535

SPLENOMEGALY, CHRONIC

Ask the following questions:

1. Is it massive? Massive splenomegaly is characteristic of Gaucher's disease, chronic myeloid leukemia, kala azar, and agnogenic myeloid metaplasia.
2. Is there jaundice? The presence of jaundice with massive splenomegaly would suggest chronic malaria. The presence of jaundice with mild to moderate splenomegaly would suggest alcoholic cirrhosis, chronic hepatitis, and hereditary spherocytosis.
3. Is there hepatomegaly? The presence of massive splenomegaly and hepatomegaly is characteristic of Gaucher's disease, chronic myeloid leukemia, kala azar, and agnogenic myeloid metaplasia.
4. Is there pallor? The presence of pallor, of course, suggests anemia and that would make one think of hereditary spherocytosis and other hemolytic anemias, collagen disease, and chronic malaria.
5. Is there lymphadenopathy? The presence of lymphadenopathy should make one think of chronic lymphatic leukemia, lymphomas, and sarcoidosis.

DIAGNOSTIC WORKUP

The diagnostic workup of chronic splenomegaly is similar to that for acute splenomegaly (page 532). A splenoportogram may be helpful in diagnosing portal vein thrombosis. Angiography may be helpful in diagnosing a splenic aneurysm. A liver biopsy, splenic aspiration and biopsy, and bone marrow biopsy may all be helpful in diagnosing the reticuloendothelioses such as Gaucher's disease.

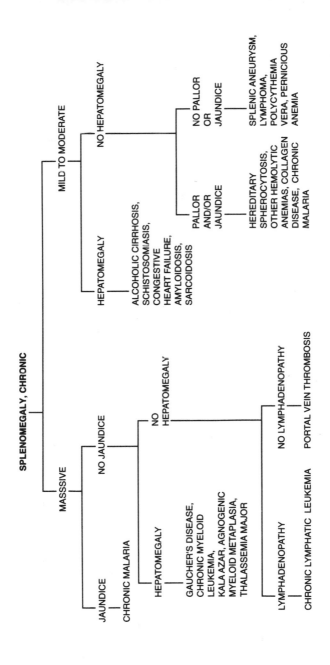

SQUINT

Squint simply means the eyes do not line up evenly. In other words, one eye deviates to the left or the right compared to the other. They may be concomitant, in which case the alignment remains the same during extraocular movements, or they may be nonconcomitant, in which case the alignment or amount of deviation changes with movement of the eyes.

Concomitant strabismus is almost always congenital and the result of birth trauma or anoxia. Rather than performing a diagnostic workup, the clinician should simply refer the patient to an ophthalmologist.

Nonconcomitant strabismus is due to paralysis of the extraocular muscles. The differential diagnosis of this disorder is discussed under Diplopia (page 142).

STEATORRHEA

Ask the following questions:

1. Is the patient a child or an adult? Children with steatorrhea may have celiac disease, cystic fibrosis, or tropical sprue.
2. Are there associated respiratory symptoms? The presence of respiratory symptoms should suggest cystic fibrosis, regardless of whether the patient is an adult or a child.
3. Is there jaundice? The presence of jaundice would suggest obstructive jaundice such as that due to biliary cirrhosis and other disorders.
4. Is there pallor and anemia? The presence of pallor or anemia suggests malabsorption syndrome, blind loop syndrome, intestinal parasites such as *Diphyllobothrium latum*, scleroderma, amyloidosis, and chronic obstructive jaundice.
5. Are there signs of systemic disease? If there are signs of systemic disease, then scleroderma, amyloidosis, and cystic fibrosis should be considered.
6. Is there an abdominal mass? The presence of an abdominal mass should suggest obstructive jaundice, pancreatic carcinoma, and hemochromatosis. Chronic pancreatitis may also present with an abdominal mass if there is a pseudocyst of the pancreas.

DIAGNOSTIC WORKUP

The basic workup includes a CBC, a blood smear for cell morphology, sedimentation rate, urinalysis, chemistry panel, serum B_{12} and folic acid, serum amylase and lipase, stool for occult blood, ovum and parasites, fat and trypsin, and a urine for 5-hydroxyindoleacetic acid (5-HIAA).

A sweat test should be done if cystic fibrosis is suspected. A D-xylose absorption test will help differentiate primary diseases of the small intestines.

An abnormal yield of labeled carbon dioxide after ingestion of a meal with radioactive ^{14}C-glycocholate will help diagnose bacterial overgrowth. An upper GI series and small bowel follow-through may be helpful. Intubation and analysis of pancreatic secretion of enzymes after pancreozymin or secretin injection will help differentiate pancreatic disorders. A CT scan of the abdomen and endoscopy may be useful. Intestinal biopsy with a Crosby capsule may help differentiate primary intestinal diseases also. Consult a gastroenterologist before ordering many of these expensive diagnostic tests.

A therapeutic trial with pancreatic enzymes, antibiotics, or even a gluten-free diet may also assist in the diagnosis.

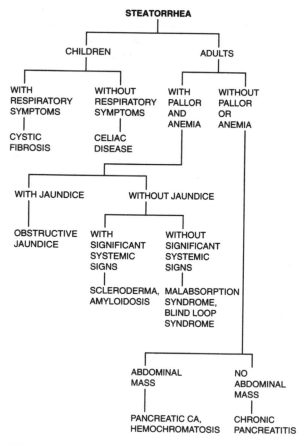

STRESS INCONTINENCE

Stress incontinence occurs most commonly in women who have had many pregnancies or who are in the menopause. The patient loses control of their bladder when they cough, laugh or sneeze and consequently leak small amounts of urine. Nocturia is rare in stress incontinence. There is often an associated cystocele. In postmenopausal women there is often an atrophic vaginitis due to the deficiency of estrogen. Men occasionally develop stress incontinence following a prostatectomy.

DIAGNOSTIC WORKUP

In most cases the diagnosis will be obvious. You can ask the patient to cough during a vaginal examination and the urine will trickle out. If that does not establish the diagnosis, have the patient drink a lot of water and not void until they return to the office. Then you can have them cough in the recumbent or erect position and the urine will be released. This is called the *stress test*. In the Q-tip test, a Q-tip is inserted in the tip of the urethra and the patient is asked to cough or strain. The Q-tip will move at least 30 degrees above the horizontal in cases of stress incontinence. For further discussion of incontinence, see page 318.

STRETCH MARKS
(STRIAE)

Stretch marks are common in obese patients or during pregnancy, in which case they are of no pathologic significance. However, purple striae of the abdomen, especially when they are associated with moon facies or a buffalo hump, should immediately call to mind Cushing's syndrome. Patients on prolonged corticosteroid therapy also develop purple striae. The workup is the same as for Cushing's syndrome (page 410).

STRIDOR

Ask the following questions:

1. Is the patient an adult or a child? If the patient is a child, then acute epiglottis, acute laryngotracheitis, foreign body, congenital laryngeal stridor, laryngismus stridulus, and a retropharyngeal abscess should be considered. Diphtheria is rarely found nowadays. If the patient is an adult, then myasthenia gravis, bulbar and pseudobulbar palsy, recurrent laryngeal palsy, pharyngitis, laryngotracheitis, carcinoma of the larynx or trachea, angioneurotic edema, foreign bodies, thyroid disorders, and disorders of the mediastinum should be considered.
2. Is it acute or gradual onset? The presence of stridor of acute onset would suggest acute epiglottitis, acute pharyngitis, laryngotracheitis, angioneurotic edema, retropharyngeal abscess, laryngismus stridulus, and foreign body.
3. Is there fever? The presence of fever would suggest acute laryngotracheitis, diphtheria, subacute thyroiditis, retropharyngeal abscess, and mediastinitis.
4. Are there abnormalities on the ear, nose and throat examination? On ear, nose and throat examination, the clinician may find pharyngitis, acute epiglottitis, a foreign body, tenderness of the thyroid suggesting thyroiditis, and thyroid masses.
5. Are there neurologic abnormalities on examination? Neurologic abnormalities may be found in myasthenia gravis, bulbar and pseudobulbar palsy, bilateral recurrent laryngeal nerve palsy, and comatose states.

DIAGNOSTIC WORKUP

Routine tests may include a CBC, sedimentation rate, smear and culture of material from the nose, throat and sputum, x-ray of the chest and sinuses, and in adults an EKG. In adults also, it might be wise to order a chemistry panel, thyroid profile, and VDRL test depending on the clinical picture. Direct laryngoscopy can now be done in the office with the fiberoptic laryngoscope. In addition, fiberoptic bronchoscopy may be valuable. A Tensilon test may need to be done. An ear, nose and throat specialist should be consulted before ordering expensive diagnostic tests. If there are neurologic signs, a neurologist should be consulted.

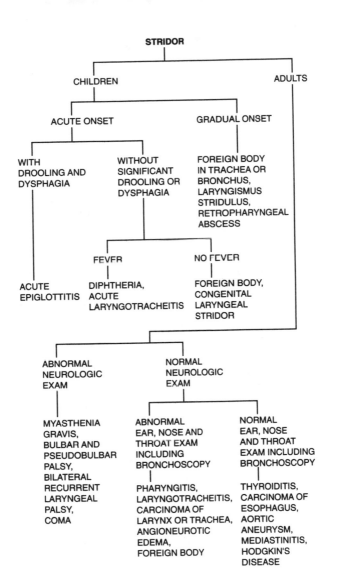

STRIDOR

CHILDREN — ADULTS

CHILDREN:
- ACUTE ONSET
  - WITH DROOLING AND DYSPHAGIA
    - ACUTE EPIGLOTTITIS
  - WITHOUT SIGNIFICANT DROOLING OR DYSPHAGIA
    - FEVER
      - DIPHTHERIA, ACUTE LARYNGOTRACHEITIS
    - NO FEVER
      - FOREIGN BODY, CONGENITAL LARYNGEAL STRIDOR
- GRADUAL ONSET
  - FOREIGN BODY IN TRACHEA OR BRONCHUS, LARYNGISMUS STRIDULUS, RETROPHARYNGEAL ABSCESS

ADULTS:
- ABNORMAL NEUROLOGIC EXAM
  - MYASTHENIA GRAVIS, BULBAR AND PSEUDOBULBAR PALSY, BILATERAL RECURRENT LARYNGEAL PALSY, COMA
- NORMAL NEUROLOGIC EXAM
  - ABNORMAL EAR, NOSE AND THROAT EXAM INCLUDING BRONCHOSCOPY
    - PHARYNGITIS, LARYNGOTRACHEITIS, CARCINOMA OF LARYNX OR TRACHEA, ANGIONEUROTIC EDEMA, FOREIGN BODY
  - NORMAL EAR, NOSE AND THROAT EXAM INCLUDING BRONCHOSCOPY
    - THYROIDITIS, CARCINOMA OF ESOPHAGUS, AORTIC ANEURYSM, MEDIASTINITIS, HODGKIN'S DISEASE

STUPOR

Ask the following questions:

1. Is it intermittent? Intermittent stupor should suggest epilepsy, chronic illicit drug use, transient ischemic attacks, migraine, and insulinoma.
2. Is there a positive drug or alcohol history? This finding would suggest cocaine, barbiturate, alcohol, morphine, LSD, or PCP abuse.
3. Are there focal neurologic signs? The presence of focal neurologic signs may mean cerebral vascular disease, advanced brain tumor, cerebral abscess, encephalitis, subdural hematoma, central nervous system lues, Wernicke's encephalopathy, and subarachnoid hemorrhage or meningitis.
4. Is there nuchal rigidity? The presence of nuchal rigidity would suggest a subarachnoid hemorrhage or meningitis, but it could occasionally indicate an intracerebral hemorrhage.
5. Is there a distinguishing odor to the breath? Besides alcohol, uremia, diabetic acidosis, and liver failure may be suggested by a characteristic odor to the breath.

DIAGNOSTIC WORKUP

Routine tests may include a CBC, sedimentation rate, urinalysis, chemistry panel with electrolytes, arterial blood gas analysis, blood and urine drug and alcohol screen, electroencephalogram, and CT scan of the brain. A spinal tap may be done if the CT scan is negative for a space-occupying lesion. A neurologist or neurosurgeon should have been contacted by this time. A cerebral vascular disease may need further investigation, including carotid duplex scan and cerebral angiography.

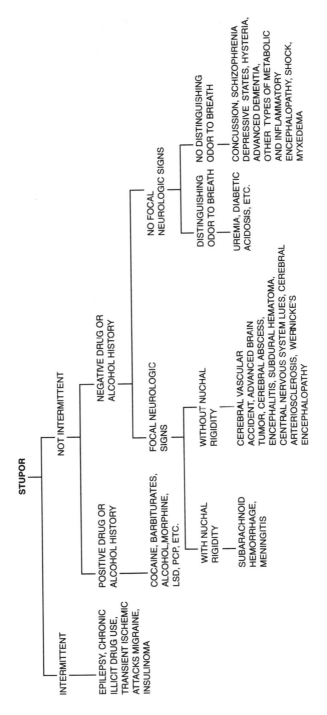

STUPOR

- INTERMITTENT
  - EPILEPSY, CHRONIC ILLICIT DRUG USE, TRANSIENT ISCHEMIC ATTACKS MIGRAINE, INSULINOMA
- NOT INTERMITTENT
  - POSITIVE DRUG OR ALCOHOL HISTORY
    - COCAINE, BARBITURATES, ALCOHOL, MORPHINE, LSD, PCP, ETC.
  - NEGATIVE DRUG OR ALCOHOL HISTORY
    - FOCAL NEUROLOGIC SIGNS
      - WITH NUCHAL RIGIDITY
        - SUBARACHNOID HEMORRHAGE, MENINGITIS
      - WITHOUT NUCHAL RIGIDITY
        - CEREBRAL VASCULAR ACCIDENT, ADVANCED BRAIN TUMOR, CEREBRAL ABSCESS, ENCEPHALITIS, SUBDURAL HEMATOMA, CENTRAL NERVOUS SYSTEM LUES, CEREBRAL ARTERIOSCLEROSIS, WERNICKE'S ENCEPHALOPATHY
    - NO FOCAL NEUROLOGIC SIGNS
      - DISTINGUISHING ODOR TO BREATH
        - UREMIA, DIABETIC ACIDOSIS, ETC.
      - NO DISTINGUISHING ODOR TO BREATH
        - CONCUSSION, SCHIZOPHRENIA DEPRESSIVE STATES, HYSTERIA, ADVANCED DEMENTIA, OTHER TYPES OF METABOLIC AND INFLAMMATORY ENCEPHALOPATHY, SHOCK, MYXEDEMA

Stupor   547

SUCCUSSION SOUNDS

Most of us have heard these sounds on ourselves after consuming a large quantity of liquid. If they are heard with the stethoscope in a patient with abdominal disturbance, they are of pathologic significance. When there are associated hyperactive and/or high-pitched bowel sounds, intestinal obstruction should be considered. When there are hypoactive bowel sounds, paralytic ileus or peritonitis should be considered.

Succussion sounds coming from the chest are due to hydropneumothorax or hemopneumothorax. The chest x-ray should make the diagnosis obvious. Other rare causes of succussion sounds are acute gastric dilatation, chronic pyloric obstruction, subdiaphragmatic abscess, and pneumoperitoneum. The diagnostic workup will be determined by associated symptoms and signs (vomiting, page 391; abdominal pain, page 6; abdominal mass, page 11).

SYNCOPE

Ask the following questions:

1. Are there convulsive movements? The presence of convulsive movements should suggest convulsions, and the differential diagnosis of this is discussed on page 107. Convulsive movements can occur with other forms of syncope, however.
2. Is the pulse slow or absent? The presence of a slow or absent pulse would suggest heart block, vasovagal syncope, and carotid sinus syncope.
3. Is the pulse rate normal? The presence of a normal pulse rate would suggest anemia, aortic stenosis, aortic insufficiency, and cyanotic congenital heart disease.
4. Is the pulse rate rapid? The presence of a rapid pulse would suggest the various types of ventricular and supraventricular tachycardias, including auricular fibrillation and flutter, and it should also suggest heat exhaustion or heat stroke.
5. If the pulse is rapid, is it regular? The presence of a rapid regular pulse should suggest supraventricular or ventricular tachycardia, heat exhaustion, or heat stroke.
6. Is there a heart murmur? The presence of a heart murmur should suggest aortic stenosis, aortic insufficiency, and cyanotic congenital heart disease.
7. Is there pallor? The presence of pallor should suggest shock or severe anemia and acute bleeding.
8. Are there focal neurologic signs? The presence of focal neurologic signs should suggest cerebral vascular insufficiency, hypoglycemia, and transient ischemic attacks.

DIAGNOSTIC WORKUP

The diagnostic workup includes a CBC, sedimentation rate, urinalysis, chemistry panel, VDRL test, thyroid profile, glucose tolerance test, EKG, and chest x-ray. Several blood pressure recordings in the recumbent and upright positions should be made. If hypoglycemia is suspected, then a 72-hr fast and a tolbutamide tolerance test should be done. The drug history should always be reviewed.

Most cases will require 24-hr Holter monitoring or event Holter monitoring. In addition, other cardiovascular studies such as echocardiography and His' bundle studies may need to be done. If transient ischemic attacks are suspected, a carotid scan and cerebral angiography may be necessary. If the syncopal attacks are thought to be due to epilepsy, then wake and sleep EEGs may need to be done. A CT scan or MRI of the brain may need to be done.

A cardiologist or neurologist should be consulted before ordering expensive diagnostic tests. A psychiatrist may also need to be consulted.

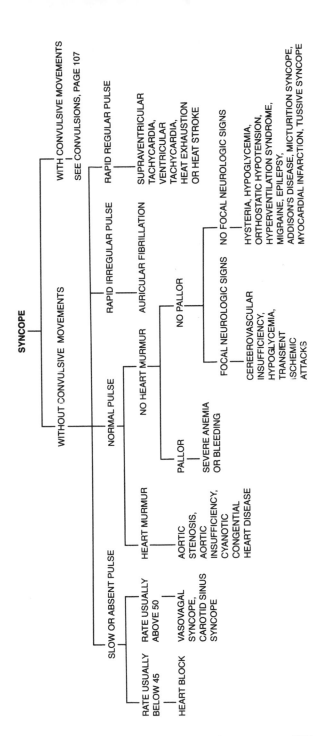

SYNCOPE

- **WITH CONVULSIVE MOVEMENTS**
  - SEE CONVULSIONS, PAGE 107

- **WITHOUT CONVULSIVE MOVEMENTS**

  - **RAPID REGULAR PULSE**
    - SUPRAVENTRICULAR TACHYCARDIA, VENTRICULAR TACHYCARDIA, HEAT EXHAUSTION OR HEAT STROKE

  - **RAPID IRREGULAR PULSE**
    - AURICULAR FIBRILLATION

  - **NORMAL PULSE**
    - **NO HEART MURMUR**
      - **NO PALLOR**
        - **NO FOCAL NEUROLOGIC SIGNS**
          - HYSTERIA, HYPOGLYCEMIA, ORTHOSTATIC HYPOTENSION, HYPERVENTILATION SYNDROME, MIGRAINE, EPILEPSY, ADDISON'S DISEASE, MICTURITION SYNCOPE, MYOCARDIAL INFARCTION, TUSSIVE SYNCOPE
        - **FOCAL NEUROLOGIC SIGNS**
          - CEREBROVASCULAR INSUFFICIENCY, HYPOGLYCEMIA, TRANSIENT ISCHEMIC ATTACKS
      - **PALLOR**
        - SEVERE ANEMIA OR BLEEDING
    - **HEART MURMUR**
      - AORTIC STENOSIS, AORTIC INSUFFICIENCY, CYANOTIC CONGENITAL HEART DISEASE

  - **SLOW OR ABSENT PULSE**
    - **RATE USUALLY ABOVE 50**
      - VASOVAGAL SYNCOPE, CAROTID SINUS SYNCOPE
    - **RATE USUALLY BELOW 45**
      - HEART BLOCK

Syncope   551

TACHYCARDIA

Ask the following questions:

1. Is there a positive alcohol or drug history? It is well known that alcohol can cause a myocardiopathy. Atropine, caffeine, and many other substances can cause a tachycardia.
2. Is the heart rate below 160 and/or reduced by carotid sinus massage? This finding would help confirm the diagnosis of sinus tachycardia and lead to a consideration of fever, thyrotoxicosis, shock, anemia, myocardial infarction, and other disorders as the cause of the tachycardia.
3. Is there fever? The presence of fever and tachycardia should make one suspect acute infectious diseases, rheumatic fever, and thyroid storm.
4. Is there a tremor, neck mass, or systolic hypertension? These findings suggest thyrotoxicosis.
5. Is there chest pain? The presence of chest pain should make one suspect myocardial infarction, pulmonary embolism, and acute pericarditis.
6. Is there pallor or sweating? The presence of pallor or sweating should make one think of anemia and shock.
7. Are there crepitant rales, an enlarged liver, or peripheral edema? These findings suggest congestive heart failure.
8. Is there hypotension? The presence of hypotension should make one think that there may be a pathologic tachycardia such as supraventricular tachycardia, auricular flutter, or auricular fibrillation. Auricular fibrillation is especially likely to be associated with significant hypotension.
9. Is the rate irregular? The presence of an irregular heart rate should make one suspect auricular fibrillation, or alternating flutter and fibrillation.

DIAGNOSTIC WORKUP

Routine diagnostic tests should include a CBC, sedimentation rate, urinalysis, chemistry panel, thyroid profile, antinuclear antibody titer, VDRL test, chest x-ray, and EKG. If there is fever, then an antistreptolysin-O titer and cross-reacting protein (CRP), febrile agglutinins, and serial blood cultures should be done.

If a myocardial infarction is suspected, serial EKGs and cardiac enzymes need to be ordered. If a pulmonary embolism or infarction is suspected, arterial blood gases and lung scans need to be ordered and ultimately pulmonary angiography may need to be done.

If congestive heart failure is suspected, a venous pressure and circulation time and possibly pulmonary function studies may be done.

If the tachycardia is paroxysmal, 24-hr Holter monitoring or admission to the hospital for ambulatory telemetry and observation may be necessary. A cardiologist should be consulted. Ultimately, a psychiatrist may need to be consulted also.

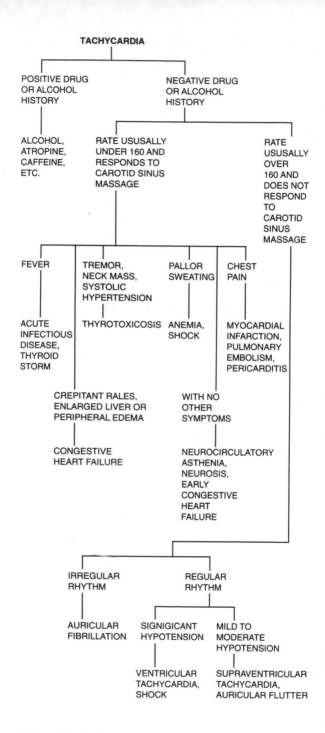

TACHYCARDIA

- **POSITIVE DRUG OR ALCOHOL HISTORY**
  - ALCOHOL, ATROPINE, CAFFEINE, ETC.
- **NEGATIVE DRUG OR ALCOHOL HISTORY**
  - **RATE USUSALLY UNDER 160 AND RESPONDS TO CAROTID SINUS MASSAGE**
    - FEVER
      - ACUTE INFECTIOUS DISEASE, THYROID STORM
    - TREMOR, NECK MASS, SYSTOLIC HYPERTENSION
      - THYROTOXICOSIS
    - PALLOR SWEATING
      - ANEMIA, SHOCK
    - CHEST PAIN
      - MYOCARDIAL INFARCTION, PULMONARY EMBOLISM, PERICARDITIS
    - CREPITANT RALES, ENLARGED LIVER OR PERIPHERAL EDEMA
      - CONGESTIVE HEART FAILURE
    - WITH NO OTHER SYMPTOMS
      - NEUROCIRCULATORY ASTHENIA, NEUROSIS, EARLY CONGESTIVE HEART FAILURE
  - **RATE USUSALLY OVER 160 AND DOES NOT RESPOND TO CAROTID SINUS MASSAGE**
    - IRREGULAR RHYTHM
      - AURICULAR FIBRILLATION
    - REGULAR RHYTHM
      - SIGNIGICANT HYPOTENSION
        - VENTRICULAR TACHYCARDIA, SHOCK
      - MILD TO MODERATE HYPOTENSION
        - SUPRAVENTRICULAR TACHYCARDIA, AURICULAR FLUTTER

TASTE ABNORMALITIES

Ask the following questions:

1. Is there distortion of the taste? Distortion of the taste occurs episodically in uncinate fits of epilepsy and is persistent in hysteria, pregnancy, schizophrenia, glossitis, and jaundice.
2. If there is distortion, is it constant or intermittent? If the distortion of the taste is episodic, one should look for the uncinate fits of epilepsy.
3. Is there a positive history of drug or poison ingestion? This finding should suggest penicillamine, mercury, bismuth, iodine, or bromide toxicity.
4. Is the ear, nose and throat or oral examination abnormal? Abnormalities that may be found on an ear, nose and throat or oral examination include glossitis, gingivitis, stomatitis, dental caries, rhinitis, and hay fever.
5. Is the neurologic examination abnormal? Abnormalities on the neurologic examination may suggest Bell's palsy, temporomandibular joint syndrome, petrositis, and brain stem lesions.

DIAGNOSTIC WORKUP

Routine diagnostic tests include a CBC, sedimentation rate, chemistry panel, urinalysis, urine drug screen, and a chest x-ray. If the ear, nose and throat or oral examination is revealing, the patient should be referred to an ear, nose and throat specialist or oral surgeon. If the neurologic examination is abnormal, referral to a neurologist should be considered. A wake and sleep EEG with nasopharyngeal electrodes as well as a CT scan of the brain may be necessary to determine the cause or the diagnosis of uncinate fits. A psychiatrist may need to be consulted if the patient is suspected of a neurosis.

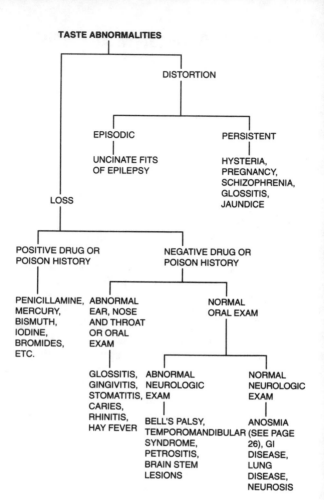

TASTE ABNORMALITIES

DISTORTION

EPISODIC

UNCINATE FITS
OF EPILEPSY

PERSISTENT

HYSTERIA,
PREGNANCY,
SCHIZOPHRENIA,
GLOSSITIS,
JAUNDICE

LOSS

POSITIVE DRUG OR
POISON HISTORY

NEGATIVE DRUG OR
POISON HISTORY

PENICILLAMINE,
MERCURY,
BISMUTH,
IODINE,
BROMIDES,
ETC.

ABNORMAL
EAR, NOSE
AND THROAT
OR ORAL
EXAM

NORMAL
ORAL EXAM

GLOSSITIS,
GINGIVITIS,
STOMATITIS,
CARIES,
RHINITIS,
HAY FEVER

ABNORMAL
NEUROLOGIC
EXAM

BELL'S PALSY,
TEMPOROMANDIBULAR
SYNDROME,
PETROSITIS,
BRAIN STEM
LESIONS

NORMAL
NEUROLOGIC
EXAM

ANOSMIA
(SEE PAGE
26), GI
DISEASE,
LUNG
DISEASE,
NEUROSIS

TESTICULAR ATROPHY

Ask the following questions:

1. Is it unilateral? The presence of unilateral atrophy would suggest hernia surgery, previous orchitis from mumps, gonorrhea, syphilis, tuberculosis or elephantiasis, varicocele, hydrocele, and undescended testicle.
2. Is there a history of trauma or surgery? A history of surgery would suggest that the testicular atrophy is related to hernia surgery or surgery for undescended testicle, vasectomy, or prostatectomy. History of trauma may suggest that the patient had an acute orchitis or hemorrhage from trauma.
3. Is there a history of an infection? A history of infection would suggest mumps, gonorrhea, syphilis, tuberculosis, or elephantiasis.
4. Is there a loss of secondary sex characteristics? These findings would suggest Klinefelter's syndrome.
5. Is there an enlarged liver? The presence of an enlarged liver or other signs of hepatic dysfunction would suggest cirrhosis or hemochromatosis.
6. Are there abnormal neurologic findings? The presence of abnormal neurologic findings would suggest myotonia atrophica.

DIAGNOSTIC WORKUP

Unilateral testicular atrophy usually requires no workup as long as there are no complaints of sexual infertility or impotence. A smear and culture of any urethral discharge should be done. Sometimes prostatic massage may be necessary to obtain a good specimen.

The workup of bilateral testicular atrophy may include a serum testosterone, FSH, urine gonadotrophins, and chromosome studies to rule out Klinefelter's syndrome; liver function tests and liver biopsy to rule out cirrhosis and hemochromatosis; and electromyography and muscle biopsies to rule out myotonia atrophica. A testicular biopsy may be necessary ultimately. A urologist will be consulted long before most of these tests would be performed.

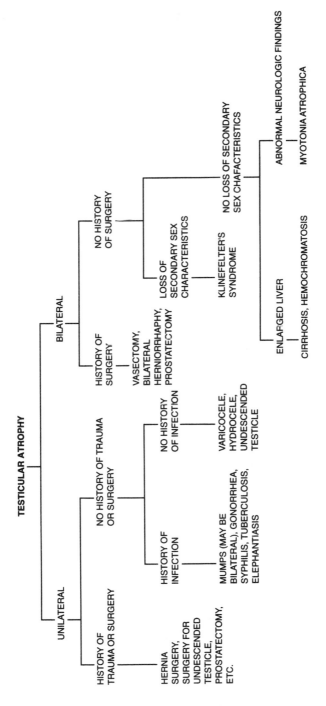

TESTICULAR PAIN

It is rare for pain in the testicle to occur without a mass. Therefore, the algorithmic diagnosis is essentially the same as that of testicular swelling (page 561). Keep in mind that there are cases of orchitis, epididymitis, and torsion not associated with testicular swelling. Also, in cases of renal colic (nephrolithiasis, etc.) and herniated lumbar disk, pain may be referred to the testicle.

TESTICULAR SWELLING

Ask the following questions:

1. Is there pain or tenderness of the testicle? The presence of pain or tenderness should suggest torsion of the testicle, orchitis, epididymitis, and a strangulated inguinal hernia.
2. Is the testicle retracted or does elevation of the testicle aggravate the pain? These findings would suggest torsion of the testicle.
3. Does the swelling transilluminate? If the swelling transilluminates, the mass or swelling is most likely a hydrocele or spermatocele.
4. Is the swelling reducible? If the swelling is reducible, the mass is probably an inguinal hernia or varicocele. A mass that does not reduce could still be an incarcerated inguinal hernia.

DIAGNOSTIC WORKUP

A CBC, sedimentation rate, urinalysis, chemistry panel, and VDRL test should be done routinely. If a tumor of the testicle is suspected, 24-hr urine gonadotrophins may be ordered. If there is a urethral discharge, a smear and culture should be made. If a hernia is strongly suspected, a general surgeon should be consulted. Testicular scans with technetium-99m will help distinguish torsion of the testicle from orchitis or epididymitis. Scrotal ultrasound may be useful in differentiating a hematoma, abscess, or rupture from orchitis. It may also be helpful in evaluating testicular tumors.

The expense of some or all of these tests may be avoided by consulting a urologist early in the diagnostic workup.

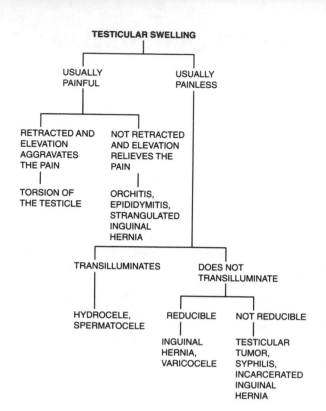

TESTICULAR SWELLING

USUALLY PAINFUL

USUALLY PAINLESS

RETRACTED AND ELEVATION AGGRAVATES THE PAIN

TORSION OF THE TESTICLE

NOT RETRACTED AND ELEVATION RELIEVES THE PAIN

ORCHITIS, EPIDIDYMITIS, STRANGULATED INGUINAL HERNIA

TRANSILLUMINATES

DOES NOT TRANSILLUMINATE

HYDROCELE, SPERMATOCELE

REDUCIBLE

INGUINAL HERNIA, VARICOCELE

NOT REDUCIBLE

TESTICULAR TUMOR, SYPHILIS, INCARCERATED INGUINAL HERNIA

THIRST

Ask the following questions:

1. Is there a positive drug or alcohol history? Alcohol, amitriptyline, diuretics, and many other drugs may cause excessive thirst.
2. Is there fever? The presence of fever would make one suspect an infectious disease (see page 218).
3. Is there pallor or shock? Pallor or shock should make one think of gastrointestinal bleeding, ruptured ectopic pregnancy, trauma, and other disorders associated with anemia or shock.
4. Is there significant polyuria? Polyuria that is either significant or massive would suggest diabetes insipidus, diabetes mellitus, or thyrotoxicosis. Mild or insignificant polyuria may be due to hypercalcemia, hyperparathyroidism, and excessive salt intake.

DIAGNOSTIC WORKUP

Routine tests include a CBC, sedimentation rate, urinalysis, chemistry panel, thyroid panel, glucose tolerance test, blood alcohol level, and 24-hr urine collection for sodium, potassium, and calcium. If pituitary diabetes insipidus is suspected, then a CT scan of the brain, the Hickey-Hare test, and vasopressin (Pitressin) injection test may need to be done. If hyperparathyroidism is suspected, a serum parathyroid hormone assay and x-rays of the skull and long bones may be done. A consultation with an endocrinologist may be necessary.

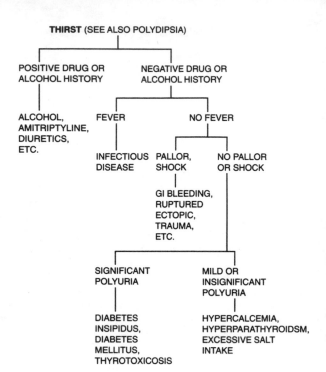

THIRST (SEE ALSO POLYDIPSIA)

POSITIVE DRUG OR ALCOHOL HISTORY

ALCOHOL, AMITRIPTYLINE, DIURETICS, ETC.

NEGATIVE DRUG OR ALCOHOL HISTORY

FEVER

INFECTIOUS DISEASE

NO FEVER

PALLOR, SHOCK

GI BLEEDING, RUPTURED ECTOPIC, TRAUMA, ETC.

NO PALLOR OR SHOCK

SIGNIFICANT POLYURIA

DIABETES INSIPIDUS, DIABETES MELLITUS, THYROTOXICOSIS

MILD OR INSIGNIFICANT POLYURIA

HYPERCALCEMIA, HYPERPARATHYROIDSM, EXCESSIVE SALT INTAKE

THYROID ENLARGEMENT

Ask the following questions:

1. Is it focal or diffuse? Focal masses in the thyroid include thyroglossal cyst, toxic adenoma, colloid cyst, Riedel's struma, nontoxic adenoma, and malignancies.
2. Is there movement with protrusion of the tongue? This is a typical finding in cases of thyroglossal cyst.
3. If focal, are there signs of thyrotoxicosis? The presence of thyrotoxicosis and a focal mass suggest toxic adenoma.
4. If diffuse, are there signs of thyrotoxicosis? Diffuse thyroid enlargement with thyrotoxicosis indicates Graves' disease.
5. Is it tender? The presence of a tender enlarged thyroid suggests subacute thyroiditis and Hashimoto's thyroiditis.

DIAGNOSTIC WORKUP

Routine tests include a CBC, sedimentation rate, urinalysis, thyroid profile with a TSH immunoassay, chemistry panel, chest x-ray, and EKG. Thyroid antibodies may be tested if Hashimoto's thyroiditis is suspected.

The most important study is a thyroid technetium-99m or iodine-123 uptake and scan. If the results of these are abnormal, then an endocrinologist or general surgeon should be consulted to assist in the interpretation. If the scan indicates a cold nodule, ultrasonography may be done to determine whether the nodule is cystic or solid. If it is cystic, generally it can be aspirated and followed. If it is solid, then a biopsy or aspiration and biopsy should be undertaken. If there are malignant cells or at least suspicious cells for malignancy, surgery should be done. If the scan reveals a hot nodule and there is clinical and laboratory evidence of thyrotoxicosis, the patient should be treated with radioactive iodine or surgery. If the scan shows diffuse uptake of radioactive materials and there is clinical thyrotoxicosis, then the patient also may be treated with radioactive iodine or surgery.

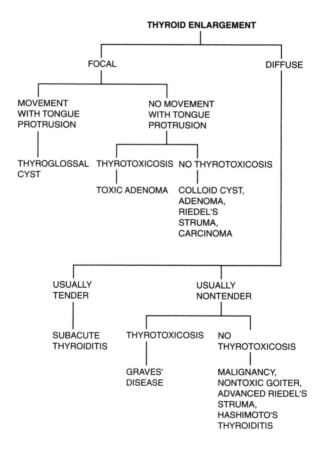

TINNITUS

Ask the following questions:

1. Is it subjective or objective? Objective tinnitus is unusual, but it may indicate glomus tumors, arteriovenous malformations, carotid stenosis, aneurysms, anemia, a patent eustachian tube, or myoclonus. Objective tinnitus means that both the patient and the examiner can hear the noises.
2. If it is subjective, is it unilateral or bilateral? Unilateral subjective tinnitus is more likely to be associated with a more serious disorder such as Ménière's disease, acoustic neuroma, cholesteatoma, or vascular disease.
3. Is there a history of trauma? A history of trauma would suggest that the tinnitus is due to whiplash, concussion, or trauma to the middle or inner ear.
4. Is there a history of the use of ototoxic drugs? Drugs that may cause tinnitus include aminoglycosides, tetracyclines, clindamycin, caffeine, and the tricyclic antidepressants. Aspirin and quinine may also be associated with tinnitus.
5. Are there abnormalities found on the ear examination? Abnormalities on the ear examination include cerumen, otitis externa, otitis media, mastoiditis, and cholesteatomas. The tympanic membrane may be red in cases of glomus tumors.
6. Is there vertigo and deafness? The presence of vertigo with deafness should suggest Ménière's disease, acoustic neuroma, and cholesteatoma, as well as multiple sclerosis, basilar artery insufficiency, and brain stem tumors.
7. Are there other neurologic signs? The presence of other neurologic signs along with vertigo and deafness would suggest multiple sclerosis, advanced acoustic neuroma, basilar artery occlusion or insufficiency, brain stem tumors, and central nervous system syphilis.

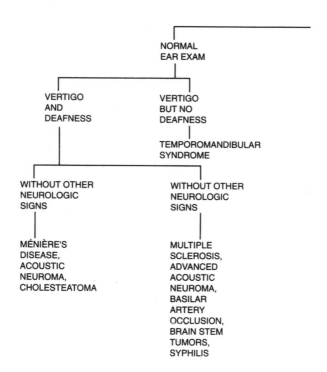

NORMAL
EAR EXAM

VERTIGO
AND
DEAFNESS

VERTIGO
BUT NO
DEAFNESS

TEMPOROMANDIBULAR
SYNDROME

WITHOUT OTHER
NEUROLOGIC
SIGNS

WITHOUT OTHER
NEUROLOGIC
SIGNS

MÉNIÈRE'S
DISEASE,
ACOUSTIC
NEUROMA,
CHOLESTEATOMA

MULTIPLE
SCLEROSIS,
ADVANCED
ACOUSTIC
NEUROMA,
BASILAR
ARTERY
OCCLUSION,
BRAIN STEM
TUMORS,
SYPHILIS

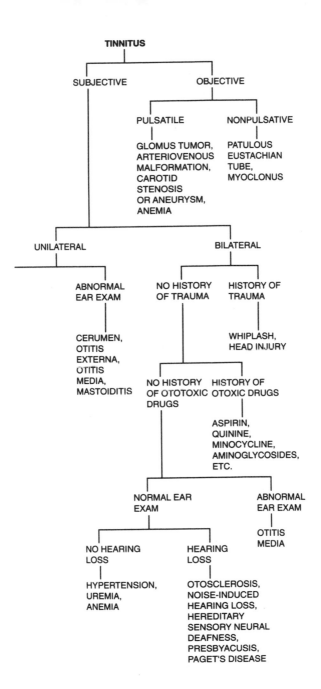

DIAGNOSTIC WORKUP

The basic workup includes a CBC, sedimentation rate, urinalysis, chemistry panel, thyroid profile, VDRL test, audiometry, caloric tests, (electronystagmography) and x-rays of the mastoids and petrous bones. Specialized audiometry may be performed, such as impedance audiometry, Békésy audiometry, and brain stem evoked potential studies.

If an acoustic neuroma is strongly suspected, CT scans with iodine infusion or installation of 4 cc of oxygen in the subarachnoid space would be indicated. Angiography and venography may help diagnose objective tinnitus. A spinal tap may be helpful in diagnosing multiple sclerosis and central nervous system syphilis. A glucose tolerance test may be indicated to rule out diabetes mellitus.

TONGUE MASS OR SWELLING

Ask the following questions:

1. Is it painful? Painful swellings of the tongue include trauma, burns, herpes simplex, pemphigus, erythema bullosum, carcinoma, Ludwig's angina, angioneurotic edema, bee stings, and hemorrhage due to coagulation disorders.
2. Is the mass or swelling focal or diffuse? Focal masses include trauma, herpes simplex, pemphigus, erythema bullosum, carcinoma, angioma, fibroma, lipoma, mucus cyst, papilloma, or syphilitic gumma. Diffuse masses include Ludwig's angina, angioneurotic edema, bee sting, hemorrhage, myxedema, acromegaly, cretinism, mongolism, primary amyloidosis, diffuse lymphoma, and riboflavin deficiency.

DIAGNOSTIC WORKUP

Focal lesions of the tongue should be referred to an oral surgeon or dermatologist for biopsy or excision. Diffuse enlargement or swellings require a workup including CBC, sedimentation rate, urinalysis, chemistry panel, thyroid panel, VDRL test, and antinuclear antibody titer. If a coagulation disorder is suspected, a coagulation profile may be done. If a vitamin deficiency is suspected, a therapeutic trial of vitamins is indicated. If amyloidosis is suspected, a biopsy may be done. Other disorders may require biopsy also. A trial of antibiotics or corticosteroids may be necessary.

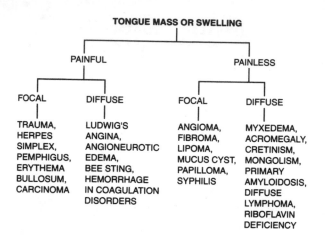

TONGUE MASS OR SWELLING

PAINFUL

FOCAL

TRAUMA,
HERPES
SIMPLEX,
PEMPHIGUS,
ERYTHEMA
BULLOSUM,
CARCINOMA

DIFFUSE

LUDWIG'S
ANGINA,
ANGIONEUROTIC
EDEMA,
BEE STING,
HEMORRHAGE
IN COAGULATION
DISORDERS

PAINLESS

FOCAL

ANGIOMA,
FIBROMA,
LIPOMA,
MUCUS CYST,
PAPILLOMA,
SYPHILIS

DIFFUSE

MYXEDEMA,
ACROMEGALY,
CRETINISM,
MONGOLISM,
PRIMARY
AMYLOIDOSIS,
DIFFUSE
LYMPHOMA,
RIBOFLAVIN
DEFICIENCY

TONGUE PAIN

Pain in the tongue is rarely an isolated symptom. There is usually a focal or diffuse inflammation of the tongue or an ulcerating lesion. Diffuse inflammation is found in antibiotic glossitis, glossitis of avitaminosis (pernicious anemia), aphthous stomatitis, thrush, streptococcal glossitis, and acute diffuse glossitis. Focal lesions include cuts and ulcerations from trauma such as the bitten tongue or burned tongue (hot pizza, etc.), or injury from a sharp tooth or jagged dental plate. Other painful focal lesions are carcinoma, tuberculosis, syphilis (often painless), and herpes simplex ulcers. When the tongue is completely normal, trigeminal neuralgia, polymyositis, trichinosis, and calculus of the submaxillary gland should be considered.

DIAGNOSTIC WORKUP

Most lesions will respond to conservative treatment and time. In patients with signs of systemic disease and vitamin deficiency, the workup includes serum B_{12} and folate level, upper GI series, ANA, and *Trichinella* antibody titer. Focal lesions that persist should command a referral to a dentist or oral surgeon.

TONGUE ULCERS

Ulcerations of the tongue are most commonly due to aphthous stomatitis (canker sore), but they may appear in various stages of syphilis, in herpes zoster, as a result of repetitive trauma from a sharp or carious tooth, in tuberculosis, and in carcinoma. The chancre of primary syphilis rarely causes severe pain, so this will often distinguish the lesion from the others. To differentiate the other causes, a smear and culture and ultimately a biopsy must be done. Most physicians will find referral to a dentist or oral surgeon is the best course of action when the ulcer persists.

TOOTH AND GUM ABNORMALITIES

As physicians, we often neglect inspection of the teeth. We seem to expect the dentist to do this part of the examination for us. Multiple cavities are found in diabetes mellitus, pernicious anemia, and multiparous women. Separation of the teeth may be a clue to *hypopituitarism*, while teeth that taper to a thin edge are typical of the screwdriver appearance of *Hutchinson teeth* in congenital syphilis. Who has not heard of the dramatic gum hypertrophy associated with phenytoin use in epileptic children? In *scurvy* the gums become swollen and the teeth get loose, drop out or become misaligned. In dental ectodermal dysplasia, the teeth may be partially or completely absent and at times there is no evidence of enamel formation. The dark blue line positioned where the gums meet the teeth is a sign of lead intoxication.

Mothers frequently complain that their children grind their teeth, but this is rarely of pathologic significance. Of course, it may be a sign of malocclusion and temporomandibular joint syndrome, especially in adults.

Yellow teeth are a sign that a child has been affected by Tetracyclines either *in utero* or early childhood.

TREMOR

Ask the following questions:

1. When does the tremor occur? Intention tremor, which means that the tremor occurs on movement, would suggest that the patient is suffering from a familial or senile tremor or multiple sclerosis, Wilson's disease, or hereditary familial ataxia. It also may suggest alcoholism. Nothing is more dramatic than the intention tremor of alcohol withdrawal. A tremor occurring at rest would suggest Parkinson's disease or manganese poisoning. A fine tremor of the outstretched hands, which is sometimes described as tension tremor, would suggest hyperthyroidism.
2. The next question to ask is are there associated neurologic findings? A tremor with long tract findings such as hyperactive reflexes or Babinski sign would suggest multiple sclerosis, while a fairly symmetrical tremor with no long tract signs or other neurologic findings would suggest a familial senile tremor. A tremor with mental deterioration would suggest Wilson's disease.
3. Are there associated systemic findings? If the patient has tachycardia and an enlarged thyroid, one should consider hyperthyroidism. However, simply tachycardia alone might indicate that the patient is very sensitive to caffeine. Kayser-Fleischer ring and enlarged liver would suggest Wilson's disease. An enlarged liver alone would suggest alcoholism.

DIAGNOSTIC WORKUP

Certainly a thyroid profile should be done on all cases that present with a tremor alone. In addition, blood tests for serum copper and ceruloplasmin should be done when Wilson's disease is suspected. A drug and alcohol screen should be done also. If multiple sclerosis, Wilson's disease, or a cerebellar tumor is suspected, a CT scan or MRI of the brain should be done. Most patients presenting with a mild intention tremor which is symmetrical and not associated with other neurologic findings will probably have familial or senile tremor and the response to beta blockers can be determined.

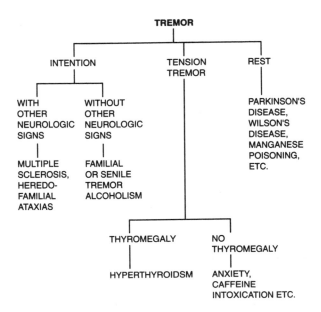

TRISMUS

True trismus or lockjaw is found in tetanus, rabies, and trichinosis. In strychnine poisoning it is a late development, as the twitchings and convulsions are well established before it appears. Intermittent trismus may be found in epilepsy and cataplexy. Trismus may be simulated by impacted wisdom teeth, temporomandibular joint syndrome, scleroderma, and malingering or hysteria. The diagnostic workup will be obvious in cases of true trismus. Cases not associated with a systemic disease should have an EEG and x-rays of the teeth and temporomandibular joints. A referral to a dental specialist is often in order.

URETHRAL DISCHARGE

Most cases of urethral discharge in both males and females are due to gonorrhea or *Chlamydia trachomatis*. When the smear and culture are negative for gonorrhea, a course of tetracycline can be given as a therapeutic trial to diagnose *Chlamydia* infection. Alternatively, the urine can be cultured for chlamydia. A prostate examination should always be done in males, as acute and chronic prostatitis are common causes of urethral discharge. In teenagers a urethral discharge may develop in prolonged abstinence or excessive masturbation. Rarer causes of urethral discharge are syphilis, tuberculosis, foreign body, and herpes. Carcinoma of the urethra is extremely rare.

URINE COLOR CHANGES

Red urine may be due to hematuria (page 267), hemoglobinuria (hemolytic anemia), myoglobinuria (muscle trauma, myocardial infarction), and coproporphyria or uroporphyria (porphyria). Phenazopyridine hydrochloride (Pyridium®) also colors the urine red or orange. Ingestion of large amounts of beets will also color the urine red. *Brown urine* is usually due to hepatitis or obstructive jaundice, but myoglobin and melanuria may also color the urine brown. *Black urine* is found in malignant melanoma. Porphyrins may also color the urine black. In alkaptonuria the urine turns black on standing. Green or blue urine may be found in patients taking methylene blue, indigo carmine, or indigo blue. *Pseudomonas aeruginosa* infection may turn urine green also. The key to the diagnostic workup is to send the urine to the laboratory for complete analysis and culture. Most of the conditions listed above will have another symptom that will offer additional keys to the diagnostic workup using these pages.

VAGINAL DISCHARGE

Ask the following questions:

1. Is it purulent? A purulent vaginal discharge suggests nonspecific bacterial vaginitis and gonorrhea.
2. Is it frothy and yellow? This type of discharge is very often due to trichomoniasis vaginitis.
3. Is it cheesy and associated with itching? These findings suggest candidiasis vaginitis.
4. Is it watery and bloodstained? This type of discharge suggests carcinoma of the cervix or endometrium, polyps, hydatiform mole, and chronic cervicitis.
5. Is it offensive smelling? An offensive smelling discharge would suggest foreign body of the vagina.
6. Is there inflammation of the cervix? The presence of cervical inflammation would suggest chronic cervicitis and gonorrhea.

DIAGNOSTIC WORKUP

The most important test is microscopic examination of a saline and potassium hydroxide preparation. This will diagnose most cases of trichomoniasis and candidiasis. Gardnerella vaginalis can be diagnosed if clue cells are found. If this is unrevealing, a Gram stain for gonorrhea and cultures for trichomoniasis, candidiasis, chlamydia, Gardnerella vaginalis, and gonorrhea may be done. A Pap smear should be done to rule out malignancy. Polyps or inflamed areas of the cervix should be biopsied. A dilation and curettage may be necessary to diagnose endometrial carcinoma and hydatiform mole. Occasionally, pelvic ultrasound and CT scans are necessary. However, before ordering these expensive diagnostic tests, a gynecologist should be consulted. Patients with documented evidence of gonorrhea should have a VDRL test and HIV testing.

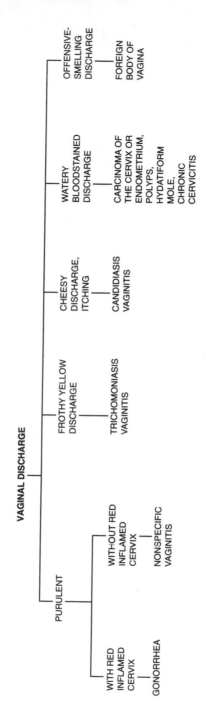

VAGINAL DISCHARGE

- **PURULENT**
  - **WITH RED INFLAMED CERVIX** — GONORRHEA
  - **WITHOUT RED INFLAMED CERVIX** — NONSPECIFIC VAGINITIS
- **FROTHY YELLOW DISCHARGE** — TRICHOMONIASIS VAGINITIS
- **CHEESY DISCHARGE, ITCHING** — CANDIDIASIS VAGINITIS
- **WATERY BLOODSTAINED DISCHARGE** — CARCINOMA OF THE CERVIX OR ENDOMETRIUM, POLYPS, HYDATIFORM MOLE, CHRONIC CERVICITIS
- **OFFENSIVE-SMELLING DISCHARGE** — FOREIGN BODY OF VAGINA

VARICOSE VEINS

Varicose veins are common in the lower extremities and are usually not a sign of other disease. Varicose veins of the rectum are called hemorrhoids and can be a sign of cirrhosis of the liver or portal vein obstruction from other causes. Distention of the abdominal veins may be due to cirrhosis of the liver, thrombosis of the inferior vena cava, or distention of the abdomen due to a large tumor (e.g., ovarian cyst), ascites, or massive hepatic or splenic enlargement. Varicose veins of the thorax and upper extremities are seen in mediastinal malignancies, (primary or metastatic) thoracic aortic aneurysms, and chronic fibrous mediastinitis.

DIAGNOSTIC WORKUP

Obviously a liver profile will be important. Chest x-rays and a flat plate of the abdomen should be routine. When these fail to identify a lesion and even when they do, it is often necessary to get a CT scan of the thorax or abdomen. Exploratory surgery may be necessary to establish a tissue diagnosis, as biopsy may be dangerous.

VULVAL OR
VAGINAL MASS

Ask the following questions:

1. Is it tender? A tender vulval or vaginal mass would suggest vulvitis, hematoma, acute bartholinitis, or urethral caruncle.
2. Is it reducible? A reducible vulval or vaginal mass would suggest pudendal hernia, varicocele, cystocele, rectocele, and uterine prolapse.
3. Is the rectal exam abnormal? The rectal exam will be abnormal when there is an impacted feces or rectal carcinoma.

DIAGNOSTIC WORKUP

Referral to a gynecologist or urologist can obviate an expensive diagnostic workup in most cases. The primary care physician may wish to treat acute bartholinitis or vulvitis, however. A culture and sensitivity is the only procedure required in those cases.

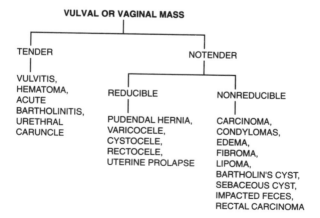

VULVAL OR
VAGINAL ULCERATIONS

Ask the following question:

1. Is the lesion or surrounding lymph nodes tender? The presence of tenderness of the lesion or the surrounding lymph nodes would suggest chancroid, lymphogranuloma venereum, herpes genitalis, and carcinoma. On the other hand, if the lesions or the surrounding lymph nodes are nontender, chancre, yaws, condyloma latum, and lupus should be suspected.

DIAGNOSTIC WORKUP

The workup includes a CBC, sedimentation rate, urinalysis, and VDRL test. A smear and culture of material from the ulceration should be done. A dark field examination may also be necessary. The Frei test may diagnose lymphogranuloma venereum, but a serologic test for this disorder may also be ordered. Biopsy may be ultimately necessary. It is wise to enlist the help of a urologist or gynecologist in difficult cases.

VULVAL OR VAGINAL ULCERATIONS

USUALLY TENDER LESIONS OR TENDER LYMPH NODES	USUALLY NONTENDER LESIONS OR LYMPH NODES
CHANCROID, LYMPHOGRANULOMA VENEREUM, HERPES GENITIALIS, CARCINOMA	CHANCRE, YAWS, CONDYLOMA LATUM, LUPUS

WEIGHT LOSS

Ask the following questions:

1. Is there fever? The presence of fever would suggest an infectious disease such as tuberculosis, acquired immune deficiency syndrome (AIDS), brucellosis, and typhoid fever, but collagen diseases and neoplasms should not be forgotten.
2. Is there anorexia? The presence of anorexia may be related to a febrile process, but if there is no fever one should consider the possibility of Addison's disease, anorexia nervosa, Simmonds' disease, drug abuse, poisoning such as arsenic poisoning, scurvy, malabsorption syndrome, uremia, and liver failure. There may also be a neoplasm.
3. Is there lymphadenopathy? The presence of generalized lymphadenopathy should suggest leukemia, sarcoidosis, and lymphoma, as well as infectious disease processes.
4. Is there an abdominal mass? An abdominal mass may be an enlarged spleen, a pancreatic carcinoma, an enlarged liver or renal mass. These masses would suggest disease of those organs. The mass also may be a carcinoma of the stomach or intestine.
5. Is there hyperpigmentation? The presence of hyperpigmentation would suggest Addison's disease.
6. Is the appetite normal or increased? The presence of a normal or increased appetite in the presence of weight loss should suggest hyperthyroidism and diabetes mellitus. The patient also may be taking thyroid hormone medication in increased quantities.
7. Is the thyroid gland enlarged? The presence of an enlarged thyroid would suggest hyperthyroidism. One should also look for a focal thyroid mass which might be a toxic adenoma.
8. Is the chest x-ray abnormal? Abnormalities found on x-ray that may induce weight loss are carcinoma of the lung, tuberculosis, congestive heart failure, pulmonary emphysema, and fibrosis.

DIAGNOSTIC WORKUP

Routine diagnostic studies include a CBC, sedimentation rate, urinalysis, chemistry panel, thyroid panel, serum amylase and lipase, febrile agglutinins, tuberculin test, antinuclear antibody titer, serum protein electrophoresis, serum B_{12} and folic acid, chest x-ray, EKG, and a flat plate of the abdomen. An HIV antibody titer needs to be done in selected clinical circumstances.

A stool for fat, trypsin, occult blood, and ovum and parasites should be done. If these tests are within normal limits or are unrevealing, it is best to refer the patient to a gastroenterologist or oncologist for further evaluation. Sometimes clinical clues suggest the need for an endocrinologist as well. However, if the primary care physician wishes to proceed further, he may order an upper GI series and esophagram, a small bowel series, barium enema, and a sigmoidoscopic examination. A CT scan of the abdomen and pelvis may be useful, but it is an expensive procedure.

Twenty-four hour urine collection for 17-ketosteroids and 17-hydroxysteroids or rapid ACTH stimulation test will diagnose Addison's disease. Quantitative stool fat and D-xylose absorption or a simple glucose tolerance test will diagnose some cases of malabsorption syndrome. Endoscopic procedures including laparoscopy and even an exploratory laparotomy have their place in the diagnostic workup. However, it is always best to enlist the help of specialists before considering these procedures, even if one is in an isolated community.

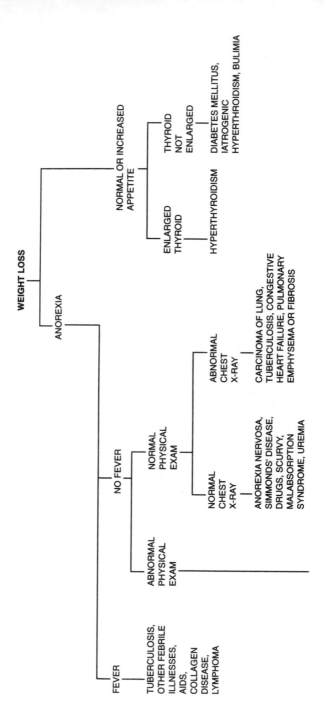

WEIGHT LOSS

NORMAL OR INCREASED APPETITE

ENLARGED THYROID
HYPERTHYROIDISM

THYROID NOT ENLARGED
DIABETES MELLITUS, IATROGENIC HYPERTHROIDISM, BULIMIA

ANOREXIA

NO FEVER

NORMAL PHYSICAL EXAM

NORMAL CHEST X-RAY
ANOREXIA NERVOSA, SIMMONDS' DISEASE, DRUGS, SCURVY, MALABSORPTION SYNDROME, UREMIA

ABNORMAL CHEST X-RAY
CARCINOMA OF LUNG, TUBERCULOSIS, CONGESTIVE HEART FAILURE, PULMONARY EMPHYSEMA OR FIBROSIS

ABNORMAL PHYSICAL EXAM

FEVER
TUBERCULOSIS, OTHER FEBRILE ILLNESSES, AIDS, COLLAGEN DISEASE, LYMPHOMA

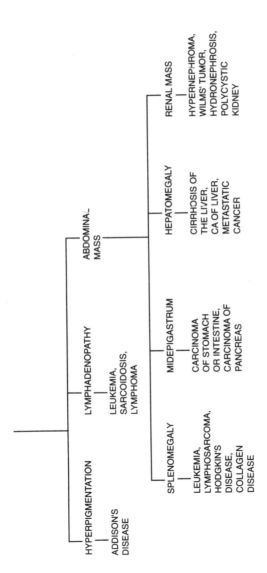

HYPERPIGMENTATION
ADDISON'S DISEASE

LYMPHADENOPATHY
LEUKEMIA, SARCOIDOSIS, LYMPHOMA

ABDOMINAL MASS

SPLENOMEGALY
LEUKEMIA, LYMPHOSARCOMA, HODGKIN'S DISEASE, COLLAGEN DISEASE

MIDEPIGASTRUM
CARCINOMA OF STOMACH OR INTESTINE, CARCINOMA OF PANCREAS

HEPATOMEGALY
CIRRHOSIS OF THE LIVER, CA OF LIVER, METASTATIC CANCER

RENAL MASS
HYPERNEPHROMA, WILMS' TUMOR, HYDRONEPHROSIS, POLYCYSTIC KIDNEY

WHEEZING

Wheezing is classically due to bronchial asthma, but there is a danger to jumping to that conclusion because it occurs in a few other conditions as well. The wheezing of *bronchial asthma* is heard primarily on expiration, while the wheezing of tracheal or laryngeal obstruction is heard on inspiration, such as *tracheobronchitis* in children. The wheezing of *cardiac asthma* (in congestive failure with acute pulmonary edema) is associated with pink, frothy sputum while the sputum of bronchial asthma is thick and tenacious. Acute *infectious bronchitis* may simulate bronchial asthma, but the response to epinephrine is poor. This is true also of *pulmonary emphysema*, but the history will usually differentiate this condition from bronchial asthma. A *foreign body* may often be distinguished because the wheezing is unilateral.

DIAGNOSTIC WORKUP

The CBC, sedimentation rate, chest x-ray, EKG, sputum analysis and culture, and pulmonary function testing will usually assist with the clinical diagnosis. Bronchoscopy may be needed also, especially when there is hemoptysis (see page 276).

Index